DOG DAZE AND CAT NAPS

DOG DAZE AND CAT NAPS

A VET STUDENT'S ODYSSEY

by

Mark E. Burgess

THE BORGO PRESS

An Imprint of Wildside Press LLC

MMIX

CONTENTS

DEDICATION

To my forever funny and supportive mom,

BETTY,

Who always told me that I could

ACKNOWLEDGMENTS

My thanks go to my brother Mike, whose lifelong pursuit of writing and publishing gave me the crazy idea of trying it myself; to my angel Denise, who has lovingly played the role of cheerleader and patient partner through these long months (thank you for understanding); and to my parents, who provided an education and taught me that hard work pays off in the end.

Additional thanks to Drs. Heidi Buehner and Thomas Reibold for their technical advice; to Drs. Tom Terbeck and Doug Phillips who long ago showed me the right way to practice; and finally to Dr. Jim Hardesty in Grand Terrace, California, whose example on a warm summer's night inspired a college kid to go and do likewise.

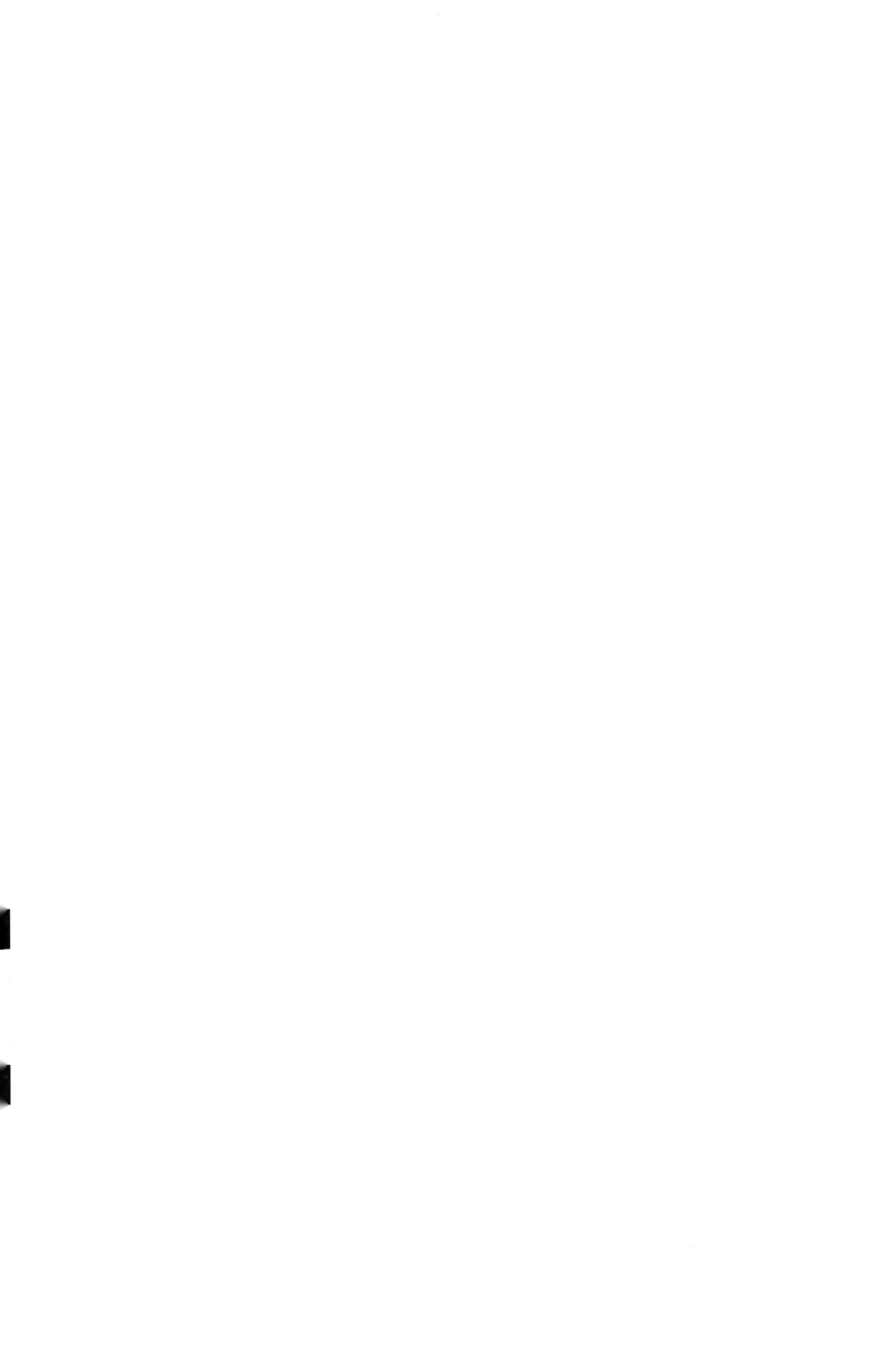

DOG DAZE AND CAT NAPS

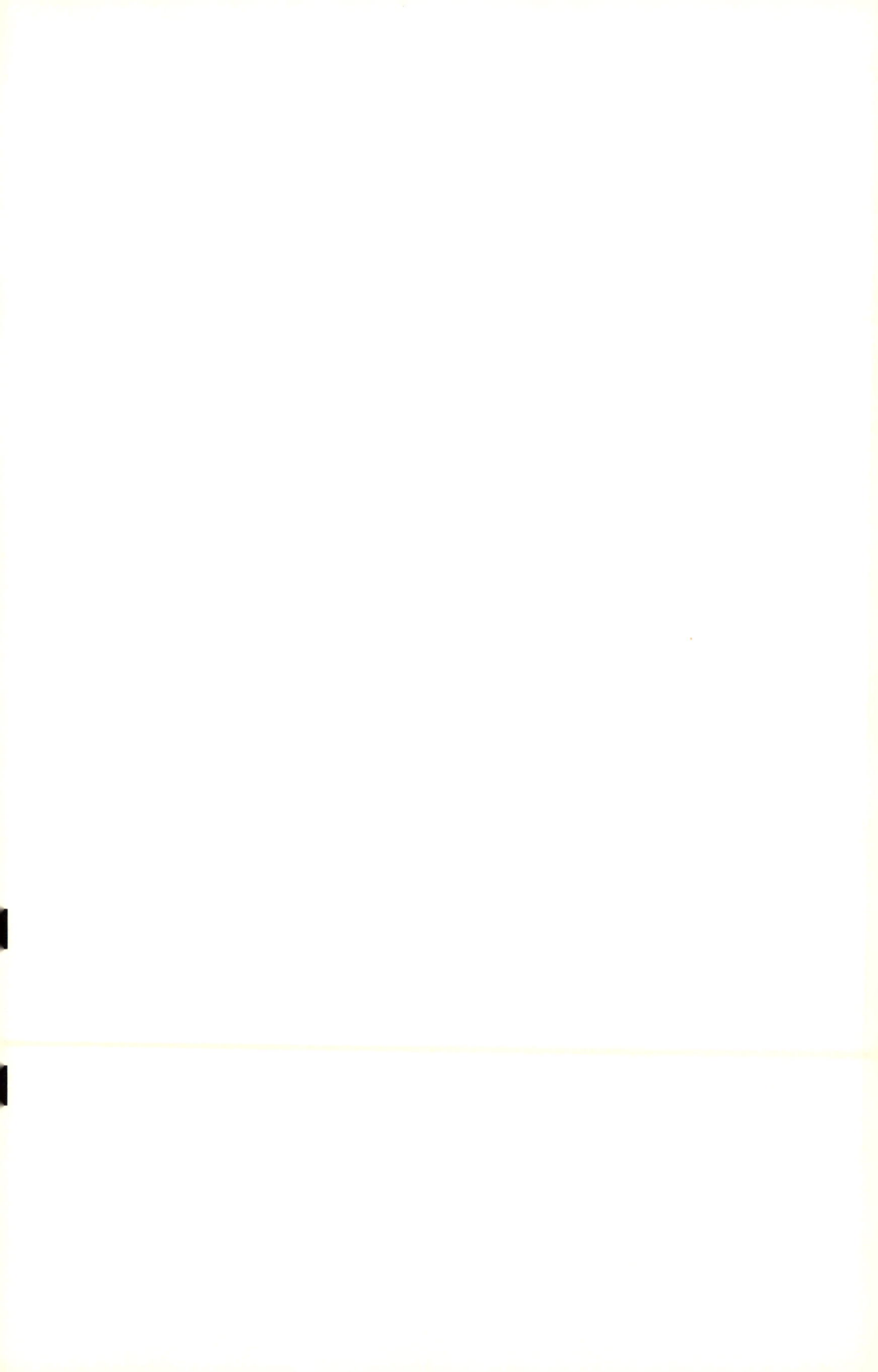

PROLOGUE

CHAPTER ONE

I held the scalpel poised over the naked skin of the dog as I simultaneously held my breath. All of my veterinary courses covering anatomy, anesthesiology, and the principles of surgery had culminated in this moment. My heart was pounding and my mouth felt like it was stuffed with dry cotton. In addition, the adrenaline rushing through my body had strangely heightened all my senses. I could clearly hear the rhythmic click and hiss of the gas anesthetic machine to my left, as the female Golden Retriever on the table breathed oxygen and halothane gas in and out, in and out through the black rubber tubes connecting patient to machine. Cutting through the soft rush of her respirations was the sharp, high-pitched *"beep, beep, beep"* of the cardiac monitor, assuring me that my patient's heartbeat was strong and steady.

The seven-month-old dog was lying on her back, belly shaved smooth and scrubbed with povidone iodine soap, which had left its characteristic yellow-brown stain on her skin. Leather cords resembling long boot laces held her wrists and ankles tied spread-eagled to the stainless steel table. The dog's prone body was mostly covered by a sky-blue paper surgical drape. A long narrow hole had been cut in the drape's middle to expose the area of skin I was about to incise.

Looking down, I saw the clean, mirror-bright surface of the scalpel blade glittering in my grip. The tiny reflections it cast were jumping and jittering over the surface of the drape, mercilessly exposing the fact that my hand was trembling just a little.

The heat of the two focused surgical lights bore down on my head and shoulders from close above. I hadn't even begun the procedure, and already moisture was trickling down the back of my neck and under the collar of my scrub top. The green cotton surgical cap and gown felt oppressively heavy, and the stifling mask that covered my face forced me to re-breathe my own oxygen-poor air. With a healthy dose of tension added to the mix, I found myself perspiring like a mobster in a tax audit. Funny I had never foreseen these distractions when imagining being a surgeon.

I took a deep breath and glanced around me. My three student team members clustered close about the table, each with their assigned duties. My surgical assistant Jason Thomas, also gowned, stood directly across from me, ready to hand me instruments and wipe up any flowing blood (hopefully not mine). Danielle Peterson, the "anesthetist," stood to my left near the machine; her job was monitoring the patient's stability and depth of anesthesia. The fourth member of our team sat in a chair to my right. Dan Alderman had the uninspiring task of studiously taking surgical notes for the patient's chart. His head was bent over as he jotted something in the small notepad on his lap. Right about now I was envying him his low-key role in this little venture. As for me, I had the dubious honor of being designated head surgeon for today's procedure, which was the challenging and groundbreaking surgery known as the dog spay.

All around the huge instruction arena similar scenarios were playing out. Eight surgery tables stood arrayed there, each with an anesthetized male or female dog, each with its complement of four rigidly alert veterinary students in caps, masks, and green surgical clothing, attempting their first procedures on living, breathing patients. Eight tense tableaus vividly outlined in bright islands of halogen lighting. In our third year of veterinary school the moment we had all yearned for was upon us—and it seemed way too soon.

One could feel the apprehension as a palpable cloud hanging over the room. I sincerely believe that if someone had broken wind right then, half a dozen students would have hit the floor in dead faints. Thankfully, the only blood pressure monitors in this room were being used on the patients, and not the people tending to them.

My scalpel seemed frozen in place and I desperately searched for something to take my mind off the task at hand. "Where do you suppose they get the dogs for these surgeries?" I asked as I gazed around at my teammates.

Danielle looked up from her post at the anesthetic machine and responded, "They come from the local animal shelter."

"Oh, really?" I glanced over at her, surprised. "How did they manage that?"

"Well, the shelter needs animals neutered, and the vet school needs surgery patients," Danielle answered. "So they give us dogs and cats to work with, and in turn we provide free sterilization services. The animals are easier to place in homes if they are already neutered. Plus it helps curb pet overpopulation."

"It sounds like a win-win arrangement," I said, nodding. "I don't know if I would have thought of that."

I also couldn't think of anything more to say, and as the conversation died away the suffocating silence pressed in once again around our table. I stood looking down, scalpel in hand, summoning up the nerve to make that incision. Meanwhile, my teammate Dan, the surgery note-taker, had taken notice and was obviously relishing my unease. "I'd say our surgeon is enjoying a sphincter factor of about ten," he chuckled, adding. "Just close your eyes and make a slash! It's not the first time you've handled a scalpel. We've all dissected our share of animals by now."

I scowled and waved the blade in his direction. "Easy for you to say! Cadavers don't tend to become any more dead if you slip up. Plus they don't do disturbing things like, well, *bleeding.*"

There was also the little matter of performing the surgery correctly. In real-life practice, it just wouldn't do to remove Muffy's small bowel instead of her uterus. Her chronic obesity problem might finally be solved, but her longevity could be a bit less than desired. Long experience has shown that, oddly enough, most pet owners seem to place a fair amount of importance on the longevity issue. These were not pleasant things to contemplate on my first day as a surgeon, not at all.

Nevertheless, it was time to take the plunge. I called to mind that old surgical mantra, *"Grab a Knife and Save a Life,"* and lowered my blade to touch the dog's abdomen.

I envisioned a confident stroke with the scalpel, sliding through the skin so that it would part magically, practically inviting me into the abdomen. The result would be a moderately long, three-to-four-centimeter arrow-straight line, a shining example of surgical prowess. No blood, just gleaming pink tissues glowing with health, as if they were thanking me for treating them with such professional competence. Emboldened by the image, I swept the blade down the dog's midline, then I leaned in to view my work, and I saw...nothing.

What the...?! Puzzled, I bent to look closer, squinting. No, there was not a mark on the dog. There might have been a slight scuff line on the skin there where the blade had grazed it, but certainly no incision.

While pondering this development, I heard a muffled snort from across the table, and looked up at my assistant. Jason's face was half hidden behind his mask, but his eyes were crinkled and his shoulders shook. It suddenly struck me that he was laughing!

Before I could think of a retort, he said, "Better watch it there, Mark: you might slice clear through her spine." I immediately felt my face flush hot, but he had a point. Despite the razor-sharp edge of my freshly opened scalpel blade, I had managed to be so tentative with my first stroke as to avoid cutting the skin at all.

I couldn't help it, and broke into sheepish laughter as well. "Hey, if surgery doesn't go well, it's always the assistant's fault," I retorted.

That bit of humor had a relaxing effect, and things actually became easier after that. I bore down on the blade on my second attempt, amazed at how much pressure it really did take to cut through the tough skin of a dog. The skin parted, revealing the glistening white layer of fat beneath. I used blunt forceps to push apart the soft adipose rather than cutting it, causing less bleeding that way. Finally, beneath a centimeter of fat I saw the red muscle fibers of the abdominal wall. This was the important layer, the one that held in all the organs, that provided strength to the abdomen.

Along the very midline where the left- and right-sided belly muscles meet, there is a thin line of connective tissue called the linea alba (Latin for "white line"). This was what I was looking for. An incision made there was nearly bloodless and less painful to the patient. If I missed to the left or the right, the muscles I would encounter would be much heavier, and would bleed profusely when cut.

But I was having a devil of a time seeing where the linea was. It sounded easy enough in the textbooks, a wonderfully clear white stripe against the red muscles. A heaven sent signpost saying, "cut here!" So where was the damned thing hiding?

"Wipe that for me, will you?" I asked Jason, and he used a gauze square to dab up a bit of blood that had oozed onto the exposed abdominal wall. With a freshly cleaned surface, I finally saw it, a faint white streak running down the center of the exposed muscle layer. Hardly a signpost, but I had nothing better to aim at, so I laid the scalpel along this line and cut. I was rewarded with the gratifying sight of a dark hole leading into the dog's abdominal cavity. With a sense of relief I quickly enlarged the slit until it was about three centimeters long. We were in!

As good as it felt, I had only accomplished the easy part of the procedure. I needed to find the uterus and ovaries and remove them. I knew in theory how to do this, and had watched the procedure performed more than once by experienced surgeons. The dog uterus was like a thick rubber band, long and narrow and flexible, shaped like a "Y." The base of the Y was the uterine body which connected to the vaginal canal; in front were the two "horns" which made the arms of the Y. Just off the end of each horn was an ovary.

Because the uterus was narrow and flexible, the idea was to use a long slender spay hook to catch hold of the organ, and pull it up and out through a relatively tiny skin incision. Then most of the work of suturing and cutting would be actually done outside the body. How short you could make your incision and still successfully remove uterus and ovaries was a matter of pride among many vets. More than once I had seen an experienced practitioner do a spay via an opening smaller than my fingertip. To my mind it seemed like pulling a boa constrictor through a keyhole, but somehow they did it.

Our instructors had told us to not worry about incision length if things weren't going well. "Open them up so you can see," they advised. "You'll save time in the long run, and long incisions heal just as fast as short ones." Yes, but long incisions took more time to suture closed too—hence the desire of most surgeons to make as small an incision as possible.

I had begun with a three-centimeter opening, more than enough space for anyone who knew what he was doing. The problem was, I didn't. Theory was fine, but as I fished the steel hook into the dog's abdomen again and again, I quickly realized how much skill was involved in making it look easy. The endless loops of small intestine seemed eager to come out and play. Sadly, the uterus had more anti-social tendencies. Time and again I pulled out a bowel loop on my hook, only to stuff it back and try again.

After about ten minutes of this, I could feel my frustration mounting. My fellow students were watching the proceedings with keen interest, and I desperately wanted to perform well in front of them. I also knew that there are limits to how long one can safely keep a dog anesthetized.

I looked around to see if a professor was handy nearby. The surgery course instructors were wandering casually here and there between the tables, observing, calmly offering advice or encouragement, and occasionally handing out a sharp word of correction when they spotted a problem. For all their relaxed demeanor, they could have been overseeing a grade school penmanship class, nodding and smiling tolerantly at each young pupil's crude attempts to control the pencil's trajectory. This was indeed child's play to them. I would look like a moron if I had to call for help.

What to do? My mind began to race with dire possibilities. Perhaps I might never find the evasive uterus. Maybe the dog had been spayed already, and I would spend the entire surgery session fruitlessly searching for the missing organ. No, I was convinced the uterus was there, hiding deep inside, mocking me. I would simply miss it, again and again, until my futility caught the attention of an instructor. He would approach and say loudly (so that everyone in the room would hear), "Why is it taking you so long to find that uterus, Mark? Everyone else is having an easy time of it. You must be doing something wrong!"

Yes, I could see it clearly. He would stand over me as I struggled, and lecture me once again on the basics of using the spay hook, as if I had forgotten everything I had heard in class. Meanwhile, I would blush deep red and continue searching without success, until finally he would throw up his hands in exasperation and proclaim, "Oh, enough of this, let ME do it!" After quickly donning gown and gloves, he would slip the spay hook in and retrieve the uterus on his first try. A nice big mature organ, the easiest type to find. The other professors and students (who had completed their surgeries by then and were enjoying soft drinks and cookies) would applaud and laugh as they watched the whole affair.

The image made my colon twinge. But what if the instructors insisted that I complete the spay myself? I could picture the surgery extending into the late evening hours, all of the professors now crowded around my lone team in the otherwise empty room. They would glower down disapprovingly as I fished the spay hook in and out endlessly. My fellow team members would be swaying on their feet, faint from exhaustion and from missing their evening meals. It would go on and on and on....

What would happen if I never completed a spay during veterinary school? Would they even let me graduate? Would I be expelled in shame?

My dismal musings were interrupted by a calm voice from just beyond the table. "How goes it, people?" I looked up to see Dr. Brakel, one of the course instructors, and one of the best-liked doctors in the school. He was a stocky, energetic man with a broad face and unruly blond curls. Whenever I saw him, he always had a bounce in his step and a smile on his lips, even when struggling with difficult cases that would give most surgeons ulcers. His irrepressible optimism and active sense of humor made him fun to be around, and I had taken a liking to him from the first time we met. He took in my situation in a glance, and as his eyes met mine, he winked and said, "Not finding the uterus yet, hmmm?" I shook my head silently, and he clapped his hands briskly together and said, "Well, open her up more then, don't be proud. Let's get in there!"

I grabbed my scalpel and dutifully extended the incisions through the skin and abdominal wall. "C'mon, a bit more, make it longer!" Dr. Brakel insisted, so I kept cutting. When at last he was satisfied, I had created a gaping hole large enough that I could have crawled into the abdominal cavity myself and looked for the uterus that way. I stared at the wound, wondering how many days it was going to take me to suture that closed again.

Dr. Brakel nodded with satisfaction. "Now you can see what you're doing," he proclaimed. "The uterus is located fairly dorsally, up near the spinal column, so when she's on her back like this, it is often 'under' the small intestines. Move the bowel loops off to the side now, and see if you can find the uterus." I did as he said, and there, snaking out from between the bladder and colon, was a tiny, immature-looking pink noodle that forked as it extended forward. It was hardly bigger than a cat uterus, and Dr. Brakel whistled, saying, "She must be a bit younger than we thought! It's so small I doubt you could have stretched it up out of her even if you'd hooked it. Well, go on then, remove it."

I grabbed the uterus and pulled it up a bit to allow easier access, and began the process of performing an ovariohysterectomy. The main attachments and blood vessels to the uterus were at its front and back ends; once these were cut, the entire organ would come free. Using absorbable suture which would later dissolve on its own, I ligated the forward blood vessels near the ovaries, and then cut the tissues to free the ovaries and adjacent uterine horns—and then to the back end of the uterus, ligating the uterine arteries and the uterine body. Once all vessels had been tied off, I severed the base of the uterus. With front and back ends now free, the skinny little organ easily came up and out in my hands.

I held it dangling for a proud moment, beaming like a fisherman with a prize catch, to a chorus of *"Yeah!" "That rocks." "Another one bites the dust!"* from my surgery teammates. Finally I dropped the little strand of tissue in the medical waste can on the floor. Dr. Brakel smiled and nodded at me before heading off toward another table.

I checked for blood inside the abdomen and was gratified to see none. My vessel ligatures were holding. I sighed with relief; it was time to get this lady closed! Grabbing more absorbable suture, I began the tedious process of closing the layers of the abdominal incision. First the linea alba, then the fatty subcutaneous layer, and finally the skin. The skin sutures were external and were of monofilament nylon; they would need to be removed in ten to fourteen days when healing was complete.

The incision was long enough that I had ample opportunity to practice suturing technique, and as I worked I was gratified to find that I had a knack for instrument handling and knot-tying. It occurred to me that I might have made a good seamstress. I lost myself in the rhythm of grabbing tissue, thrusting the needle through, pulling and tying suture, holding the ends out so my assistant could cut them short, and repeating the process.

Before I knew it, the incision was closed and the dog was recovering from anesthesia, sporting a nice neat (if rather long) row of skin sutures. Equally gratifying was the realization that we had finished nearly forty minutes ahead of the other surgery teams. I was grinning like a fool as we carried our patient to the recovery room and placed her in her kennel, covered by warm blankets. She was groggy and droopy-eyed, feeling the aftereffects of anesthetic and the injection of opiate pain killer she had received. But she was conscious and her tail wagged weakly when I stroked her head.

The following day I anxiously walked (okay, it was more of a run) to the kennel to see my patient. I opened the door to her dog run, and was almost bowled over by an exuberant whirlwind of golden fur. To my delight she was bouncing and energetic, eyes alight, tongue lolling, tail lashing furiously side to side as if oblivious to what had happened to her the day before. She was a happy dog, typical of her breed, and I had to grin as I watched her.

When I checked her incision, it was clean and dry, with minimal redness and no swelling or discharge. As I crouched down examining her, I felt the hot wet slurp of a tongue across my cheek. Right then it felt incredibly good to be a veterinary student. I had survived my very first surgery. More importantly, so had my patient.

CHAPTER TWO

It is an amazing fact of life that a single small event can radically alter the entire course of your future. In my case, the birth of my veterinary career happened during the summer of 1980, while visiting my oldest brother, Rob, in Southern California. He and his wife both worked, leaving me to fend for myself during much of my two-week stay. Their house was nestled in a quiet old suburb of San Bernardino, and without a car I was stranded there, isolated from any fun activities the area might have had to offer.

After the novelty of the visit wore off, I gradually grew bored with day after day of swimming in the backyard pool, reading paperback novels from the battered bookcase in the living room, watching TV, and listening to the slow tick, tick of the old Regulator clock on the fireplace mantle. The summer heat was unrelenting, the days blurred together, and then in the midst of my ennui Julia came to the rescue.

Julia was my niece and lived not far from my brother's house. She was close to my age; if that sounds odd, consider that my brother was nine years older than I, and his wife a decade older than he, with a daughter from a prior marriage…so do the math and it sort of made sense that Julia was twenty. She had long, brown, wavy hair nearly matching her tawny skin, with a slender petite figure, quick bright eyes, and a ready smile. At that time she worked as a technician at a veterinary emergency clinic, and one evening she stopped by the house to say hi to her mom on her way to her job. When she spotted me on the sofa reading she cocked her head thoughtfully, then she smiled and asked, "Say Mark, would you like to come into work with me, to see what I do?"

My pulse leaped at the suggestion. Compared to another night of thumbing tattered sci-fi novels and watching my toenails grow, this sounded absolutely thrilling. "Sure, that would be fun!" I replied, trying to sound less than desperate.

Julia grinned at me knowingly. "Good, we'll head out shortly if you're ready." I nodded and thus it was set.

A half hour later we were driving through downtown San Bernardino. Julia's old Toyota lacked air-conditioning so we had the windows rolled down. When I closed my eyes, the warm sweet evening breeze blowing through my outstretched fingers called up images of sunny beaches and California surfer songs. We wound our way through the city and eventually approached a single-story wood and brick building fronting the street on our right. Julia pulled her car around back to the employee parking area and we went inside.

On entering the building Julia gave me a quick tour, first showing me the exam rooms, each with a stainless steel table where pets would sit while the doctor evaluated them. Then we moved on to the radiology room with its large X-ray machine, and the surgery room, sporting a gleaming adjustable table and two large overhead lights suspended on jointed arms from the ceiling. We toured the pharmacy, stocked with row after row of medications in bottles, jars, and tubes, all sitting neatly on the shelves. A kennel room in back contained steel cages of various sizes, plus some large runs for bigger patients. A few of the enclosures housed cats and dogs who stared out at us anxiously as we passed.

Our last stop was the treatment room, where pets could be medicated, anesthetized when needed, prepared for surgery, and so forth. This room was the nerve center of the veterinary hospital, and during busy times most of the activity was focused right here.

The treatment area was large and spacious, maybe twenty feet on a side. Two shiny metal procedure tables stood in the open center of the room. On the wall opposite us were arrayed banks of stainless steel kennels of varying sizes. Directly to our right I saw a counter top upon which stood a microscope, a centrifuge, and other equipment. Julia explained that this was the laboratory area, where the hospital could perform simple blood tests, fecal exams, and so forth.

Some of what I saw that night has blurred over the years, but the important things still stand out clearly in my mind's eye. I remember meeting a young personable veterinarian only recently out of school, named Steve Harding. I also remember Kiki.

Dr. Harding was bent over the microscope at the laboratory counter when Julia and I first entered the treatment room. He looked to be in his late twenties, smooth-faced and fit, with dark brown hair. He wore a nicely cut, light blue doctor's smock with tan slacks. As we came in the doctor straightened up and smiled, saying, "Hi Julia. Who's your friend?"

Julia replied, "This is Mark, my dad's younger brother. He's been visiting at my parents' house for this past week, and I thought I'd show him what we do for fun in the evenings."

Dr. Harding came forward flashing a boyish grin, saying, "Hi Mark, nice to meet you!" We shook hands; the veterinarian had an easy way about him, and I liked him immediately. "Feel free to look around while I finish this fecal cytology," he said, so Julia and I made a tour of the hospitalized patients while the doctor again bent his head to the microscope.

Several cages had animals in them, and we looked at them one by one. A small Schnauzer sat forlornly in a floor level kennel, his front leg completely encased in a bulky splint. Julia read his case history from the file in her hand and said, "This little guy was hit by a car earlier this evening and fractured his radius and ulna, the bones of the forearm. We put a Robert Jones bandage on to temporarily stabilize it, but he'll need the fracture repaired at his regular vet tomorrow."

She pointed to the cage above the Schnauzer, which contained a tabby cat lying on its side, unmoving. "This kid is really sick; we don't know if we'll save her." I noted the IV line taped to the cat's front leg. The line led to a fluid bag and a small yellow pump that thumped and chugged as it slowly pushed the clear liquid into the cat.

"What's wrong with her?" I asked.

"Antifreeze poisoning," she replied. "Her owner was flushing his radiator in his garage and left a pan of the fluid sitting there. It's sweet-tasting; dogs and cats love it. Unfortunately, it also causes severe kidney damage, and this little girl is in renal failure."

Even an untrained observer could tell the poor cat was severely ill. Her eyes were open but she stared straight ahead, not even bothering to lift her head and look at us as we stood in front of her kennel. The little bowl of canned food sitting near her appeared untouched. I felt sorry for the small bundle of life lying there miserably. She probably had no idea what had happened to her or where she was. Her family waiting at home had to be worried sick as well. I hoped she found a way to recover and be happy again.

We moved on and looked at a couple more patients, and then we came to Kiki.

Kiki was a pretty white miniature poodle who had been brought in earlier that evening after having been in a dog fight. When I first saw her standing in a kennel in the main treatment room I was shocked at her appearance. Her white curly coat was vividly splotched and stained with large gobs of bright red blood. Even more impressive were the two large flaps of skin torn and hanging loose from her left flank, exposing the raw muscles beneath. Each open wound was the size of a large grapefruit and matted with fur and dirt. Kiki appeared unfazed, panting nervously but prancing on her feet, seemingly ready to go for an evening walk.

In a short while the doctor and Julia took Kiki from her kennel to treat her wounds. Julia held the little dog snugly, restraining her head while Dr. Harding injected anesthetic into a vein on Kiki's front leg. The effect was remarkable; by the time he had finished giving the shot, the dog's head was dropping and her entire body slumped onto the table. Julia's restraint was no longer needed, so she moved quickly to grab a clear plastic tube. I watched fascinated as the doctor opened the dog's mouth and slid the tube slowly down her throat. Kiki coughed once or twice and the doctor nodded to Julia. "Tube's in, get her on gas," he said.

Julia connected the dog's breathing tube to a machine next to the table. She adjusted some knobs on the device as Dr. Harding pulled on latex gloves. Once gloved, he began to fish out instruments from a shiny steel bowl filled with bluish liquid. Glancing up, the doctor noticed me craning to see as I stood about ten feet away. He grinned and said, "You can come closer and watch if you want."

Gratefully I moved up to the table where the dog lay. The doctor pulled up a chair and sat next to his patient. After Julia had shaved most of the soiled hair off Kiki's left flank, Dr. Harding flushed and cleaned the wounds, using forceps to pick out bits of hair, grass, and dirt from the raw exposed tissues. I watched closely as he meticulously cleaned the area. He pulled the loose skin flaps this way and that, looking underneath for hidden debris that had become lodged inside the wounds during the fight. The skin was remarkably pliable, and resembled pieces of fabric loosely tacked to Kiki's body, like clothing from a careless tailor that was now unraveling.

It was disconcerting, and I felt a bit faint and flushed as I watched living flesh opened wide for the first time. I took my eyes off the ghastly wounds for a moment and contemplated the young vet. He was relaxed and humming tunelessly as he probed and cleaned the lacerations. He seemed to really enjoy his work.

I switched my gaze back to the dog as the doctor nodded with satisfaction and said, "There, that's pretty well cleaned up. Now I've got to close the skin and put a drain in."

"What's a drain?" I asked.

He looked up and smiled. "Well, this skin is torn loose from the body, only connected along one edge here. When I close the wound the skin will still be loose, and fluid will want to collect in the hollow area beneath it. I'll put a rubber tube in at the bottom of that pocket and it will allow fluid to drain out and not accumulate. Then the skin can remain flat until it reattaches to the underlying muscle."

"What would happen if you didn't put a drain in?" I asked.

"Well, probably the dog would get a seroma, basically like a giant fluid blister under the skin, and we'd have to reopen and drain it. Might as well do it now and prevent the problem."

He grabbed suture and began closing the wounds from top to bottom, pulling the skin flaps back to their original positions. The gaps slowly but surely came together, little by little. Kiki was beginning to look more like a dog and less like a Picasso painting. I watched as Dr. Harding made a small incision near the bottom of one wound and pushed the rubber drain up inside. He left about an inch of the tube protruding and sutured it to the skin.

"Next week we can cut this one suture and pull the drain right out, once it's no longer needed," he explained to me. "The drain hole will close on its own after that."

He proceeded to install a drain in the second wound as well, and while he worked he talked to me. "So, Julia has told me a little about you. Are you thinking of becoming a vet?"

"Well, I've thought from time to time that it would be interesting work, but I've never seriously considered it," I replied.

He looked up from his suturing, eyebrows raised. "Oh? Why not?" he asked.

I shrugged and shuffled my feet. "Well, my family doesn't have a lot of money. My parents are paying for college and I'm working summers to help...but I'd never be able to afford to go to vet school."

Dr. Harding laughed and waved a finger at me, saying, "That's not an excuse! Do you think I could afford it? Heck no! Just get federal student loans, let Uncle Sam pay for it! I've got several loans myself; I'll be paying on them for another eight years. It's not much per month, quite affordable really." He grinned and resumed his needlepoint on Kiki.

His words, though, continued to resonate in my mind throughout that evening and on the car ride home. Maybe I could manage the tuition for vet school after all! After what I'd seen tonight, the idea captivated my imagination. I pictured myself doing this kind of work, saving lives. "Dr. Bridges." Hmmm...I liked the sound of that!

All these years later I can still picture that young, fresh-faced veterinarian and his badly traumatized patient. Although I would never see him again, Dr. Harding had ignited my imagination with his joyful enthusiasm, his skill and dedication treating the patients that came in that evening, and his casual dismissal of my financial concerns. I don't know what path my life would have taken if it were not for that chance summer visit, on a whim, to a small emergency clinic in Southern California. I do know that I have never regretted the choice I made on that day, to become a doctor to the animals.

CHAPTER THREE

It is one thing to decide on your career path, and another thing altogether actually to accomplish it. I went home to Medford in southern Oregon, and that fall I was back at college in nearby Ashland for my junior year. I talked to my advisor who obtained the necessary paperwork and information regarding pre-veterinary curriculum. Then I began the lengthy process of meeting the prerequisites needed to apply to veterinary school.

The only vet program in Oregon was up north in the Willamette Valley, at Northern Oregon University. This was where I would apply when the time came. I really was in pretty good shape classwise. Most of the required courses were ones I was already taking for my bachelor's degree in biology.

The hardest prerequisite to satisfy was the need for practical experience. At that time the vet school required applicants to log a minimum of three hundred hours of observation in a veterinary hospital. The reasoning was simple: many prospective students had an idealized view of what it meant to be a vet. Some thought the job consisted of little more than petting a cute animal on the head while its tail wagged, and sending home pleasant tasting medicines that the pet eagerly devoured. These well-meaning but naïve individuals didn't foresee the potential stress of the job, the often long hours, the midnight emergencies. They couldn't imagine getting smeared with blood or diarrhea or urine. Most had never pictured themselves struggling to control an aggressive patient as it tried to rend them with teeth or claws. Nor had they watched the heartbreaking euthanasia of a beloved family pet dying of cancer, while the family members clustered around and wept. In short, observation in a real life practice weeded out those who discovered that they didn't *really* want to be a vet after all.

I was sure I could deal with the realities of animal practice. The challenge for me was to find a veterinarian close to home who would allow me to observe. My next door neighbor Jim Ferris was full of advice. He was an elderly retired farmer who had moved into town when he sold his farm. Jim and his wife had an old Shih Tzu dog that they took to a vet not far from us. They had been going to him for many years, and swore by him. "Ol' Doc Bailey will do right by ya, you'll see," Jim avowed. "He's always treated my animals—cows, horses, sheep, dogs, you name it. And he's very reasonably priced, never overcharges the way younger docs do. Honest guy, he is."

I didn't know much about medicine, but I did know that you usually got what you paid for. Modern medications and equipment cost money, so a vet who was "cheaper than the young guys" rang a little alarm bell in my head. But then I thought that if he was older, maybe his overhead was low, his clinic property long since paid for. He might also be doing these old clients a favor and discounting their bills. Dr. Bailey's clinic was located close to my home, so I drove over one Saturday to check him out.

The one-story white wooden building sat back from the road in the shade of several large old elm trees. The parking lot out front was dirt with a few handfuls of gravel thrown on it. I got out of my car and walked toward the front entrance, my feet kicking up small clouds of dust with each step. As I approached the building I noted the faded sign, the moss covered roof, the peeling paint on the walls.

I pushed the front door open with a loud creak of protest from the old hinges. The air from within wafted out around me, and I was hit with a distinct smell. It was hard to place, but made me think of a mix of unwashed dog fur, mildew, and possibly stale urine. I tried not to wrinkle my nose as I approached the reception desk and announced the reason for my visit. The pretty girl behind the desk looked professional enough, neatly attired in a crisp blue smock. She smiled and told me to have a seat in the waiting room while she informed the doctor that I was here.

I proceeded to the cramped little waiting area and perched on a rickety wooden chair that had seen better days. Apparently business was slow today, since I was the only person there. I looked around and decided that the last renovation this place had undergone must have been around 1960 or so. The furnishings all looked as old and tattered as the building itself, and the floors were covered in faded pea green linoleum. I saw a diploma on the far wall hung below a Norman Rockwell print. Curious, I got up to look more closely at it. The yellowed paper proudly proclaimed Edward T. Bailey as a graduate veterinarian in the year 1942. I wondered what year he was currently practicing medicine in.

Just then Dr. Bailey made his appearance, emerging from a hallway which led back into the bowels of the building. "Hello there, young man," he said, offering his hand. As I shook it, I sized him up. He was about my height, stocky, with a craggy face and short-cropped hair that was grey shading into white. He wore a brown doctor's smock, but it was loose and rumpled and seemed one size too large. Worn corduroy pants and old tennis shoes completed the ensemble. Seeing him, I was struck by how closely his appearance mirrored that of his practice.

I pasted a smile on my face and said, "Nice to meet you. My name is Mark Bridges. I'm here because I am applying to vet school next year. They tell me I need to have a lot of hours of practice observation before I can qualify. I was wondering if you would be willing to let me observe on weekends and maybe this coming summer."

"Ah, yes, they require that now, don't they?" he said, nodding. "When I was in school no one needed any of that; you simply went and applied. If your grades were OK, you could usually get in." I nodded earnestly as if in appreciation for the good old days.

Then he peered at me intently and asked, "Are *your* grades OK? You're applying yourself in school? Taking it seriously?" I said yes, I was a good student and always got high marks. He asked me a few more questions about my background, my education, where I currently went to school, and so forth.

Finally the doctor nodded, apparently satisfied with his first impression of me. He said gruffly, "I don't mind if you come and observe. I can't pay you, but you're welcome to watch, and maybe you can eventually help out with some of the easier procedures. Will that suit you?"

"Yes, that's fine by me," I answered, nodding.

"Well then, let's not stand out here all day; come on back." He stumped off down the hallway and I followed uncertainly. I noticed that the unidentifiable odor seemed to intensify the further we moved back into the building.

The doctor turned right abruptly, into a doorway off the main corridor. When I entered the room, I was surprised to see that this appeared to be the surgery suite. It was small and cluttered, and lacked the swinging doors I had seen in my visit to the San Bernardino clinic. Such doors closed automatically behind you to reduce possible airborne contamination during surgery. But here there was just a standard entryway from the hall outside. The door was apparently left open at all times, based on the stack of boxes on the floor which blocked its movement.

Dr. Bailey went to the antique looking surgery table and brushed some papers aside, clearing a space on the table top. He looked at me and a smile briefly cracked his rough features. "Well lad, you're in luck. I was just about to do my morning surgery, a cat spay. You can watch if you wish."

"Yes, I'd like that," I replied, interested to see the doctor in action.

"I'll call for my tech to get the cat then." I thought he would use an intercom, but instead he put his head out the door and bellowed down the hall, "DIANE! GET THE THOMAS'S CAT!"

Bemused by this sophisticated communication system, I waited with the doctor until Diane the tech appeared carrying a small black cat. She placed the animal on the surgery table and the doctor grabbed a syringe filled with clear liquid off a shelf. "Is that the anesthetic?" I asked.

"Yes it is," Dr. Bailey replied. As Diane held the cat he slid the needle into a vein on the animal's front leg. Then he slowly gave a dose of anesthetic, only a fraction of what was in the syringe, stopping when his patient relaxed and went limp. He then taped the syringe to the leg, needle still inserted in the vein. The tech turned the animal on her back and began shaving the belly for surgery. Watching this, I was puzzled.

"Why did you leave the syringe on the leg?" I asked the doctor. "Aren't you going to put a tube in the cat for the gas anesthetic?"

"Naw, this is just a spay," Dr. Bailey snorted. "It's a quick surgery, no need for gas. Gas anesthetics are expensive. It's much more efficient to just use intravenous Surital and give her more as she needs it. People want cheap spays; we don't charge enough to use gas on these." So saying, he gave the plunger on the syringe a little nudge as the cat's legs had started to move. She quickly became immobile again.

I was flabbergasted. As little as I knew about medicine, I had still picked up a few pointers at the emergency clinic and during my pre-vet studies in school. I knew that gas anesthetics were safer and offered quicker recovery times than most injected drugs. Injectables were usually used only to initiate anesthesia so that a breathing tube could be placed. Dosing an intravenous drug over and over would build up high levels of the compound in the body, greatly prolonging recovery. This cat could end up being asleep for half a day.

I also knew that having a tracheal tube in place meant that if an animal stopped breathing, you could pump oxygen through the tube and breathe for her. Without a tube it was difficult to ventilate a patient when they needed it.

As if on cue, I noticed right about then that the patient, in fact, did not seem to be breathing. I pointed this out to the doctor, who said, "Oh, not to worry, she'll breathe when she's ready. Meantime we can pump her chest." He proceeded to use one gnarled hand to squeeze the cat's ribcage four or five times, then stopped and watched for a moment. After about ten seconds the little feline took a deep breath, and I realized I'd been holding mine as well.

"There, you see? She's fine," Dr. Bailey pronounced with a satisfied grunt.

The technician had finished her shaving of the cat's belly and began to scrub the surgical site. "Do I need a mask to stay in here with you?" I asked. I thought that sterile surgery should require something of the sort.

"No, no, just don't touch the cat after she's scrubbed and you'll be fine," the doctor retorted. He pulled out a package of surgery gloves and prepared to don them. Neither he nor his tech seemed to be worried about the lack of surgical caps, masks, or for that matter, sterile gowns.

Just as he was reaching for the gloves, a loud male voice bellowed down the hall from the direction of the waiting room. "Say Ed, are you back there?!" the voice inquired.

"Ah, Tom, how have you been?" Dr. Bailey responded heartily, leaning his head out the door so he could see up the hallway.

"Not so good, I'm afraid, doc," the faceless voice echoed down the hall. "I found one of my sheep dead this morning, and she's all bloated up like she's been down awhile, but she seemed okay yesterday. I'd like you to take a look at her and see what you think."

Dr. Bailey frowned, successfully distracted from the surgery at hand. "Yeah, might be Clostridium that killed her, I can come by this afternoon maybe." The patient on the table stirred a bit, and the doctor leaned back in and injected a bit more anesthetic. He hesitated a moment, apparently torn between watching his patient and chatting with his client. Then he grabbed the cat by the rear feet and carried her with him into the hall as he continued to talk to the farmer standing at the other end. They conversed for awhile about sheep, the weather, family, and the like. All the while Dr. Bailey casually held the anesthetized cat by the legs dangling head down at his side. When the conversation became animated he swung his arm back and forth, the feline's limp forelegs and head flopping against his knee. Apparently the farmer down the hall was totally unfazed by this rather bizarre sight. Finally the doctor noticed that the animal in his hand was beginning to stir, and he said to his friend, "Well, I've got to get this spay done. I'll be around to see you later then."

The farmer took his leave and Dr. Bailey came back into the surgery, casually flipping the cat back onto the table. A bit more intravenous anesthetic was given, then he proceeded to drape the cat and perform the spay. Diane occasionally reached under the surgical drape to squeeze the cat's chest whenever it hadn't taken a breath in awhile.

After observing at the clinic the rest of the afternoon, I got in my car and drove away, staring numbly ahead. I had just come out of a time warp, that was it. Old farm practices from the 1940s and '50s would have been exactly like this. What a contrast to current veterinary medicine! No wonder the doc was reasonably priced. With practically no modern equipment or medications, Bailey's overhead must have been negligible.

To be fair, I realized that the old doctor had probably seen many things in nearly forty years of practice that I could not imagine. He had ministered to the needs of countless animals in his time. No doubt he had saved more than one farmer's prized livestock, and had mended many a child's furry best friend. But his ways were not those of the modern practitioner. Medical progress had simply left the aging vet behind.

Needless to say, I soon found another practice to observe contemporary medicine at. But there are two sides to every coin, and one other anecdote needs telling here. One of the procedures I observed during my day with Dr. Bailey was the euthanasia of an aggressive dog. I remember it clearly because it was the first time I had seen an animal put to sleep. The dog in question was a large Airedale mix who had bitten people several times. When finally he attacked a young girl in his family, severely lacerating her face, his owners had had enough. The dog's unpredictable aggression had signed his death warrant, and they had dropped him off earlier in the day to be euthanatized.

We walked back to the kennel where the dog sat quietly in a run, and I watched the doctor and his tech carefully get the dog out and muzzle him. As the large brown eyes looked at me over the rim of the muzzle, I saw no aggression there now, only fear of the unknown. The doctor inserted a needle into the dog's forelimb and gave a lethal dose of pentobarbital into the vein. Standing there, I watched the light go out of those frightened eyes as the dog slumped to the concrete floor, never to rise again.

This story bears telling because after he had given the injection, the doctor sat a moment, his shoulders slumped, his head bowed. When at last he looked up I saw an expression of sadness softening the lined face. It was in that moment that I saw the other side to Edward Bailey. After decades of practice performing uncounted euthanasias, and near the end of his long career, the old doctor still *cared*.

Dr. Bailey retired a few years after, and I heard that the young vet who purchased the practice upgraded everything, eventually demolishing the old building and erecting a new state-of-the-art facility on the same site. Of course his fees were considerably higher than those of his predecessor. Some of the old-time clients probably left in search of cheaper services. But an era was ending, and the times, they were a-changin'.

CHAPTER FOUR

The practice where I eventually did my clinical observation was, by contrast, a modern facility with a sterling reputation. The hospital in North Medford was a sturdy red brick building on a tastefully landscaped lot. Inside there was no odor other than the faint aroma of disinfectant. The equipment was modern and well-maintained, the floors spotless, the supplies organized.

The practice was owned by two partners, Drs. Thurman and Strom. As I got to know them, I thought they were the quintessential odd couple. Douglas Strom was the senior partner. Slender and fit, he looked to be about fifty years old. He epitomized the successful medical professional: dapper, smooth and well-spoken. Dr. Strom was active in veterinary associations both locally and statewide, and was well respected by his peers. At home he had a pretty wife and two lovely daughters. When not working he could often be found on the nearby golf course, "having a go."

His younger partner, by contrast, was what we in casual parlance would call a redneck. Thomas Thurman was tall and clean shaven, but wore his hair long in the fashion of the late 1970s. He spoke with a slight drawl and often used modern slang vernacular. He also loved to dispense old country wisdom whenever the opportunity arose. One of his favorite expressions was, "I've seen a lot of things…and this is one of them." I was surprised that he wasn't making a living doing rural farm calls. Yet here he was practicing cutting-edge small animal medicine in the city.

Particularly fascinating to me was Tom Thurman's creativity when confronted with a client whose pocketbook couldn't cover a pet's expenses. True to his small town origins, the doctor knew that a lack of cash didn't mean the client had nothing of value. Over the time that I observed there, I saw him accept nearly every type of service or object of value in trade for veterinary care. He once did a tumor removal on a black Lab, and the owner couldn't pay the bill. The man in question was an unemployed contractor skilled in tile work. Before I knew it, the clinic sported a new white tile tub-surround in the dog grooming area. I also saw Dr. Thurman accept an old rifle as payment for medications dispensed for a dog with liver disease.

Such unconventional economics played havoc with the bookkeeping and drove the senior veterinarian to distraction. More than once I heard Dr. Strom in his office spewing epithets at Dr. Thurman's fiscal innovations. "What the heck are we going to do with a rifle, for Pete's sake?! How do we even assign a dollar value to that?" And so it went.

Watching these two vets with their disparate personalities and mannerisms, one could wonder why they ever ended up being partners. The answer became clear whenever I heard them animatedly discussing a case. They shared one unifying common ground: a love for medicine and for the animals they applied it to.

Both vets made me feel welcome at their practice and I soon felt right at home. I observed examinations, treatments, and surgeries, asking questions and taking notes. As time passed and I learned more, my duties slowly expanded. I was allowed to assist in restraining some animals, and to perform simple procedures like nail-trimming or temperature-taking. Although I was in school, my classes often ended by two P.M. On those days I made the quick drive from Ashland to Medford to observe at the clinic until closing time. The hospital was open a half day on Saturdays, and I was usually there. At the end of each week, I turned in a notebook documenting my hours at the practice, with a brief summary of what I had observed. The book was signed by one of the doctors and given to my college advisor.

These were fun times, my first prolonged exposure to the profession I was falling in love with. I could tell both vets had taken a liking to me. Not too surprisingly, each had different ways of showing it. Dr. Strom adopted a rather fatherly attitude, and made time to explain various aspects of medicine as he treated his patients. He was quick with encouragement and tolerant when I slipped up.

Dr. Thurman, on the other hand, delighted in posing questions that I could not answer. He must have felt that learning by trauma was the most effective way to make knowledge stick. At first the questions were extremely simple, such as what the "DHLP" acronym stood for on the dog vaccines. Once I could recite "Distemper/hepatitis/leptospirosis/parainfluenza" without missing a beat, he would find something else to ask. It was embarrassing to stumble and admit I didn't know the answers, especially in front of clients. Every time he stumped me, he'd grin smugly. Then he'd give a succinct answer to the question, and remind me of the importance of knowing basic facts before daring to aspire to vet school.

This went on for months. Of course, Dr. Thurman always had the upper hand. No matter how much I learned, there were a dozen more unanswerable questions he could rattle off. I think he really enjoyed playing the omniscient professor. At times Dr. Strom would chastise him for his merciless grilling, saying "Give the kid a break, Tom. He's not even in vet school yet, and you're asking him stuff that they put on Board Exams." But the inquisition continued relentlessly.

Only one time did I manage to turn the tables on Thomas Thurman. Ironically, it happened with the most difficult question he ever asked. It was, in fact, a question I'm sure he thought impossible to answer.

One day when I arrived at the clinic, Dr. Thurman was standing at the pharmacy counter. I saw him there in the hallway just behind the exam rooms, and he called to me as I came in. "Hey, Mark, come tell me what you make of this," he said.

As I approached, he held up a small empty jam jar. "A client brought this in. What do you think it is?" he asked, a trace of a smirk playing about his lips. I looked closer and saw what appeared to be a slender, threadlike brown worm, about three or four inches long, coiled in the bottom of the jar.

By a freak coincidence, a one in a million chance really, that worm actually looked familiar to me. Unbeknownst to Dr. Thurman, my younger brother and I had grown up with a fascination for insects, and when younger we had spent countless hours in the summer with butterfly nets and jars. I had contemplated a career in entomology before I chose the veterinary profession instead.

As part of our natural curiosity, my brother and I had once dissected a dead cricket to see what lay within. We were shocked to find an amazingly large parasitic worm coiled up inside that little insect. A worm that looked just like the one in this jar.

I was sure this creature was something different, some animal parasite that an owner had found in his pet's stool, but I had no idea what type. So I said what I knew: "Well, it really looks like a parasite I've seen in an insect before."

This statement caused a remarkable change in Dr. Thurman's facial expression. The smug smile disappeared, replaced by an odd look I couldn't quite place. His lips twisted spasmodically for a moment, and then he hoarsely croaked, "What kind of insect?"

"Well, a cricket."

The facial spasms intensified and finally the doctor managed to say, "Yes, well, a client found their dog chewing on a cricket, and when they pulled him away from it they found the worm on the ground nearby. They were worried it may have come from the dog."

With this revelation I finally identified his odd expression as a mixture of dismay and disbelief. He must have been wondering how the hell I could possibly have known the answer to that question.

Truthfully, I was probably the only pre-vet student on the planet who did.

During this conversation Dr. Strom had paused nearby, listening curiously. Now he erupted in laughter, pointing his finger at his younger partner. "Aw, Tom, you thought you'd trip him up with that question, didn't you? You had three books open trying to identify that worm! You'll never live that one down. Oh, the expression on your face when Mark actually knew the answer! That was priceless!" He walked off down the hall to his office, still chuckling loudly as he went. The devilish part of me took great pleasure in the deep red blush covering Thomas Thurman's face.

From that day onward, whenever Dr. Thurman became a bit too condescending with his questions, I could simply smile and say, "Well, at least I can tell a cricket parasite from a dog worm, unlike some of us." And he would scowl and leave me in peace for awhile, because he never did come up with a good answer to that.

CHAPTER FIVE

If ever there was a time where veterinary practice could test the mettle of a budding student, then the era of the first canine parvovirus outbreak was it. I had observed at the vet practice through my junior year in college, and now summer had arrived. To my delight, Dr. Strom had pulled me aside as the school year was ending, and had offered me a summer job as "kennel boy." The pay wasn't great, but the job allowed me to observe forty hours a week while saving toward tuition. I accepted his offer with profuse thanks.

During that summer my main task was keeping the clinic clean. Every day I stocked the exam rooms with supplies such as ear swabs, cotton balls, and paper towels. I made sure the alcohol dispensers in the rooms were always full, and that supplies were organized in their assigned spots. I even swept the parking lot, baking in the hot summer sun as it steamed off the black asphalt.

One of my biggest and dirtiest chores was kennel cleaning. Each morning and evening I scrubbed out cages and dog runs containing both healthy and ill pets. Over the weeks I gradually grew inured to the odors of feces, urine, and vomit. I thought that now I could withstand any mess that an animal could throw at me. Then the parvo epidemic hit town.

Canine parvovirus was a new disease that had suddenly appeared in the eastern U.S. in the late 1970s. Attacking the intestines, the devastating illness caused severe bloody diarrhea, vomiting, dehydration, and often death. Dogs at that time had no resistance and we had no vaccine to protect them. The deadly epidemic rolled across the country, killing thousands of adult dogs and puppies alike.

When sick dogs began appearing in the hospital that summer, the two vets recognized what it was. Most owners told us their pets were suddenly lethargic and losing appetite. The dogs quickly developed foul bloody diarrhea and often vomited if they attempted to eat or drink. By the time we saw them some were semiconscious and spewing rotten fluid from both ends. Most of them barely resisted when we drew blood samples or installed an IV line to get them hydrated.

There was no cure for parvovirus, and there still isn't. The only treatment was aggressive supportive care, keeping the dog strong so that the immune system could fight off the infection. With time, if the dog survived, the virus could be defeated and the bowel lining would regenerate.

Being a kennel person during the height of the outbreak was a miserable job. The hospital possessed a large isolation ward where contagious animals could be kept. All of the canine parvo cases were housed there. The stench as I entered was overwhelming, consisting of a uniquely aromatic mix of vomit, watery diarrhea, and decomposing blood that only parvovirus produced. Occasionally I caught the smell of death overlying the other odors. Searching the kennels I would find a patient cold, stiff, and lifeless, the still-open eyes gazing sightlessly ahead. Such was the final end of many parvo cases.

The living patients often had liquid projectile stools. Even when too weak to stand, many dogs had an uncanny ability to coat the entire walls and sometimes even ceilings of their kennels with the foul stuff. If you've ever seen video footage of an Apollo rocket on take-off, then picture the dog as the rocket and you'll get the general idea. Worse yet, the dried excrement clung to the stainless steel like hardened enamel. I found myself having to spray and remoisten the diarrhea to soften it, then scrape and scrub at it vigorously. The bleach we used to disinfect the kennels added its pungent odor to the mix, burning my eyes and nose.

Despite my wearing gloves, the powerful reek of the dogs' waste penetrated right through the latex and became ingrained in my skin. Hours later I'd be eating in the staff room, and as I brought my sandwich up to my mouth I'd catch a whiff of bloody diarrhea and bleach. I should have patented that scent as a sure-fire way to curb appetite. Just apply it to the hands and I could have made a fortune producing miraculous weight loss in the chronically obese.

Through all of this I kept a positive attitude, and my enthusiasm for veterinary medicine remained undiminished. Well...maybe temporarily dimmed. Medical practice can be a messy business, but I learned early on that it's a necessary part of healing the sick. Seeing one of our parvo patients walk out the door a happy survivor was all the reward I needed.

CHAPTER SIX

In the fall I reluctantly left the clinic and headed back to college for my senior year. I had accumulated enough hours over the summer to meet the prerequisites for applying to vet school. Now all that remained was finishing my undergraduate course work and sending in my application. Oh, and one minor detail—I had to get accepted.

There were, on average, about 150 applicants for the thirty-six positions in the freshman class; only one in four would make it. I hoped that Dr. Strom's endorsement of my application would count for something. Doug Strom was known and respected statewide, and he was serving on the veterinary examining board that tested graduating vet students.

I sent off the application in December of 1981 and waited. Christmas break came and went, the weeks passed, and every day when I returned home from classes, I anxiously checked the mail. Then one cold afternoon in early February I arrived at the house to find my mom excited and smiling. "You have a letter here from the vet school!" she said. "Open it and see what it says!"

I didn't need any encouragement. With trembling hands I quickly tore open the thick envelope. My veterinary career might start or stop here. I opened the stiff folded paper and read:

Dear Mr. Bridges,

Thank you for your recent application to the Northern Oregon University School of Veterinary Medicine. We have reviewed your application, and are pleased to inform you that an interview has been scheduled on Saturday, March 13, at two P.M. The interview will be conducted at McNairy Hall in Room 205; included is a map with directions to the school. If you have any questions, you may contact us at the phone number above. Please reply to this letter on receipt. We look forward to seeing you in March.

Sincerely,

Dr. Mark Hudson,
Veterinary School Dean

My mom was watching me as I read the letter, and she knew the answer from the grin spreading across my face. "They accepted your application!" she said, and I nodded yes. She let out a whoop and we laughed and hugged, practically dancing around the kitchen. I had successfully jumped the first hurdle.

It seemed like an eternity before March 13th finally arrived. On the morning of the interview I was up early. After breakfast I fretted in front of the mirror trying to be sure I was presentable, my tie neatly knotted, my hair combed, and my clothes reasonably wrinkle-free. After awhile I gave up and contemplated the image reflected back at me: a young man slender of build and slightly taller than average, chiseled narrow face framed by medium-length brown hair which was just wavy enough to be unruly. A neatly-trimmed mustache adorned an otherwise clean shaven visage, and deep-set brown eyes gazed back at me with calm intensity. At least my nervousness didn't show, but then again the day was young. With a last glance in the mirror I admonished my reflection, "Whatever you do, don't forget to smile!"

My mom and dad had suggested making the trip a family outing. We packed sack lunches and began the journey north to the Willamette Valley. Dad drove and I spent much of the trip staring unseeingly out the window. My thoughts raced in restless circles. How many people would be in the interview room? What they might ask me? How could I make a good impression? Not having been in this situation before, there was in truth no way to predict what I would encounter.

The vet school was located in the town of Corvine in the central Willamette Valley, a few miles west of the freeway. My watch read 12:30 P.M. when we arrived in town. We followed directions the school had provided, and eventually located the veterinary building, a large multistory brick structure standing alone on one corner of the college campus. We slowly approached the front, and my dad dropped me off not far from the main entrance. I heard my mom say, "Impress the heck out of them!" as I closed the car door. A few moments later my parents drove off down the road and I was on my own.

I walked from the curb across an expansive grey flagstone courtyard fronting the building. As I approached, I gazed up at the modern architecture, the tan brick-and-glass edifice sculpted into graceful sweeping curves. The school was only a few years old, and everything had a fresh, clean look to it. To my right was a large open pasture with a few pine trees scattered here and there across it. The lush spring grass was a deep vibrant green, dotted with small yellow wildflowers. The sun shone bright, and I caught the scent of moist soil and living plants carried on the warm breeze. Such a pastoral setting seemed perfect for a school dedicated to helping animals. I breathed in the sweetness one last time, and then I pushed open the heavy glass door and stepped into the building.

Just inside the entrance was a large vaulted lobby with an attractive red-tiled floor. Prominently displayed on the wall facing me was a large bronze sculpture of a woman cradling a lamb in her arms. I spotted a reception desk across the lobby from me, enclosed behind glass near the foot of a stairway. Approaching, I announced myself to the lady at the desk. She had long brown hair and wore what looked like a green medical smock. I told her the reason for my visit and said I was looking for Room 205. She smiled and directed me up the stairs. "When you get to the top go straight across the hall, to Room 203," she said. "That's the Dean's office; they'll show you where to go from there. Oh, and—good luck!"

When I found the room in question, I paused a moment, then willed myself through the door. Inside I encountered a large polished wooden desk with another receptionist seated behind it. When I gave her my name, she said, "Oh yes, they're expecting you. It will be just a few minutes; why don't you have a seat?" I found a cushioned chair against the wall and waited.

My pulse was racing and my palms felt wet and sticky. This was my moment of truth. If I nailed this interview, I would be in, and if not…well, I didn't want to dwell on that. I wiped my hands on my pants and tried to slow my breathing.

Looking around I noticed two doors on the back wall of the office. My eyes leapt to the one on the left, labeled 205. Soon I would be in there, doing my best to impress. I hoped it was an informal setting, maybe a small table with a couple of people lounging in easy chairs asking me friendly questions. *"Please,"* I thought, *"don't let it be some inquisition-style session, with a long boardroom table and me at the head of it, a dozen pairs of eyes glaring at me and a dozen voices barking questions."*

Just then the door to Room 205 opened and a young, clean-cut man attired similarly to me stepped out. He was tall and ruggedly handsome, but he looked tired and a bit dazed as he made his way past me and out the door. Gazing at him I wondered if I were seeing a future classmate.

Then an older gentleman in a suit came out of the interview room and I forgot all about the unknown passerby. The older man had short cropped silver hair and startling blue eyes. Those eyes fixed on me and he smiled. "Are you Mark Bridges?" he asked.

I quickly stood and smiled back, trying my best to look confident and relaxed. "Yes, I am," I replied, and I was thankful that my voice sounded steady. The man came forward and we clasped hands in the middle of the room.

"I'm Dr. Hudson, the Dean of the Veterinary School," he said. "Please come this way." He led me into Room 205. There my eyes beheld a long boardroom style table, with maybe ten or so men and women occupying seats around it. They all looked up as I came in. I tried to smile as Dr. Hudson took his seat, leaving one empty place which, of course, was at the head of the table.

I inhaled deeply and sat down. Dr. Hudson announced me to the members of the interview panel. Then he in turn named each of the individuals seated at the table. Most were school faculty members, but I was surprised to learn that some were not. One elderly man seated to my right was simply a farmer and a representative of the local agricultural community.

Dr. Hudson finished the introductions and then looked at me. "Mark, let me explain how this works. Each member of the panel will ask you one question of their choosing. We'll start with Mr. Wilson on your right, and then go around the table from there, okay?" I smiled and nodded, and the interview was on.

The old farmer sitting next to me was white-haired, and I guessed him to be well over seventy. To my anxious mind his grizzled features looked as unfeeling as stone, and his eyes seemed steely shrewd as he locked them on me. "Now then, young man," he rasped in a gravelly voice. "You want to be a veterinarian. Suppose that you succeed and become one. What will you do with your degree?"

I was momentarily frozen. The question took me totally by surprise! I had been prepared to demonstrate the knowledge I had learned while observing at the clinic, showing that I was an apt pupil and had paid attention. But *this*…how did I answer *this*?

I briefly contemplated the obvious retort of, "Well, I'll practice medicine, of course! What else would I do with a veterinary degree, you daft old fool?" I quickly discarded that idea as not conducive to a long career, and thought furiously. *He must be looking for something more than a simple answer. He wants me to think about the options out there for a graduate vet. Maybe he also is interested in what I really want out of this career—why am I doing it?*

I cleared my throat and replied, "Well, I definitely want to work in private practice, and maybe have my own clinic someday. I know that government departments like the USDA employ vets, but the research and regulatory sides of veterinary science aren't my focus. I am interested in all sorts of animals, large and small, even exotic species."

Mr. Wilson nodded and grunted, seemingly satisfied with my answer. I saw several faces around the table smile. With some trepidation, I looked next to Dr. Hudson, who was seated to the right of the old farmer. The doctor asked, "Mark, you observed at a small animal hospital with Dr. Strom, correct?" When I nodded he continued, "I know Doug Strom, he's a good fellow. Tell me, what diseases do we typically vaccinate dogs for?"

I smiled inwardly. Dr. Thurman's endless quizzing was now yielding benefits. I answered, "We normally vaccinate dogs for rabies and distemper. Well, actually the distemper shot is a DHLP vaccine."

Dr. Hudson grinned and replied, "Do you know what the 'DHLP' stands for in the combination vaccine?" His smile broadened when I recited off the four diseases without hesitation. "I have no more questions," he said and looked to his right at the next panel member in line.

A dark-haired woman who I remembered was a faculty member asked me, "Mark, what is the term for when horses give birth?"

I answered immediately, "Foaling."

"What is the term for when a dog gives birth?"

"Whelping," I replied.

"And for sheep?"

"Lambing."

"And cattle?"

"Calving."

"And how about for cats?" she asked.

I started to answer and then realized I had no idea what the term for cat birthing was. How could I not know that? I racked my brain, but there was nothing. I reminded myself that they did not expect me to know everything. Might as well show them that I could be cool and calm even in defeat. So I grinned and said, "It's not just 'giving birth,' is it?"

"No, it's not," she replied. But I noticed she was smiling too.

"Truthfully, I have no idea," I said. "I don't recall ever hearing a term used for cats in all the time I've spent in clinics."

With that the female doctor turned to the person next to her and said quietly, "I told you none of them would know it."

I can't describe how good it felt to overhear that comment. I then said to her, "I'm curious: what *is* the term for cat birthing?"

She grinned and said, "It is queening."

Thinking back on it, I wonder if maybe my merciless mentor Dr. Thurman had it right, and learning by trauma was indeed effective. For I never have forgotten the term "queening" in the many years since that interview, despite rarely if ever hearing it again.

Feeling more relaxed, I focused on the next person at the table. He was a tall, jovial man with sandy hair, round cheeks, and a big grin. When he spoke it was with a distinct Irish accent, and I remembered his name was Dr. O'Brien. He looked at me with a twinkle in his eye and said, "Your application form says you totaled 522.5 hours of clinical observation. My only question is this: how the heck did you come up with the 'point five'?"

I heard several people around the table laugh, and found myself smiling as well. It was hard not to like Dr. O'Brien. Feeling more at ease I said, "Well, I multiplied the average hours I worked each day by the total number of days I observed, and that's what it came out to. I just wrote down the number rather than rounding it off."

Dr. O'Brien laughed and said, "Oh. Okay, I was just curious!"

The rest of the interview went by in a blur, each of the remaining panel members taking their turn asking me a question. Most of them I answered correctly, and I was relaxed and confident toward the end. My friendly, candid approach yielded ever more smiles on the faces of the panel members. It all felt pretty positive to me.

A short while later I was standing on the sidewalk in front of the vet school, soaking up the sun and waiting for my parents to show up. I breathed in deeply and stretched, and it felt really good to be alive. With my jitters totally gone I became aware of a deep rumbling in my stomach. I was ravenous!

Eventually the family car came into view and pulled over. When I got in the back my mom turned around and asked eagerly, "Well, how did it go? Did you do all right?"

I nodded and grinned, feeling almost giddy. "Yes, I think I did pretty well," I replied. "I've got a good feeling about my chances. I really think they liked me."

We spent much of the drive home discussing the interview. My parents laughed at Dr. O'Brien's silly question, and were sympathetic when I told them of the answers I didn't know. But they agreed with my assessment that the substance of the questions wasn't always the key. Some were asked simply to elicit stress and see how I dealt with it. All in all, I thought I had done well. The question was, would the interview panel agree?

I had been told that the school would send a letter advising me of their decision by April 10th at the latest. As week after week went by, I waited anxiously for some word as to my fate. I had no idea yet what my future held. If I was turned down by the vet school, what would my alternatives be? The uncertainty wore on me.

The tenth of April came and still I received no letter. My spirits sagged as I realized that the school would have informed me if I was accepted. The rejection notices were probably a lower priority, so might be slower in coming. Everyone had told me from the start how hard it was to get into veterinary school. It seemed they were right. Still, I had felt so good about my chances, and had allowed myself to hope. Now I began to consider alternate careers. Reluctantly I talked to my advisor about applying to other programs. It was not a happy time for me.

On Friday, April 16th I came home from school and helped my mom set the dining room table for dinner. While I finished the place settings the phone in the kitchen rang. My mom answered it. After a moment she looked at me and said, "Mark, it's for you. I'm not sure who it is."

I took the phone from her and said, "Hello, this is Mark."

"Hello Mark," a woman's voice spoke in my ear. "I'm Gail Armstrong from the Dean's Office at the veterinary school. We hadn't heard back from you. I was calling you to find out if you were still interested in being in this year's freshman class."

I felt a surge of excitement shoot through me. "What do you mean?" I asked, afraid to believe what she seemed to be saying.

"Well, we sent you a letter two weeks ago and hadn't heard back," she continued. "Most of the other students have contacted us already to confirm their places in the class."

"I never received any letter!" I blurted in a daze, as her words began to really sink in. My heart felt like it was going to beat its way right out of my chest. "So…this means I've been accepted into the vet school?"

"Yes, if you are still interested," she replied.

"Yes!! Oh, yes, I am!" I breathed. "Count me in the class! Thank you so much for calling to verify. I had no idea that you had sent a notification."

"I'm glad we checked with you," Gail replied. "Otherwise your spot in the class would have been given to another applicant. I'll let the dean know. Welcome to the program, Mark."

She hung up and I stood there frozen with the phone receiver in my hand, my mind numbly trying to grasp the truth of it all. One exultant thought kept repeating itself: I was in. I was IN!

My mom had overheard my half of the conversation and she knew. Her broad smile spoke volumes as she congratulated me and gave me a huge hug. For a tiny woman she could squeeze surprisingly hard and I had to work to breathe. My dad had come in and stood nearby, smiling at me, and when I looked his way he said, "I'm proud of you, son." Through it all I could see clearly, for the first time, my future career laid out before me. There was no doubt about it now. I was going to be a veterinarian.

YEAR ONE

CHAPTER SEVEN

I finished my senior year in college and received my diploma that June. After graduation I once again worked for Drs. Strom and Thurman at the animal hospital in Medford. They both were delighted to hear that I was enrolled in the veterinary program. Even the hard-to-please Dr. Thurman seemed more patient with me now, taking time to explain diseases and treatments as he worked on cases. I learned everything I could while performing my cleaning duties. The summer sped by, long hot days and warm nights tumbling past, and before I knew it September was upon me. I prepared to leave home and head north to Corvine.

My best friend growing up, Daniel Weidler, was also attending Northern Oregon University in the Engineering Department. Daniel and I had a lot in common; we lived in the same neighborhood, were both science geeks growing up, had attended the same grade school and enjoyed the same activities. That fall we agreed to carpool to the university; he would drive and I would pay for half the gas. I packed for a school year away from home, filling a large black trunk with clothes and school supplies. A battered suitcase held extra clothing plus odds and ends. Thankfully, I didn't have to haul textbooks with me; those would be purchased at the school bookstore after I arrived on campus.

Daniel stopped by my house after he had loaded his belongings in his car. We managed to find room for all my stuff, although it was a close fit. I said good-bye to my parents; my mom made me promise to write regularly, and I assured her that I would. After a couple of long hugs I got in the car and we backed out of the driveway. My parents stood on the front porch smiling until we turned the corner and they were lost to sight. I sighed and turned my eyes to the road ahead. We were on our way.

As we drove north my friend and I discussed life at the University. Daniel was now in his senior year there, so he was familiar with the campus layout. I picked his brain awhile and he promised to show me around when we had time.

The miles passed and our conversation twisted and turned like the road in front of us. Eventually we began reminiscing about the past and the fun we had shared growing up. With much amusement we recalled the time when we had decided to avenge all the jokes my brother Stan had played on me. Stan was nine years older than I, so when I was a child he had always had the advantage, short-sheeting my bed, lacing my shoes together, you name it and he had done it. But as I had grown into my teens I had gotten more creative. Daniel and I had finally concluded that Stan was due some payback.

My brother had moved away to work up north in Portland at that time, but he and his wife Angie came to visit regularly. Daniel and I began to put bumper stickers on Stan's rear car fender whenever he was in town. Not just *any* bumper stickers, oh no. These were special ones that we made ourselves. When my brother was about to end his visit with my family I would slap one of our creations on his car. Then I would stand smiling with my parents and wave goodbye as he drove off.

Daniel and I were chuckling with twisted glee as we recalled the slogans Stan had unwittingly carried on his fender. "Remember the '*Porn Star on Board*' sticker?" I offered as we both laughed fiendishly.

Daniel grinned and said, "Do you think your brother ever noticed people looking at them strangely as cars passed?"

"Speaking of getting odd looks," I replied, "how about the one that said '*Rhino Molester*'?" This started another paroxysm of laughter from both of us.

Daniel chortled, "Oh, my, he drove all the way to Portland with that one. That's nearly three hundred miles!"

We were laughing so hard that tears rolled down our faces, and it was all we could do to blurt out each slogan as we recalled them. "*I Smoke Navel Lint*," Daniel managed as we both cackled with delight.

"Oh wait!" I gasped between breaths as I wiped my streaming eyes. "Remember the one about kids?"

"You mean '*Kids Taste Like Chicken*'?" he choked out, and I simply nodded as I shook helplessly, unable to pull enough air to form words. My cheeks hurt from laughing and I rubbed them futilely as I tried to regain control of my breathing.

When we could speak again, Daniel shook his head and said, "It's amazing you got away with it for so long before Stan figured out it was you! But when he did...."

The sobering memory effectively cut through the hilarity I had been enjoying. "It was pretty obvious when he finally knew, wasn't it?" I replied ruefully. One time after Stan had visited I had started to get in my car and glimpsed something odd out of the corner of my eye. Walking around the back of the vehicle I beheld...well, it more closely resembled a banner than a bumper sticker. It must have been a meter long, and stretched clear across the sloped back of my Volkswagen Beetle. Right up at eye level, too. "*My Bra Snags My Chest Hair.*" I looked around and quickly tore it off, thanking my lucky stars I had seen it before I went driving around town. That ended the bumper sticker shenanigans, but oh the fun at Stan's expense had been sweet while it lasted.

Daniel and I drove along in silence for awhile, each of us lost in amused reflection. But now and then we looked at each other, and the snickering would start again.

The freeway eventually led us out of the mountainous country of Southern Oregon and down onto the flat expanse of the Willamette Valley. The view opened up as the hills fell away. Far off to our right I could see the rugged peaks of the Cascade Range, extending to the north and south like an immense wall of stone erected by titans. On the horizon to our left we could see the gentler emerald humps of the coastal mountains. In front of us stretched the smooth flatness of the valley floor, its farms and crop fields extending hundreds of miles north to Portland. The freeway arrowed straight ahead like a line from a surveyor's map, eventually losing itself in the far hazy distance. Traffic was light and the miles rolled effortlessly by.

We arrived in Corvine around two in the afternoon, and slowly made our way through neighborhoods of modest old homes, their well-kept yards sporting green lawns and colorful flowerbeds. Up ahead the brick and concrete buildings of the university reared high above the surrounding residences. Our campus map guided us through the maze of multistory structures. Eventually we arrived in front of the graduate student dorm that I would call home for the school year. I got out of the car and stretched my stiff legs. Looking around, I was pleased to spot the familiar bulk of the veterinary building only a block away across a green field. Fortune had smiled upon me; it would be a quick walk to and from classes.

We unloaded my belongings on the sidewalk, and then Dan said, "Well, here's where we part ways." He squinted appreciatively up at my new residence and commented, "Looks like you'll be in decent housing at least." Then he turned and extended his hand. "Good luck with vet school, my friend. It will be great having you on campus this year. Come see me at my dorm soon, okay?"

"You can bet on it," I replied with a grin. "You're the only person I know up here! Thanks for giving me a ride, Dan." He nodded and smiled before getting back into his car. Watching him drive away, I was struck with the realization that our long friendship as we knew it was coming to an end. As undergraduates Daniel and I had attended different schools, but we had always come home to enjoy summers together in Medford. Soon that would change. Daniel would graduate after this year and would move away to wherever he found work. Never again would we spend endless hours doing anything or nothing, as only young friends can. We would live in different cities leading separate lives. During the holidays we would send each other Christmas cards, and once in a while we might get together and reminisce about old times. But it would be a friendship set in the past, and we would grow gradually apart with the distance between us.

Daniel was a symbol of all that I was leaving behind: my home town, my family, the life I had known. All this I saw in a flash as I watched his car shrink into the distance, and it saddened me to know that things could never be the same again. My heart full of memories, I turned to face the weathered brick front of the dormitory. I bent down and grabbed the handles of my trunk and my suitcase. Then I walked toward the doors and the unknown future ahead.

CHAPTER EIGHT

As I strode up the sidewalk to the dorm, I noticed a blue wooden sign set in the middle of the front lawn. The dormitory name was displayed in block yellow letters, "Wayne International House." The name suggested the nature of the dorm: it not only housed graduate students but also had a strong foreign student contingent. Looking at the sign I did a double-take. Someone had attached a second piece of wood below the main frame, painted to closely mimic the original color scheme. Below "Wayne International House" the words "of Waffles" had been added. I stared for a moment and then began chuckling. Someone here had a sense of humor. I shook my head and pushed through the double glass doors, entering the main lobby of the dorm.

The lobby was large and floored in faded brown tiles. The building had that faint musty smell of age I had come to expect on college campuses. Off the left end of the lobby I saw a carpeted student lounge with sofas, chairs, and a large television mounted on one wall. Several students were sprawled on the furniture watching a college football game. Directly ahead of me was a large reception window with an office behind it. To my right I saw stairs and an elevator leading to the upper floors.

I dragged my luggage over to the reception area and checked in. The young man behind the window gave me an information packet about the dorm, including a map and meal schedules. My papers said I would be sharing a room with someone named Daryl Dorland. I got my room key, labeled "232." The key also opened a numbered mailbox on the wall near the counter.

I walked over to the elevator and thumbed the worn call button. With considerable shuddering and grinding the ancient elevator car deposited me on the second floor. I exited into one end of a wide carpeted hallway. Room doors dotted the walls at regular intervals. I walked along reading the numbers over the doorsills. Room 232 was about halfway down the hall on the right side. I stopped in front of the door and tried my key. The lock opened and I entered the room.

My dorm room was built for double occupancy; it contained two single beds, one to each side of the doorway. A floor-to-ceiling storage closet stood at the foot of each bed. The far wall sported a long built-in desk with two chairs and reading lamps.

My roommate had apparently arrived before me. A red suitcase lay on the bed to my left, and a variety of clothes hung in the adjacent open closet. I went to the window over the desk and peered out. The room overlooked a brick courtyard below; directly across from me was the cafeteria building which served this dorm. Meals would at least be convenient, if somewhat uninspiring.

As I turned from the window, I noticed a glass terrarium perched on the left end of the desk. Peering closer, I saw a small coiled snake nestled in the pebbles at the bottom. It had an attractive orange-brown diamond pattern down its back and a sharply turned-up nose. Having an interest in all sorts of animals, I recognized this as a hog-nosed snake. I had never seen one in person before. Fascinated, I crouched down and watched awhile. The snake's small forked tongue flicked in and out as the unblinking yellow eyes stared back at me. I grinned thoughtfully; based on this pet I suspected my roommate might prove to be an interesting character.

After unpacking my things, I lay back on the bed and closed my eyes, relaxed in the knowledge that I had found my new home successfully. The air was warm and still and the dorm relatively quiet. I heard the footsteps and voices of other students occasionally passing by my room, and once in a while the soft whine of the elevator down the hall.

Graduate student housing did have its advantages. Students here were generally older and more serious about their studies than in the average undergraduate dorm. My neighbors would not likely be wild partiers, so I would have time undisturbed to handle the heavy coursework the vet program would throw at me. I pondered the upcoming school year, my thoughts wandering aimlessly. Eventually the warmth and quiet of my room worked their magic and I dozed off for awhile.

I was awakened abruptly by the noise of the door opening. I sat up groggily and saw a young man in blue jeans and a white T-shirt pulling his key out of the open door. He had light brown hair cropped very close. Even lying on my back I could tell that he was shorter than I and slight of build. Overall he appeared well-groomed, and his smooth, even-featured face wore an amiable grin. He stepped forward and held out his hand. "You must be Mark," he said.

I smiled back and shook his hand, saying, "And you must be Daryl." He had a good grip for a small guy, and his brown eyes looked me steadily in the face. I thought he had an honest, open feel to him. I blinked my eyes, trying to shake off the remnants of sleep, and asked him, "When did you arrive?"

"Oh, a couple of hours ago. I brought my stuff up and then went out with some friends," he replied.

We introduced ourselves a bit more, talking about where we came from, what we were majoring in, and so forth. Daryl hailed from Eugene, Oregon and was pursuing a master's in business. His face lit up when I asked him about his pet. "Oh yeah, isn't she a beauty?" he said. "Her name's Roseanne. You don't have a problem with snakes, do you?"

I assured him I didn't and he looked relieved. We went over to the tank and peered inside. Daryl removed the top and reached in to grab the little animal. She didn't react much at all, just coiled placidly around his fingers and sat there, tongue tasting the air as she alertly looked around. I asked if I could hold her and he offered the snake to me. I took her gently in my hands. Many people envision snakes to be slimy like an earthworm, but the opposite is true. Roseanne was warm and dry, and soft like supple leather.

I held her for a minute or two, enjoying the chance to handle and see her up close, then gave her back to Daryl, who replaced her in the cage. He carefully attached the lid, saying "She's an escape artist; if this top isn't secure all the way around she'll find an opening and be gone. Once it took me two weeks to find where she'd hidden in my room."

I whistled. "Wow! Where'd you find her?"

Daryl laughed. "In the bottom drawer of my dresser, curled up inside a pile of underwear." We both had a good chuckle at that image, and I found myself liking this roommate already.

That evening there was an outdoor barbeque in the plaza between the buildings, to welcome the students on their first day in the dorms. As the sun fell toward the horizon, scores of young men and women mingled and feasted on the bounty of food and drink spread on the long tables in the courtyard. I eagerly helped myself to a plateful of food. Chatting students formed small impromptu groups, and I joined one after another as I wandered slowly around. Eating and sharing small talk with various people, I grew restless after a while. Everywhere I looked were friendly faces, but I knew no one. I suddenly knew what it meant to feel alone in a crowd. In time I hoped I would find companions in this unfamiliar place.

Later in the evening I lay awake in my small bed staring up into the dark. It had been a long day. The building was quiet and still other than an occasional muffled voice or the thud of a door closing. Daryl's slow, regular breathing was barely audible from across the room. The new strangeness of everything kept my thoughts racing ahead of slumber's grasp. I closed my eyes, my mind full of the day's events and wondering about the challenges ahead. Past, present, and future began to merge and spin together in a hazy blur. I had time to wonder what my family might be doing at that moment, and then the sweet oblivion of sleep finally claimed me.

The following morning was Sunday. When I awoke, I dressed casually in jeans and T-shirt and went down the hallway to the second-floor bathroom. This dorm was coed, but each floor was unisex, either men or women. The men's room turned out to be quite busy this time of day. I would have to get used to sharing space with a dozen other guys in the morning. After shaving and showering, I dressed again and went to the dining hall next door. Inside the door was a line of students selecting food from a buffet-style counter. I grabbed a tray and joined the line. The dining area consisted of rows of long tables, each with about ten chairs on a side. Toting my loaded plate, I found an empty seat and dug into my food. It wasn't too bad for institutional fare.

After breakfast I grabbed my campus map, and hiked to the school bookstore to procure my required textbooks. Each was an impressively thick heavy tome, sporting equally heavy titles like *Canine Anatomy*, *Animal Physiology*, *Histopathology*, and *Animal Neurology*. I paid for the texts and walked back to the dorm. My overloaded backpack made the return trip a bit more arduous. As I labored along, I pictured myself at eighty, hunched over and walking with a pronounced limp, telling my grandkids in wheezy voice, "Yes, young ones, the weight of knowledge did this to me." The image made me straighten my back a bit more as I continued on to the dorm.

Once I dropped off my books at my room, I had time to wander the campus. The university was an attractive mix of old brick and concrete architecture and tree-lined streets. Everywhere was greenery, courtesy of the heavy annual rainfall here. As the day wore on, I kept one eye on the clock. The veterinary school had scheduled a welcoming dinner that evening for the incoming freshman class. We were to gather at McNairy Hall at six P.M. From there we would drive to the Thompson Arboretum just outside of town.

When the hour drew near, I donned a nice shirt and slacks and made my way over to the vet school. As I approached the front of the building, I recalled my first visit there as a timid outsider hoping for admission. Seen up close, the beautiful teaching hospital with its flowing lines still impressed. But today there was no question in my mind as I walked up to the heavy doors, no self doubt. I possessed a confidence born of the certainty that I was now part of all this. I belonged!

Inside the doors, a group of young men and women milled around in the spacious lobby. I had my first glimpse of my new classmates, the people with whom I would share the next four years. I guessed about twenty were here already, so more were coming after me. Our class size was listed as thirty-six, with about equal numbers of male and female students. I looked around and had to smile when I recognized one face. It was the young man who had passed by me in the dean's office the day of my interview. He had been accepted as well. For some reason that made me feel good, even though I didn't know him. Perhaps it was because I had glimpsed in his eyes the same hopes and doubts that had consumed me that day.

Students came through the door one by one until it looked as though the entire class must be there. I introduced myself to a handful of my new classmates as we waited. The student I had seen interviewing was named Stan Hulbert. He was tall and strong-jawed, with medium-length, curly black hair and light blue eyes. His voice was deep and his smile engaging. His striking looks and his confident bearing gave him an undeniable charisma. My first impression of Stan was that he would have done well in public office or posing for a statue of a Greek god. But once I began talking with him, I was taken by his modesty and total lack of self-importance. He humbly expressed how anxious he was about handling the difficult curriculum ahead. Listening to him, I could tell that he was in the habit of saying what he felt, with no games and no pretenses. His laugh, which came easily and often, was contagious. You just couldn't help but like Stan, and I knew right away that I would enjoy spending time with him.

Around ten minutes past six, Dr. Hudson came down the stairs from his office and greeted the assembled students. "Hello everyone," he said, smiling broadly. "I want to formally welcome the Class of 1986 to the Northern Oregon University School of Veterinary Medicine. Whew, that's a mouthful!" A trickle of laughter ran through the students, and then he continued, "I think everyone is here, so we'll head over to the arboretum for the dinner. This will be chance for each of you to get to know your classmates a bit, as well as meet some of the professors. Some of you may not have cars, so it would be great if we can carpool. Anyone who can't find a ride, let me know and we'll figure something out."

With that announcement students began turning to each other, discussing rides and driving arrangements. I had no car, so I asked Stan, who immediately invited me to ride with him. A petite blonde woman standing near us overheard our conversation and rather timidly said, "Excuse me, is there any chance I can come along with you guys? I'm sorry, but I don't have a ride. I'm Amy Baker, by the way!" She offered her hand, and we made introductions all around, and Stan told her that of course she could ride with us.

As a group the students began heading out to the parking lot across the street from the vet school. Stan's car was a faded blue Chevy sedan with more than a few miles under its wheels. He sheepishly apologized for the shabby appearance of the ride, and for the tattered veterinary journals piled on the back seat. "They're my dad's old ones; he's a vet too. Just throw them on the floor to make room," he said as he casually waved his hand at the stacks. I displaced a few dog-eared issues of *Veterinary Medicine Monthly* and got in the back, giving Amy the front passenger seat. We began the drive out to the arboretum, following directions that the school had included in our orientation packets.

The Thompson Arboretum was nestled in old growth forest not far from the outskirts of town. I asked Stan why we were heading there, and he explained that the facility possessed conference rooms where dinners and other functions could be held. Out of town and into the countryside we drove, past farm fields and into the heart of McClain Forest. Here a multitude of evergreens, dozens of species in all, vied for space and light along the roadside. They grew so densely that nowhere could I see more than ten or twenty meters into the woods. Dominating the forest, both in numbers and in sheer size, were the Douglas firs. Their straight, smooth trunks, many well over a meter in diameter, stretched fifty meters (160 feet) and more into the deepening blue of the sky overhead. Down at ground level a medley of shrubs, ferns, and grasses added their delicate textures and hues as they crowded around the feet of their massive cousins.

At dusk we arrived at the arboretum, a large attractive building nestled in the trees at one edge of a clearing. Its single-storied frame appeared to be constructed entirely of cedar, with steeply peaked gables and long wall planks that sloped diagonally. Large windows provided grand views of the natural beauty all around. The stylish yet rustic structure almost seemed an outgrowth of the forest itself.

Other cars were pulling into the parking lot as we exited Stan's vehicle. We made our way together toward the arboretum. Pathways laid with crushed grey rock led through a landscaped collection of native trees and shrubs. Beautiful wood and glass doors ushered us into the arboretum, and Dr. Hudson directed us toward a conference room off the main lobby. Inside the large room were nine square dining tables with white tablecloths, each set for four guests. In front of each place setting was a small placard with a student's name in flowing script. At the front of the room were longer tables with a buffet of wonderful smelling foods. There were also additional place settings at the end of one table, which I guessed were for attending faculty.

Dr. Hudson told us to grab food from the buffet and seat ourselves where we found our names. By contrast to the previous night's barbeque, this was a tastefully catered affair, with white porcelain plates and a nice selection of entrées. I found baked salmon and chicken cordon bleu, plus steamed vegetables, baby red potatoes and wild rice as side dishes. Fresh salad greens with several types of dressing complemented the other offerings. Drink selections included ice water, sparkling cider, and a couple of bottles of chardonnay. Nothing extravagant, but a very nice presentation. The school was showing us its appreciation, and with our small class size the evening felt quite intimate.

I filled my plate and found my seat. A pleasant surprise was seeing that Amy Baker had the place to my left. "Wow, this is nice," she murmured appreciatively. "Seeing your name on the place setting makes it seem personal, you know?"

"Exactly," I agreed with a smile. "It feels like we matter, that we're not just numbers on an enrollment list."

She nodded eagerly. Just as we were getting settled, I heard the chime of a utensil on a glass and I looked up. Dr. Hudson was standing at his place at one of the front tables, and he announced, "Greetings everyone. This dinner is to welcome and congratulate all of you for making this year's class. As you can see, you are seated in groups of four, arranged by alphabetical order. This will also be the seating arrangement in your classroom. You will be grouped together at your workstations, and much of your anatomy lab coursework will be done as a team. We felt that seating you thusly tonight would give you a chance to know your teammates a little."

He paused, and then turned to the several men and women who were seated beside him. "I'd like to introduce some of your course instructors now. This fair lady seated next to me is Dr. Marsha Tobin; she'll be teaching the freshman neurology course." The doctor in question was tall, slender, maybe in her late thirties, with long, reddish-blond hair and an open smile. She nodded and waved at the class, her freckled face blushing a little.

Next Dr. Hudson introduced the anatomy professor, Dr. Hank Warner. He was short and stocky, powerfully built, and had a close-cropped, military-style crew cut atop a rather stern face. He nodded slightly when introduced, and offered only the briefest of smiles before returning to his dinner. Contemplating him, I decided that Dr. Warner might be wound a bit tight. Apparently I was not alone in that assessment. Just as I reached to take a drink from my glass, Amy leaned over to me and said under her breath, "Gee, do you think he'd feel better if he pulled the corn cob out?" I spent the next few seconds trying desperately not to spew sparkling cider out my nose.

When I regained my composure, the physiology professor was being introduced. Dr. Dan Lawson was a large burly man with thick ebony hair and a full beard. He bore an eerie family resemblance to Blackbeard the Pirate. When his name was called, he grinned broadly, flashing white teeth. His voice boomed through the room even when directed at the person next to him; he didn't appear to have a low volume setting.

Dr. Hudson informed us that our other professors were not able to make tonight's dinner. We would meet them in class on the first day of school. With that, he told us to enjoy our meals and get to know one another, and he resumed his seat.

I turned my attention to the two students seated with Amy and me, and we made our introductions. Across from me sat a wiry guy whose face was all angles and hollows. His straggly brown hair fell randomly about his head; I had to wonder if he owned a comb. The name placard said he was Mike Callahan. Mike exuded sheer energy and enthusiasm, and he talked so fast it was a challenge to follow him. At any moment I expected him to come unglued from his seat in defiance of gravity and go bouncing around the room like a ping pong ball. He seemed to find humor in almost everything, but despite his casual levity, he did not come across as dull or goofy. His alert expression and lively repartee hinted of an acute intelligence at work behind those darting eyes.

The fourth member of our group was Molly Boyer, a quiet, thirty-something mother of two who had decided to go back to school. Her dark brown hair was cropped above her shoulders and she dressed conservatively in a tan pant suit. She was friendly but more reserved than Amy or Mike. I debated whether this might be due to age and maturity, or if she was simply shy.

The four of us chatted the evening away, each of us learning something of the others' backgrounds and interests. Mike and Amy both came from rural communities and had majored in animal husbandry in college. Mike in particular would prove useful to our lab group, I thought. He had taken animal anatomy as an undergraduate. My college hadn't even offered that course, and I felt completely ignorant when it came to dissecting a cadaver. I was glad to have him on board.

After we finished dinner, I mingled with classmates and eventually introduced myself to the professors in attendance. They seemed open and personable, with the possible exception of Hank Warner, the anatomy instructor. My initial impression of him as a strict drill sergeant was reinforced when face to face. His manner was curt and humorless, and I suspected his class would be a real challenge to excel in. Still, classmates had told me that his reputation was solid, and students came out of his course possessing an excellent grasp of anatomy. I could overlook a gruff personality if he was a dedicated teacher.

All in all, the evening was uniquely memorable, an inviting beginning to my time at the veterinary college. I had to pinch myself as I gazed around at the elegant accommodations, the intimate setting, and the small group of bright-eyed men and women that comprised my class. There are more prestigious veterinary programs to be sure, older and with storied traditions. But none of those schools could have made their incoming students feel more welcome than I felt that night.

CHAPTER NINE

The next morning came early, and the shrill beep of my bedside clock was an unwelcome intrusion into the warm cocoon of sleep. Awkwardly I groped until I found the alarm shutoff, and I dragged myself down the hall to shave and shower. My first class was scheduled for 7:30 A.M., which in my opinion was not an hour for sane people to be conscious. I made my way to the cafeteria and ate on autopilot, then headed for McNairy Hall.

The morning air was crisp with autumn's chill and I pulled my light jacket closer around me as I strode up the sidewalk. After walking about one block, I crossed railroad tracks and found myself skirting the meadow adjacent to the veterinary building. On my first visit here, wildflowers had flaunted their vivid colors in counterpoint to the greens of spring. Now the grass had browned and gone to seed, the flowers long since withered.

I entered the building and found the student lecture hall a mere handful of steps from the outer door. The veterinary program in Oregon was fairly new, and the facilities provided education only for the farm animal portion of the curriculum. The school had a cooperative arrangement with Washington University in Tullville. Students spent their freshman year in Oregon, then went to the vet school in Washington for their small animal medicine and surgery training. We would return to Corvine in the middle of our junior year to finish our degree here.

Because the school was small and half the students were at another location, only one lecture hall had been provided to serve both the freshman and upper classes. But what the school lacked in quantity, it made up in quality. The auditorium was visually impressive, and I paused in the doorway as I took it all in. Shaped like a pie wedge tapered toward the front podium, it was steeply tiered and widened progressively as you climbed up toward the back. Each rising tier sported a long, curved, continuous desktop that stretched across the entire width of the room. Comfortable swiveling chairs were lined up behind each row's stretch desk at about one meter intervals, giving students plenty of working room for books and notes. Dual slide projectors, banks of adjustable lighting—this place had it all.

Many of my classmates were already seated along the desks, notebooks at the ready. I took a seat up high near the back of the room and waited. Glancing around, I picked out Stan Hulbert down near the front, smiling and chatting with a woman seated to his left. Even from behind Stan's height and black curly hair made him an easy mark.

After a few minutes Mike Callahan came bouncing into the room and I waved him up to where I sat. He took the steps two at a time, and dropped his narrow frame into the seat to my left. Amy Baker came in a short time later and also joined us. Molly, the fourth member of our team, sat way down near the lecture podium. From my vantage point above, I saw that she placed a small tape recorder on the desk top next to her notebook.

Around this time I became aware of a rapid thumping noise, and looked down to see Mike Callahan's foot steadily bouncing off the floor. He saw me looking and his foot stilled, but a few seconds later I heard the *tap, tap, tap* of his pencil drumming on the desk surface. Apparently Mike could not hold all his body parts immobile at the same time. I tried in vain to comprehend how someone could have that much energy this early in the morning.

Dr. Lawson the buccaneer look-alike taught the animal physiology course, which was our first lecture of the day. At 7:30 A.M. sharp he came bustling in and plunked his notebooks on the podium. He was neatly attired in dark slacks and a blue, short-sleeved dress shirt, and with every movement there seemed to be a battle raging between the tightly stretched clothes and the huge frame they had been called on to cover.

He scanned his eyes over the assembled students, and with a big smile he boomed, "Good morning, class! Welcome to your first day in the veterinary program." He disdained using the microphone, his deep voice easily filling the room clear up to the back rows where my companions and I sat. He continued, "Today will not involve a lot of class work. Mostly we'll be doing orientation, including a tour of the teaching hospital so you all know your way around."

He paused, stroking his beard thoughtfully, and said, "For my part, I want to congratulate you all for getting here. As you know, that in itself is quite an accomplishment. Now I want you to forget what you've seen on television shows about med schools, where classmates ruthlessly compete for the best grades or top standing. Our approach is in fact quite the opposite. You all have shown that you have the requisite gray matter to succeed. The competition ended when you were accepted into this school. You no longer need to worry about pulling straight A's; just concentrate on learning the material so that you can become proficient practitioners of medicine. Potential employers want a good clinician, with medical aptitude and good people skills. That isn't necessarily the student who gets the top grades in a class."

He paused and extended his hands outward to encompass everyone in the room. "You are also not on your own. We strongly encourage you to work together and help each other. Your class is small and you will be side-by-side for the next four years. Best to do it as friends, yes?" He smiled and nodded as if in answer to his own question.

"Oh, and one last thing," he said, and his dark eyes narrowed as he spoke slowly and intently. "This program is strenuous and there is a lot of material to learn. We do not recommend that you try to hold down a job or take other classes while you are enrolled in the veterinary program. If you stretch yourself too thin you won't do justice to your studies, and you will probably burn out.

"Also, on a more personal note, I would caution each of you to take care of your home life. Becoming a veterinarian is very exciting, and it can be overwhelming at times, but you also need a life outside of your work. Please do not neglect relationships and those that matter to you. The medical professions have some of the highest divorce rates of any lines of work. Take my advice and don't become a statistic."

His words had everyone's attention. You could have heard a flea pass gas in the stillness that followed. Apparently everybody looked suitably serious, because Dr. Lawson abruptly slapped the podium and said, "Okay, enough heavy talk! Let's show you the building and our lovely teaching hospital. First we'll head upstairs to the anatomy lab which will serve as your main classroom for this year." With that he headed for the door, waving for us to follow him.

I grabbed my notebooks and filed out with my classmates. As a group we headed up the broad stairway that I had first climbed on the day of my interview. This time when we reached the top we turned away from the Dean's office and headed left down a long corridor. Eventually we came to a doorway on the right which was open; we entered single-file and had our first view of our classroom.

The sign above the door designated this place as the anatomy lab. It was certainly equipped for that, with multiple steel sinks and a large vault-like door to a refrigerated cold room on one wall. A long countertop ran against another wall, with a row of gleaming white microscopes arrayed along its length. Below the counter were burgundy cupboards and drawers, each labeled to show what supplies were contained within.

We had been told the seating arrangement would be similar to that used during our welcoming banquet. Sure enough, here were multiple work stations, each station comprised of four interconnected desks. Each group of desks had adjacent storage cabinets for students' supplies.

In one corner of the room I found the workstation that housed the desks for Mike, Molly, Amy, and me. We each took our seats and checked out the desks. Amy was seated to my left and Mike was across from me. My desk looked shiny new, with a generously large working surface. I opened my cabinet and found a small array of dissecting instruments, plus a wooden box full of bones, including what looked like a small dog skull.

My inspection was interrupted by Dr. Lawson's voice once more calling for our attention. I looked up to see him standing in the open area at the center of the room. He swept his arm around him and said, "This will be your main classroom while you are freshmen. Inside your cabinets you will find your dog bones and dissection instruments. This is also where you will store your microscopes. Each student is responsible for his or her equipment. Be sure that everything is cleaned and put away at the end of each day.

"Your anatomy and histology labs will be held in this room. The first labs begin tomorrow as scheduled. For now let's make a tour of the hospital. Please follow me." So saying, he lumbered back toward the door and we quickly closed our cabinets and followed.

The teaching hospital was primarily a large animal facility, so everything here was built on a grand scale. Oversized rooms provided ample space for both the patients and their attending veterinarians. The ceilings were very high, so even a bucking and kicking horse could not strike them. All the flooring was smooth concrete with inset drains, allowing rooms to be hosed down when soiled.

We visited the surgery suite, equipped with a table that looked large enough to neuter an elephant on. The anesthetic machine was awe inspiring in itself, a hulking conglomeration of pumps and tubes, its black oxygen hoses nearly the diameter of my leg.

Just off the surgery area we walked through a large, empty room with soft padded walls. When the doors were closed it was dimly lighted, and there were huge rubber mats strewn across the floor. I could not imagine what this room would be used for, other than perhaps confining psychotic cattle in straight jackets. It made more sense when Dr. Lawson told us that this was a post-surgical recovery room. I had seen dogs coming out of anesthetic, careening drunkenly around their cages when half awake; I didn't want to imagine a two-thousand-pound horse in a similar state.

Next we toured the main radiology room, sporting a high-power X-ray machine that could create a film exposure even through the thickness of a horse's thorax. This room was nearly seven meters (over twenty feet) across, and the machine's imaging head could be lowered from above and positioned at almost any height or angle around the patient. Dr. Lawson explained that horses and cattle were too large to easily place them on a standard radiology table even if anesthetized. Instead, the mobile X-ray head would be aimed horizontally at the standing patient, with the film placed on the other side of the animal's body. This allowed images of legs or body to be obtained with the patient wide awake and minimally restrained.

We moved down the hall to a central treatment area. As in small animal hospitals, much of the important activity was focused here. Hospitalized patients could be examined, given daily medications, have blood samples drawn, and such. Several squeeze chutes stood in the open center of the spacious room. Each could hold a horse or cow immobile while they were treated, maximizing safety for both doctor and patient. An amazing array of white cupboards and cabinets lined the walls of the room; to my eyes it seemed that they must contain every medication and piece of equipment known to veterinary science.

The last area we visited was the inpatient housing, consisting of a series of large stalls around the periphery of the hospital. They were not the dark, cramped accommodations you might encounter on an old farm, wooden cells riddled with dry rot and foul odors. Instead, these animal holding rooms were light, airy, clean and spacious. They also looked impressively solid. The front of each stall was constructed of vertical iron bars as wide as my forearm, extending at least three meters (nine feet) high. The walls between adjacent stalls were thick concrete, painted an attractive antique white with tan trim. These were equal in height to the stall fronts, but still ended well short of the lofty ceiling twelve feet overhead. Buckets containing feed and water hung from the bars on some of the occupied stalls. Sturdy industrial hoses attached to spigots in front of the chambers, allowing easy washing down of the walls and floors.

Here and there we encountered veterinarians and senior students in the wide hallway fronting the stalls. They were clad in light blue head-to-toe coveralls, and wore identification badges on their collars or breast pockets. Dr. Lawson introduced some of them to us. I met Dr. O'Brien for the second time, and watched him treating a large grey mare in one of the stalls. I had to grin when I recalled his humorous question during my interview. Today he was as jolly and outgoing as ever, joking boyishly with the senior students who were assisting him.

Dr. Lawson pointed out their clothing to us, remarking, "You might want to invest in some coveralls like those. Freshmen don't get to do much hands-on work with the patients. Nonetheless, you may learn some basic handling techniques, and your neurology class will include doing neuro exams on horses, cattle, and sheep. In doing so, you'll get plenty dirty and you'll want something to cover your street clothes.

"Buy coveralls with plenty of pockets for items like thermometers and bandage scissors. I'd advise getting one that zips right down the middle for easy removal if you catch a bucketful of cow dung down your front." With that he let out a rumbling laugh and waved us onward down the hall.

One thing I saw that day stands out in my mind, because it impressed upon me the awesome power that our patients possessed, and the respect that one must always accord them. We had come to the end of the animal stalls and encountered large, barn-like doors which opened to the outside. A set of chutes ran from these doors to an indoor holding pen area, allowing cattle or sheep to be funneled in from the outdoor corral.

One of the chutes led to a large holding device which resembled an open pair of hands with curved fingers pointing upward. The animal would be directed to walk between the wide open halves of the device, and then large hydraulic pistons would drive the two halves together, closing the "hands" around the patient. It allowed a large, fractious animal to be immobilized while standing, without the need for heavy sedation.

Though impressive, the hydraulic squeeze machine seemed a supreme example of excess in design. The bright yellow steel beams that made up the clamps of the device resembled a double row of small tree trunks. The hydraulic units driving the arms looked like they could jack an eighteen-wheel truck off the ground. A nice piece of hardware to be sure, but it hardly seemed likely that all that bulk was really necessary. Such was my thinking until Dr. Lawson pointed something out to us.

"See that unit there?" he asked us, pointing to the machine. "That's one of our favorite toys; we call her Big Bertha. Quite impressive, isn't she?" Murmurs of assent arose from the assembled students, and he grinned and said, "Hard to believe she almost isn't strong enough to do the job, eh?"

He laughed out loud at the astonished looks on the students' faces, and said, "Look here and you'll see what I mean." He pointed to the base of the steel arms on one side of the unit. "We had a large Red Angus bull in here a few months ago, a prized breeding animal with a lacerated penis. We brought him in to examine and treat his wound, and he wasn't too happy about being here. After we tightened Bertha down on him, he threw a major tantrum and heaved the entire machine around. You can see where he bent the arm there all to hell." Sure enough, when I looked closer, I could see the massive steel rods had unbelievably been twisted awry near the base. What kind of force it would take to do that, I could not conceive of. That must have been some show. I vowed to never again think small when dealing with patients who could mangle me without breaking a sweat.

We finished the day early, but despite the light schedule I felt exhausted by evening. At the cafeteria I had a quick dinner, Sloppy Joes and cornbread, no less. If you want to embrace the college dorm food experience, it just doesn't get any better than that! I hit my bed by ten P.M. and was unconscious within minutes. My last waking thought was that despite the hard work ahead, this year could prove to be quite fun.

CHAPTER TEN

The following morning I was again seated in the back of the auditorium, in the very first lecture of my veterinary curriculum. The room was quiet, the class hushed with anticipation. Dr. Lawson's large frame filled the doorway as he entered the room. He made his way to the lecture podium and opened his notebook. Looking out over the class, he rubbed his nose and bid us "Good morning," smiling broadly. After consulting his notes for a moment, he looked up and began an introductory overview of animal physiology.

As I listened, I realized that the material sounded reassuringly familiar. I'd had similar coursework as an undergraduate, so I expected that some of this class would be review for me. I settled back in my chair and began to take down notes as he talked. The lecture hall was familiar ground and I knew this routine well.

After fifty minutes with Dr. Lawson we had a ten-minute break, and then histology class began. Histology is basically the study of tissues under the microscope. The two things we needed to learn were how to recognize the various structures of the body micro-scopically, and also how to recognize pathology when present.

I had never seen the histology professor until now, so I looked up with interest as he walked in. Dr. Ted Smythe was young, maybe thirty-five or forty, with short, dark hair and a pale complexion. His build was as slight as Dr. Lawson's was large. He was attired quite dapperly in a sports jacket and dress slacks. Soft-spoken and soft-skinned, wearing small gold-rimmed glasses, he seemed more of an academician than someone who worked in the field. I'd have bet money that he didn't own coveralls or a thermometer.

Dr. Smythe's first lecture introduced histology, and showed some projected color slides of how tissues looked under the micro-scope. He also discussed the common types of stains used in prepar-ing specimens. His knowledge of the subject seemed solid, and he fielded questions from the students with the ease of someone stroll-ing through his own back yard.

Another break, then the gross anatomy lecture began. Dr. War-ner marched in promptly on the hour, thumped his notes down, and began speaking without preamble. He posed stiffly erect behind the podium, his buzz haircut bristling as it too stood at attention. His lecture was dry but easy to follow, and he didn't mince words, stick-ing to the subject at hand with few deviations. I was surprised to find that I liked his speaking style, even if the concept of amusement seemed foreign to him.

Once morning lectures concluded, we dispersed for our lunch break and I walked back to the dorm cafeteria to eat. Outside in the midday sun I breathed in deeply, listening to the soft rustle of the fall breeze in the trees over the sidewalk. After sitting indoors for hours, the fresh air was like a tonic, and I felt an extra spring enter my step.

In the cafeteria I ran into my roommate Daryl, and we ate lunch together. We hit the buffet line, then found adjacent seats at a long lunchroom table and attacked our sandwiches. The cafeteria was packed, and around us swirled the din of a myriad of voices in friendly conversation, punctuated by the clatter of plates and silver-ware.

Before long a couple of girls sat down across from us, one blonde and one brunette. Daryl was smooth with the ladies and soon he had struck up a conversation with the blonde girl across from him. Her companion looked at me and smiled. I smiled back, and then dropped my gaze back to my plate, feeling suddenly shy. The girl was quite attractive, and I didn't really know what to say to her. An uncomfortable silence grew as I picked at my food. Her blonde friend was seemingly engrossed in Daryl and vice versa, leaving us with no one else to talk to. I had never been very confident around women, especially cute ones, but I knew I should do something. Finally I swallowed the lump in my throat, looked across the table, and introduced myself. Our gazes met, and when she smiled again it went all the way to her eyes, warm and genuine.

I learned that her name was Cindy. She was studying organic chemistry, rather an uncommon pursuit for a woman at that time. I thought that she must possess a fairly keen mind. But her brain wasn't all I was noticing. Cindy had lovely brown eyes matching her long hair, and full lips that framed her pretty smile perfectly. Beneath her snug-fitting sweater her build was slender, but with curves in the best places. I had to fight to keep my gaze focused above her neck.

Then she asked me what I was studying, and when I told her I saw her face light up. Seeing her obvious interest gave me some added confidence, and I relaxed and began to enjoy myself. We chatted about how our classes were going, the ups and downs of dorm life, even the vagaries of cafeteria cuisine.

Cindy was quick and witty, and her laugh sounded like music in my ears. She also acted genuinely interested in what I was studying. Most people, Daryl included, would inquire about what a vet did on the job, then when I began to answer they would screw up their faces in revulsion and say, "Please, not while I'm eating! Forget I asked!" But Cindy seemed fascinated, often asking questions that required fairly graphic answers. It was a joy being able to freely share my experiences, and the entire conversation was a truly pleasant diversion.

After what seemed like only a few minutes lunch was over, and Daryl and I said goodbye to Cindy and her friend. As I walked out with Daryl, he grinned at me and said, "I saw you putting the moves on that cute lady, you smoothie, you!" I probably blushed every shade of red in the spectrum, and he laughed at my discomfort. He held up a slip of paper and said, "I got Trish's dorm room number; did you get anything from your girl?"

My heart sank as I realized I had no idea which dorm Cindy lived in, much less what her room number was. I hadn't gotten her last name either, so I had no way of looking her up. I had to admit I just wasn't proficient at the dating game. I'd been having such a good time that it hadn't occurred to me to think about seeing her again. Boy, had I blown it! I couldn't count on our paths crossing; the college was a big place and so was the cafeteria. My thoughts were in a jumble as Daryl and I parted to head back to class.

Fifteen minutes later I was sitting at my desk in the anatomy lab with my three team members. All around the room my classmates clustered in their groups, everyone wearing long white lab coats that shone spotlessly clean. Dr. Warner introduced the laboratory portion of the course, outlining our goals for the quarter. We would be learning the anatomy of the dog and cat, with exams being held every four weeks or so, plus some unannounced pop quizzes thrown in along the way. I cringed inwardly when I heard that. Anatomy was sounding more fun by the minute.

Before I knew it I was staring at a preserved dog carcass sitting in a flat plastic bin on my desk. There were two dogs for our work group, one that Amy and Molly would work on, and one for Mike and me. My dog was small, weighing maybe nine kilos or twenty pounds. It was a male, rigidly frozen in the rigor of death, eyes open but clouded an opaque milky blue.

Our first assignment was to dissect the front limb, exposing the muscles, arteries, and veins. I pulled on my latex gloves and picked up a scalpel hesitantly, unsure of where to start.

Mike dived right in, slicing the skin across the leg near the shoulder, then beginning to peel it off down the limb. I grabbed the lower leg and began to work on removing the skin there. It was surprisingly tough, like furry leather, and the flesh was cold and unyielding under my fingers.

We had to work close to our subject to see the finer points of anatomy beneath our blades. I quickly discovered that such proximity had unpleasant consequences. The bodies of the dogs had been saturated with formalin to preserve them. When we bent over our specimen, the chemical fumes emanating from the tissues were almost overwhelming. We would work for awhile, then step back to gulp fresher air before diving in again.

As we whittled away Mike grinned at me over the carcass, and said, "Have you taken anatomy before?" When I shook my head, he nodded and continued, "Well, patience is the key. It takes awhile to get anywhere dissecting, and you have to be careful, otherwise you'll damage the structures we're supposed to be exposing. Of course, it helps to know where they're actually located." With that he laid his scalpel aside and grabbed his canine anatomy book. He pawed through it rapidly, seemingly oblivious to the greasy smears his soiled gloves were leaving on the expensive text. After a moment's thumbing he found the page showing the arteries and veins of the forelimb.

With the colored illustration alongside the dog, I could see better where the vessels should be situated. Sure enough, as the skin was slowly flayed back, I saw the twisting lines of blood vessels running over the reddish brown surfaces of the muscles.

While we worked side by side I observed my partner out of the corner of my eye. I noted that despite his restless energy Mike had a steady hand and didn't rush the work. He was quick but not hasty, and he made no careless strokes. Amy and Molly were less sure of themselves, and occasionally Amy would glance over at my desk to see what Mike and I had done. Finally she asked us if she and Molly could come over and watch. For awhile, all four of us poured over the one specimen together. After a bit the girls nodded to each other and went back to dissecting their dog.

Thanks mostly to Mike's efforts, we made good time. By the end of the two-hour lab, we had the entire front leg freed of skin and had removed most of the connective tissues that hid the larger vessels. I was able to identify the brachial vein, the cephalic vein, the radial artery and nerve, and various muscle groups. Even Dr. Warner pursed his lips and nodded in apparent approval when he stopped by to check our progress. At the end of the lab we cleaned our instruments and put the specimens back into the cold room.

Looking back on it now, I am glad we had classes like gross anatomy and histology in our freshman year. There is the obvious need to cover basic subjects first. But the other advantage is that we dealt with the most tedious tasks while we were still flush with enthusiasm. Most of that first year we spent doing rote memorization and pouring over anatomy specimens as we wiped our watering eyes. Nonetheless, we were all so glad just to be there that we took it in stride.

Years later when we returned as juniors, we would see the current crop of freshmen in the lab, backs bent as they painstakingly dissected out tiny structures on their anatomy dogs. Despite our own heavy course work, we would look at each other thankfully and say, "Well, it could be worse. At least we aren't doing *that* any more!"

The weeks passed, and we settled into the routine of sitting in the lecture hall and working in the lab. I came to enjoy spending time with my study partners as we gradually got to know each other better. It turned out Mike had a warped sense of humor and loved to play practical jokes. Amy was bubbly and outgoing, with a fun, vivacious personality that made everyone smile. Her petite figure and blonde good looks had many of the guys in the class eyeing her, and I was surprised she was still single.

Molly became less reserved as we interacted and was actually quite interesting to talk with. Vet school was harder on her than the rest of us, because she had a family to think of amidst all the coursework. Sometimes when we had a break in our studies, she and I would tour the hospital together. It kept us in touch with the real reason we were there, the living animal patients and the illnesses that afflicted them.

Our first big exams came about four weeks after classes started. The instructors had devised a diabolical plan wherein the tests for all the courses were scheduled together: two on a Friday, and the other two on the following Monday. Friday's examinations took most of the day to complete. The gross anatomy midterm included material from both the lecture and lab sections of the course. First we tackled page after page of surprisingly challenging questions in the written portion. This was immediately followed by a trip to the lab, where the students were called upon to identify a myriad of structures on the anatomy specimens laid out on various tables.

The physiology test was a relief by comparison, being a fairly straightforward sampling of the lecture notes. Nonetheless, the two subjects in one day covered a lot of ground, and it wasn't until late afternoon that I left the veterinary building and trudged wearily back to my dorm.

That weekend I studied each day from morning until night in preparation for the histology and neurology tests. Come Monday morning, my classmates and I were once again wading through pages of questions, each designed to challenge our mastery of the material, revealing every weakness, every gap in our knowledge of these difficult subjects.

The lab portion of the histology test consisted of multiple microscopes set up with various tissues displayed. Next to each scope was a card with a question, such as, "What organ is this? What structure is this? What lesion is shown here?" I had poured over the preserved tissue slides just the day before, so nearly everything I saw was familiar. I felt pretty good about my performance, but by the end of the last exam I was utterly drained.

I didn't even have time to worry about the test results, because classes resumed the next day and there was ever more to learn. When I eventually retrieved the exam scores from my mailbox several days later, I breathed a sigh of relief. In all four classes I had pulled marks in the high eighties to low nineties.

In those first weeks of school I discovered that my favorite subject was neurology, not because it was the easiest, but because the instructor made it interesting. Dr. Marsha Tobin attacked her teaching with the enthusiasm of one in love with her work. She was easygoing and personable, and her face usually carried a smile. Her sky-blue eyes would open very wide when discussing something that interested her. She dressed in nice pant suits during lectures, and wore a white doctor's smock during clinical rounds. Despite her conservative dress style, she reminded me most of an educated hippie. She wore minimal makeup and her unstyled hair hung long and straight. When something met her approval she would often exclaim, "Cool!"

Her passion rubbed off on her students, and studying neurology was surprisingly fun. During gross anatomy class I had found learning the locations and names of nerves to be an exercise in monotony. In neurology Dr. Tobin took that knowledge and gave it meaning in the real world. We learned how to test reflexes on live patients and determine whether specific motor nerves were functioning. Other nerves were sensory, and when damaged caused numbness in certain areas. Pinprick skin testing could determine which sensory nerves were intact. A good neuro exam was sometimes enough to diagnose a horse lameness without any other tests being done. Anatomy remained my least favorite subject, but Marsha Tobin made us see the benefit in knowing where the nerves ran and what their functions were.

Through all the hard work and early challenges I remained supremely grateful that I was part of the veterinary program. I know that all of my classmates felt similarly. Each of us had strived for years and had overcome stiff competition to be one of the thirty-six in our class. That made the unexpected news of a classmate dropping out even harder to bear.

I must confess I never knew Theresa Downey well. Her team mates said she seemed to love veterinary school, always studied hard and never complained. Thus it came as a shock when she abruptly resigned early that October. The official word was that she left for personal reasons. Rumor in the classroom had it that her husband was an overbearing sort and had become frustrated with her spending time and energy on something other than him. She'd had to choose between her career path and saving her marriage. I hoped that she didn't live to regret her decision; it would be tragic if she gave up her one chance of following her dream only to be mired in an unhappy relationship, or alternatively to find herself divorced and without a career some time later. Over the years I have often wondered what path her life took. I hope that she found happiness along the way.

CHAPTER ELEVEN

With the opening created by Theresa Downey's absence, an opportunity arose for one more applicant to be accepted. Theresa's replacement was Ed Martinelli. Though short in stature, he was handsome and athletic in build, with a solid tan and a head full of blond curls. He looked more like a frat boy than a vet student. I had a good chuckle when I learned that indeed, he was the sole student in our class who belonged to a fraternity. Because of his name and the unusual circumstances of his arrival, he quickly was dubbed "Special Ed." He seemed to take the jesting without offense and was really quite a likable guy. He was also the source of much amusement to his classmates, though not by intent.

Every morning when we arrived for our first class, Mike and I would climb to the back row of the lecture hall. There we could talk quietly to each other without disrupting the class. And every morning Special Ed would come dragging in wearing sweat pants and take a seat in the very front row. Why he didn't sit in the back we never understood, but up front wasn't the place for him to be. I think that combining veterinary studies with fraternity life was not conducive to getting a lot of sleep.

Each day the lecture would begin and soon the warmth of the room, the muted lighting, and the drone of Dr. Lawson's voice would have their effect on Ed. You could set a clock by it. Maybe ten or fifteen minutes into the lecture, his head would start to nod, at first just slightly, like he was agreeing to something the professor had said. Mike would elbow me and point, and we would fight laughter as we watched. You could see Ed's cranium weighing more as the minutes dragged on, until it became an unbearable burden. He would fight it valiantly, wrenching his head up again and again, the nods becoming steadily deeper and more violent. But in the end the outcome was always the same, and Ed would be sprawled out on the desktop for all the class to see, his face plastered against the smooth surface, drool pooling by his slack jaw. Occasionally he even snored.

At first Dr. Lawson took offense at his student's lack of consciousness. A sharp rap on the desk would temporarily revive Ed and he would jolt upright, sitting bleary-eyed but with a serious expression as he tried to focus on the lecture. Ten minutes later he would be nodding off again and the cycle would be repeated. As the days went by the doctor waved his hands in exasperation and left Ed sleeping, commenting, "Well I assume one of you will give him your lecture notes."

Ironically, I encountered one circumstance where it didn't really matter if you stayed awake or not, and that was when Dr. Biddle lectured. Nathaniel Biddle was the second instructor for the histology class, assisting Dr. Smythe mostly in the lab portion. He was white-haired and close to retirement, with jowls that flapped when he talked and a quaver in his voice. Despite his apparent fragility, he dressed impeccably and held himself with an air of dignity. He could easily have played the role of an aristocratic butler, holding out a cup and inquiring with a proper British accent, "More tea, suh?"

In the lab Dr. Biddle was a godsend, as he could identify minute objects under the microscope with consummate ease. He also had a knack for explaining what we were looking at in the simplest of terms. Lecture was a different story. Usually Dr. Smythe handled this portion of the course, but on occasion he would have Dr. Biddle step in for him. The first time this happened I had my notebook open, pen at the ready as usual. The venerable professor took the podium, his gaze sharp and focused as he gazed out at us, full of wisdom and the commanding "look of eagles"—and then he started to speak. I began writing, but after a moment I paused. There had been no conclusion to the sentence Dr. Gribble had just uttered; it had abruptly changed course and veered in an entirely different direction. Thrown a bit off balance, I crossed out the words I had written and started again, only to find that once more he changed subjects before completing his first thought. It was a stream of consciousness in verbal form as I had never experienced it before. It went something like this: "We'll begin by discussing the liver and its pathology this morning…the liver has a characteristic appearance when stained with a standard H&E stain…but of course many protocols now use other stains that yield similar colors…I still prefer standard H&E, but others might argue otherwise, I'm a bit of a traditionalist I guess…some stains are more technique sensitive than others, such as gram stains used with bacteria…if you decolorize too long, then gram positive bacteria may look gram negative…but you can visualize bacteria in the liver, for instance, using standard tissue stains like H&E as well…now, if bacteria were present in the liver you would also expect to see a suppurative hepatitis consistent with bacterial infection…neutrophils would be the primary white blood cells seen in that case…neutrophils of course can be distinguished from mononuclear cells such as lymphocytes by their distinctively segmented nuclei...."

On and on he went, spewing a multitude of little factoids only loosely related to each other. I looked around and grinned as I saw even the most rabid note takers in the class with their pens frozen, looking at each other, totally at a loss as to what to write down. Eventually we all just sat back, put our pens aside, and went along for the ride. I tried to commit a few tidbits to memory, occasionally jotting down an item. Afterward I walked out of the auditorium feeling like I had killed a few thousand brain cells.

The weeks passed, autumn slowly deepened and the days grew shorter and colder. My roommate Daryl and I saw surprisingly little of each other after the first week or two of school. We were both occupied with our classes, and while Daryl sometimes studied in our dorm room, I found the anatomy lab had fewer distractions and spent more time there. I also learned that Daryl had started spending considerable time with Trish, the blonde girl he had met in the cafeteria. Often he would disappear for hours, returning very late to collapse into his bed. Once he offered to ask Trish about Cindy for me, as the two girls had seemed to be friends, but I was too embarrassed to let him do so.

Halloween approached, and with it came the opportunity for my classmates and me to exercise our creative scalpel skills. Someone bought a dozen or so medium sized pumpkins and one afternoon the anatomy lab turned into Ghoul-Carving 101. Mike and I managed to etch a ghastly face into our gourd and I was quite proud of our achievement, until I beheld what some of my classmates had conjured up out of their twisted imaginations. I saw pumpkins carved to resemble our professors, one fitted with glasses, another with a surgical cap. Several creations were hideously adorned with pieces of dog skeletons; leg bones sprouted from the base of one like some bloated orange spider. Another had a dog's jawbones extending out from its carved mouth in a skeletal grimace.

My classmates' comic tendencies manifested in other ways as well. Even a subject as dry as gross anatomy was fodder for amusement-making. One of the more obscure bits of trivia we learned about during our fall quarter was the cremaster muscle. There are two of these, and their function is to pull the testicles up close to the body to protect them in certain situations, such as in extreme cold or during a fight. Dogs, cats, and humans all possess them. One day we came to class and found a poster on the door to the lab. It pictured a young man in a white T-shirt and blue jeans, probably a clothing ad. The model had his hands jammed deep into his front pockets; one could almost imagine he was groping his anatomy. Under the picture someone had inscribed, "Advanced Cremaster Training, Room 102, 7 P.M."

Aside from humorous endeavors, one of the little pleasures of school life was getting mail. My mother wrote regularly and sent gift packages loaded with home-baked goodies. Banana bread, cookies, brownies—these were all like solid gold compared to the cafeteria food, and I savored every bite while they lasted.

When spare moments presented themselves, I would sometimes wander down to the dorm basement. They had a game room there, with a dart board and a few other diversions. The main attraction was the ping pong table. Wayne International House was home to students from all over the world, including a fair number who hailed from Asia. Table tennis was popular with many of the Chinese and Thai students, and I quickly discovered that some were highly skilled and challenging to play against. All of them seemed openly friendly and they welcomed me without question. Even when a student's English was almost as bad as my Mandarin, I could simply lift a paddle and ball and look at him questioningly. He in turn would smile broadly and nod yes, and the game was on!

As my table tennis game improved, so did my understanding of Asian cultures and points of view. One thing that impressed me about my new companions was their incredible sense of humor. I gradually became part of their circle of friends, and would be invited to sit with them in the cafeteria, often as the only American in the group. Even more enjoyable was when they were cooking food late at night in the dorm. Near the stairwell on each floor was a kitchen, really no more than a room with a dining table, a sink, and a microwave oven. I would return from an evening at the anatomy lab, taking the stairs for a little exercise. On reaching my floor, the aromas emanating from the kitchen were enough to make me weak in the knees. The Chinese and Thai students would be in there socializing and having a late night snack. Noodles and other oriental foods were heating in small cookers that they had brought with them.

I didn't want to impose, but they would see me through the open door and cheerily wave me in, insisting that I sit and eat with them. We would laugh and talk and share food into the late hours. I had never really spent time with anyone from Taiwan or Thailand before, and I found them to be truly delightful friends. To this day I consider myself privileged to have known them.

CHAPTER TWELVE

When Thanksgiving vacation arrived it was brief, only a few days' reprieve from the classroom. I hitched a ride with Daniel in his car and we visited our families in Medford. My younger brother was home as well, and we had a traditional holiday feast with turkey, stuffing, cranberry sauce, and, of course, pumpkin pie for dessert.

There was one change to the usual family rituals that year. As far back as I could remember, my mom or dad had always carved the turkey. But on this Thanksgiving Day my mom handed me the knife and said, "You're the one learning surgery, so you're better qualified to do this." Never mind that my knowledge of bird anatomy was nonexistent, or that it would be years before I performed my first surgical procedure. The way they saw it, I was in vet school studying to be a doctor, and therefore I deserved to do the blade-wielding. When I managed to produce some nice, even slabs of dark and light meat, my parents beamed, apparently satisfied that the money spent on my education was yielding results.

I returned to school after only a few days away, jumping once again into the thick of the curriculum. Final exams for the quarter were coming up just before Christmas break, and the amount of material covered for the entire three months was intimidating. I sat through long hours in class and worked feverishly in the lab, and found moments to relax whenever I could.

One day in early December I went to the cafeteria for dinner. Daryl was out for the evening and I didn't see any of my Asian friends either, so I found a mostly empty table and sat down with my tray of food. A student newspaper had been left on a chair next to me and I browsed through it as I ate.

More students were gradually filling the room around me and soon I was no longer alone at the table. I was engrossed in my meal and paper, and paid little attention until a distinctly female voice said, "Mind if I sit here?"

I glanced up and there was Cindy standing right beside me, looking down into my eyes with a friendly smile on her face. She was pointing to the vacant seat next to me. I couldn't believe my luck. A jolt of adrenaline rushed through me and I tried not to babble as I quickly said, "Oh sure, please do, I'd be delighted, sit right here!"

"Thank you," she said and sat down next to me. She was dressed in form-fitting jeans and a snug, white turtleneck shirt, and she looked fantastic. I found that once again I had to consciously lock my gaze on her face to avoid being caught ogling her figure. But there was plenty to appreciate eye to eye as well. Her thick brown hair was brushed back and glowed with a healthy shine. Those full lips were enough to keep my attention all by themselves, especially when they curved into that bright smile that she flashed as she looked over at me. I was so excited to see her that I felt jittery and on edge.

"It's nice to see you again, Cindy," I offered as we began to eat.

"I'm glad we ran across each other, Mark," she replied. "It's been awhile; I thought maybe you were avoiding me." I started to protest that nothing could be farther from the truth, and then she winked at me teasingly. I relaxed then and smiled back at her, and it struck me that she had remembered my name after all this time.

We ate and chatted, and I found that our interaction was more comfortable, more enjoyable than even the first time we had met. We learned that we had both regretted not having gotten each other's dorm addresses, and both had kicked ourselves for our lack of foresight. We had a good laugh at that *faux pas* once we knew that it was mutual.

For a while we caught up on how school life had been going, and then the conversation gradually shifted. When we had first met, our dialogue had mostly revolved around casual trivia. Now we found ourselves talking about things that people share when they really want to know each other. Starting with the ever popular "So what do you do for fun?" question, we began to explore each other's likes and dislikes, family background, plans for the future, and relationship status (I was very pleased to find that Cindy was indeed single and unattached). We also learned each other's surnames; hers was Webster.

As we talked, we found that we shared more than a superficial attraction. Cindy had grown up in a small city in Oregon, as I had. Her parents had been happily married for decades, just like mine. We both loved the outdoors and stayed active, and had compatible belief systems. Cindy's conservative upbringing had been tempered by a liberal college education, similar to my own experience. Listening to her, I found myself nodding time and again as things she said struck a chord.

While we talked the time flew by, our empty plates long since forgotten as we shared and laughed and flirted. I finally understood what it meant to experience a dance of the minds with someone. It was so easy with her, so natural, that it felt like we had known each other for a long time. I didn't want it to end.

Before we knew it the cafeteria was closing and we looked around us, startled to find that the long tables were nearly empty. My watch said it was nine P.M. We had been talking for nearly three hours!

We hurried to empty our trays and headed for the door, one of the cafeteria staff locking it behind us as we left. Once outside I hesitated, uncertain of what to say next. Cindy broke the silence by asking, "Would you like to walk me to my dorm room? Then you can see where I live. It's really near."

I nodded enthusiastically and to my surprise she led me back toward Wayne International House. All this time she had been in the same building with me! I noted with pleasure that Cindy walked close beside me, a happy smile lighting her face. We entered the dorm and took the elevator up to the fourth floor where she lived. Exiting the elevator we headed down the long corridor toward her dorm room.

As we walked we were laughing about how her friend Trish and my roommate Daryl were getting very chummy of late. According to Cindy, Trish thought Daryl was a pretty ideal guy, other than his choice of pets. I told Cindy that my roommate was an all-around nice person, from what I could tell.

Cindy then looked at me coyly and said, "So are you, Mark, from what I can tell."

I could feel my face instantly grow warm, and I smiled and looked down, managing to mumble the words, "Thank you."

We stopped in front of Room 410 and she turned to me and smiled brightly, saying, "This is my room. Thank you for a wonderful time tonight. I enjoyed it a lot."

Riding a small wave of confidence I summoned the courage to say, "I'd really like to see you again, if you're interested. Maybe we could go out for a bite to eat or see a movie sometime."

Cindy's smile widened and she answered, "Yes I'd like that very much. And...do you really need to ask if I'm interested?"

I must have looked very pleased at that last statement because it was her turn to suddenly blush and lower her gaze. We said goodnight then and she unlocked her door and went in. I stood there for a moment, basking in the warmth of that last exchange. Then I headed back to the elevator with my feet not touching the carpet, smiling to myself as I replayed the evening in my head. The future was always uncertain, but I knew two things right then. Dorm life was definitely looking up, and I was definitely falling for this girl.

CHAPTER THIRTEEN

With final exams and Christmas break rapidly approaching, the rest of December flew by, and I had little extra time to pursue Cindy. I did make sure to stop by her dorm room at least every couple days and say "hi" after classes were done. She always seemed happy to see me, and she understood my schedule, since her chemistry curriculum was pushing her hard as well. Both of us had to spend evenings studying, but we synchronized our dinner schedules when we could and met in the cafeteria. Surrounded by a crowd of diners, it was hardly a romantic setting. Nonetheless our meals together allowed us to continue to get to know each other and to share our daily experiences. I found every minute I spent with Cindy to be delightful, no matter how mundane the circumstances. Throughout those hectic but exciting weeks I could feel our bond slowly becoming closer. I was pretty sure she felt the same way.

Final exams for the quarter were, as usual, scheduled in a block around one weekend. I took my gross anatomy and physiology finals on a Friday in late December, and the neurology and histology exams on the following Monday. This time I was prepared for the concentrated barrage and had studied well ahead of time. We would not get our scores back until after the holidays, but I handed in the last test feeling confident. My feeling of accomplishment was only slightly dampened when Dr. Smythe crossed his arms and said to everyone, "Congratulations, you're one-twelfth of the way through vet school!" Then he laughed at our crestfallen expressions and walked out of the auditorium carrying the completed tests.

With the finals behind me, the pressure of the preceding weeks evaporated. School didn't resume until after New Year's, and for the first time since arriving on campus, life was free and easy. I left McNairy and walked slowly back to my dorm, enjoying the total lack of responsibilities. Outside the day was brisk, with a light cold breeze and a tumbling sky full of broken clouds. The sun peeked out at intervals, and the streets brightened and dimmed as the heavens shifted. It looked like another storm was coming in.

Later that evening I knocked on Cindy's room door, and after a few seconds she opened it. When she saw me, she flashed that ready smile I loved and said, "Mark! I was just thinking of you."

I cocked my head and replied, "Ohhhh…good thoughts, I hope."

"Always," she giggled.

"Have you eaten dinner yet?"

"No, and I'm starved," she answered.

"Want to join me in the cafeteria?" I asked.

"Sure!" She grabbed her keys and locked her door, and we walked together to the dining hall. There we shared a meal of forgettable food that was memorable for the way that it brought us closer together. We flirted and smiled and openly enjoyed each other's company. After dinner I walked her back to her room. Both of us were driving home early the next day. I would hitch a ride with Daniel to Medford down south, and Cindy would drive to Bend, which was in central Oregon. We wouldn't see each other for over a week and a half.

We arrived in front of her dorm room door, and I pulled out a Christmas card I had been saving for the right moment. "Merry Christmas, Cindy."

Her eyes widened and she said, "Aw, Mark, that is so sweet! You didn't need to get me anything...." She opened the card and read it, giggling at the silly punch line, and then she became quiet as she read the words I had written below, telling her that I would miss her while we were apart.

She looked up at me then, her eyes warm and inviting, and she said softly, "I'll miss you too, Mark. A lot." We were standing very close, and as our gazes locked, I reached out and stroked her soft hair. She didn't flinch away, and before I knew it her arms were wrapped around me and her full lips were brushing mine.

That first kiss was the best I had ever experienced, a slow, intimate, playful dance of lips and tongues, with our bodies pressed against each other from head to toe. The light scent of her perfume and the warmth of her breath on my face added to the other sensations washing over me. It only lasted a few moments but it was intoxicating, and it answered once and for all the question that had been ceaselessly running around inside my head since I had met this sweet, sexy lady. Yes, she liked me, and yes it was an affection that went beyond friendship. Now I knew that Cindy felt the same way that I did, and it was wonderful to be falling in love.

I had a hard time pulling myself out of her embrace. It had taken quite some time to get there and I wanted to stay awhile. When we did eventually pull back, we looked at each other smiling, knowing that our interaction would be more openly intimate from now on. I wished her a safe trip and a fun family holiday, and she wished me the same. Then we made our goodbye, and I walked away as she stood at her doorway. I turned and blew her a kiss, and she smiled and blew one back. She was still watching me as I got into the elevator to head to my floor.

The following morning, I was waiting by the street in front of my dorm when Daniel drove up. I hadn't had much time to get together with my longtime friend; we kept different schedules and our dorms were on opposite ends of the campus. We had only seen each other a couple of times the entire quarter. We both were excited for vacation to begin and our spirits were high as we headed out for Medford.

As the miles rolled by Daniel and I exchanged stories about the past three months. Neither of us had dated much while living in Medford, so I think each of us was a bit surprised to find that the other had a budding love life. Daniel's female friend was named Jenn. He had been seeing her for a couple of months. They were going strong, and from the way he talked I think Daniel was very serious about the relationship. He asked me about my girlfriend, and as I expounded on all of Cindy's attributes, it occurred to me that Daniel would probably conclude I was smitten as well.

We pulled into Medford just after four P.M. Daniel dropped me off in front of my home and I thanked him for the ride. After he drove off, I trod the familiar curved walkway to the front door. My family had lived in this house since I was twelve years old and it felt great to be back.

When I reached out my hand to open the door, I found myself unexpectedly conflicted. It felt awkward walking in unannounced after being away for so long. I realized this was the beginning of my establishing a life away from home. I was now visiting rather than living here. I hesitated and then rang the doorbell.

After a few moments my mom opened it, wearing an apron and a big smile. "There's our long-lost son!" she bubbled. "Come in here and give me a hug!" As soon as I stepped across the doorsill, I found myself wrapped in a motherly embrace. Dad came into the front room and greeted me, smiling and shaking my hand warmly. My younger brother Ted made an appearance too, giving me a grin and a "How have ya been?" I could smell dinner already cooking, and the sounds of a televised football game drifted in from the family room. Yes, it was good to be home.

I spent the next week and a half relaxing, visiting with friends, watching sporting events on TV with my dad, and helping out where I could. My parents were getting older, and yard work in particular was something I could do more quickly and easily than they. I raked fallen leaves from the backyard Sycamore trees and cleaned the gutters.

A baby Oregon Grape bush had volunteered in the rear corner of the yard when I was just a kid. Now towering seven feet high and nearly as wide, it was badly in need of pruning. I donned leather gloves, grabbed implements of destruction, and attacked it with vigor. It fought back bravely, its shiny holly-like leaves adorned with sharp prickles along the edges. A few choice words escaped my lips whenever a spine raked my arm or pierced a glove. In the end I conquered, and the subdued bush stood relatively small, while sporting a Dr. Warner-style haircut. I raised my arms in victory, barking out a series of man grunts until the neighbor dog began to howl. I quickly looked around to make sure no one was watching, and slunk off to clean up the trimmings.

Christmas morning came, and once the family was awake we gathered around the tree and opened presents. Everyone looked happy being together, and watching them I wished that somehow these times could last forever. Much later I would come to realize that such moments, and the people who make them, do live on as long as there is someone to hold them close to heart.

On New Year's Day we watched the tape-delayed countdown on television as the ball was lowered in Times Square and 1982 became a part of the past. I wished Cindy were there, maybe standing under that piece of mistletoe that hung on the wall by the Christmas tree. *That* would be fun!

On January 2nd Daniel and I drove back to Corvine. We were well-rested and recharged after the extended vacation. When we reached my dorm I wasted no time, heading directly upstairs to drop off my things in my room. There followed a quick trip down the hall to brush my teeth, splash on some of my best cologne, and drag a comb through my hair. Within ten minutes I was on my way to Cindy's room.

I found myself tapping my foot impatiently as the elevator wheezed its way up to the fourth floor. When I exited the car, I encountered several girls standing in the hall chatting. I tried to slow my pace so that I wouldn't draw attention. Nonetheless I could feel them looking at me as I strode by. As they resumed talking I caught the words "…Cindy's guy" just before I moved out of earshot. My ears were burning, but I smiled to myself and managed to make it to Cindy's door without tripping or running into a wall. Fervently hoping that she would be in, I reached out and knocked. There was no answer. I tried once more, and my shoulders slumped when again I received no response. Cindy was not there.

Wondering if she had made it back safely from Bend, I walked slowly to the elevator. At least the group of girls had vanished in the meantime, so I was alone with my thoughts. I pushed the call button and waited for a ride, hoping Cindy was okay.

The elevator doors finally opened and I started to enter—and nearly ran into someone coming out. I looked up and found myself face to face with Cindy! She looked startled for a second, then her face lit up with joy and she exclaimed, "Mark! Here you are! I was just looking for you to go eat din—." Her words were cut off mid sentence as I wrapped my arms around her and we shared a lingering kiss. After a moment of pure bliss, I pulled her into the elevator and punched the "down" button. For once I was truly thankful that the ride was slow.

From that time onward Cindy and I spent nearly every spare moment together. Our classes still dominated our time, but after school we would share dinner whenever possible, and I often spent most of my evenings studying in her room when I didn't have to be in the anatomy lab. As you might expect, we took regular breaks from our lessons when we were together, but it was great just to be near each other even when our heads were buried in books.

On occasion I would lift my gaze from my notes, rubbing my eyes and stretching. Then I would look over to see Cindy's lovely face bent over her work, a tiny frown of concentration creasing her brow. Eventually she would sense me watching and she would look up, her sweet smile lighting her features, and I would smile back. No words were needed; just that shared look spoke volumes. It was tonic enough to reinvigorate me, and I could dive happily again into my studies.

For the most part, my classes were a continuation of the previous term. The biggest change was in gross anatomy, as in addition to dog dissection we began to study the anatomy of the horse and cow.

As you might imagine, these species were too large for each student to have a dissection specimen. Instead there was one preserved horse and one cow. Each was rolled in from the cold room on a lumbering wheeled cart. Large metal hooks pierced the animals' flanks, suspending each specimen in a standing position. Once the carts were positioned in the center of the room, the entire class would descend on them. Different groups worked on specific parts of the animal, one group dissecting the forelimb, another group opening the abdomen, and so forth. When a team uncovered something of particular interest, Dr. Warner would call all the students to gather around as he pointed it out and described the relevant anatomy.

The abdominal cavities in these animals were massive. As organs were dissected out one by one for closer examination, students had to move further and further inside to reach the next structures. Eventually their entire torsos were buried in the animals as they worked. Such were the cavernous dimensions of these herbivores.

I had suspected that gross anatomy would be my most challenging freshman course and I was not disappointed. Dr. Warner was a tough instructor, and rote memorization made me yawn, but the challenges didn't stop there. If the exams had stuck to simple identification of bodily structures, I would have had no problems. Where it got difficult was when Dr. Warner started asking spatial relationship questions.

For example, I knew the basic anatomic structures in the abdomen by heart. But a test question might read, "The right phrenicoabdominal vein joins the caudal vena cava just anterior to the right kidney. Which lobe of the liver lies adjacent to this confluence?" I knew the liver lobes, and the veins in question, but I had never bothered to look at how they sat relative to each other. Dr. Warner forced us to have a perfect three-dimensional picture of the animal's body in our heads. Sadly, it was never something I was particularly good at. On every one of his exams there were always questions that completely stumped me.

As a diversion from the burdens of classroom work, my fellow students and I continued to make time to visit the hospital and watch patients being treated. At that time the teaching hospital was just beginning to treat llama and alpaca patients. These South American herbivores with their long graceful necks and luxuriant coats were a novelty to many students. Much smaller than horses or cattle, they posed less physical threat, but when agitated they could bite or kick. They also had another interesting attribute. They could spit, and with remarkable accuracy.

I recall one female llama named Judy Mae that was being treated for a severe chronic mastitis. Her condition was gradually improving, and with it her attitude was steadily deteriorating. Whenever you approached to check her medical chart, Judy Mae would walk slowly up to the front of her enclosure. All the while she would be staring at you and working her mouth side to side. If you didn't back off, a huge gob of viscous saliva would explode from between her cleft upper lips, invariably striking its target in the face or chest. The slime didn't wash off easily, and was often mixed with greenish bits of half-chewed food. The aroma was quite delectable and could persist for the entire day, rivaling the most expensive brands of cologne. Even other animals in the hospital would flare their nostrils at you in disgust. Getting hit with one of Judy Mae's love bombs certainly added to the flavor of the veterinary experience.

CHAPTER FOURTEEN

Winter term whirled by in a montage of studying, eating, sleeping, and spending time with Cindy. Looking back on it now, most of it is a blur, but a few experiences stand out from the rest.

One of these was the night I took Cindy out to the Green Gable Restaurant. It was one of the more upscale places in town, and I wanted to do something special for Valentine's day. She had no idea where we were going, but I hinted that it would be a place where one should dress in something nice.

When we arrived at our destination, she exclaimed, "Oh my gosh, this is where you're taking me? I've seen this place and always wanted to come here! Thank you! This is so romantic." Our exit from the car was delayed a bit as Cindy felt the need to show her appreciation of my thoughtfulness. Never one to deny a partner her wishes, I willingly obliged. Some things you just have to do for the sake of the relationship.

Inside the restaurant the décor was beautiful, the lighting was muted, and our table was private and candle-lit. It was a perfect venue for celebrating a romantic day. I congratulated myself on having done something right. We spent the evening dining on excellent cuisine, holding hands across the small table, and sharing intimate conversation. It was one of those perfect interludes that I had always pictured when dreaming of being close with someone. I still smile when I think of that night.

I can recall another incident that occurred during winter term, and this one was quite humorous. It also taught me the value of clear communication skills when talking medicine to a layperson.

In this instance I was in my dorm room chatting with Daryl, and the conversation turned to dogs and their problems. One of the things I had learned while working at the clinic in Medford was that dogs have anal sacs. These are a pair of glands near the anal opening, which store a particularly foul-smelling liquid. When the dog is scared or excited the liquid can be ejected, creating a burst of odor. Skunks have taken this to the extreme, and the glands in that species have evolved to be a potent defensive weapon.

In veterinary practice, the anal sacs are of importance mainly when they become blocked or infected. In either case they may swell and become painful, and the affected animal may scoot its rear end on the ground or lick the area, trying to relieve the pressure and discomfort. The treatment often involves manually squeezing the sacs from the outside to force them to empty. Sometimes antibiotics are given as well.

Dog groomers often empty the anal sacs as part of the grooming service, whether the glands are bothering the animal or not. Occasionally the act of squeezing the glands could actually get them inflamed, and the dog would begin scooting as a result. I always thought that the old saying "If it ain't broke, don't fix it" probably applied here.

With this in mind, I was telling Daryl one afternoon about anal sacs in dogs. I mentioned how some clients would complain that their groomers always did the anal sacs on their dog, even when the owner requested that it not be done. Then the dog would come home scooting its butt on the carpet because it was sore. I told Daryl that in my opinion groomers should leave anal sacs to veterinarians, who were trained to do the procedure properly. It probably was not necessary to mess with anal sacs in most dogs who had no symptoms of illness.

During my entire discussion of this subject, Daryl's eyes were growing wider and his expression more dismayed. Finally he blurted, "But why would anyone want to do that to a dog? What purpose could it serve? You mean vets are *trained* to do that?!"

I could not understand his degree of consternation, and I explained that when an anal sac gets blocked or swollen, it needs to be squeezed and emptied, so there are times when it is appropriate. As I used the singular form of the term "anal sac," I suddenly saw comprehension dawn in Daryl's eyes, along with a look of tremendous relief. I still was puzzled by his reaction until he spoke up.

"Wow! Okay then," he said, "that makes more sense. You said anal *sacs*. I thought you were saying *sex*!"

It took me about five minutes to stop laughing.

CHAPTER FIFTEEN

As February moved into March the weather grew gradually warmer. The mild Willamette Valley temperatures led to an early resurgence of life, and by late February the crocuses and daffodils planted around the campus had burst forth in joyous blooms. Their bright dashes of color were a welcome sight after months of brown and grey. Rain still dominated the weather pattern, but the chill of midwinter was fading.

Another big change came at us as the junior class returned from their stint in Washington. With more students competing for space we were suddenly thrown out of our plush lecture auditorium into exile in Dietz Hall. The old red brick building stood on the opposite side of the railroad tracks from the vet school, in fact nearly across the street from my dorm. The convenient location was the only good thing about it.

Hailing from the earliest days of the university, Dietz was as archaic as McNairy Hall was modern. In its heyday it had been a center for the study of chicken production. Above the main entrance the word "Poultry" was still etched in a slab of badly-weathered concrete.

The building's interior was downright dreary. Paint peeled from the walls, while the flooring had buckled and warped over the many years since it had been laid. We sat on creaky wooden chairs behind desks that were better suited to grade school-sized students. Old steam radiators wheezed and rattled, making it difficult to hear lectures in the cramped classrooms. After being pampered in McNairy this was quite a drop in our standard of living, and we were less than thrilled.

But life wasn't all bad. As I became accustomed to the demanding curriculum I was able to carve out more personal time while still maintaining my grades. I had brought my bike from Medford after Christmas, and when I wasn't spending time with Cindy I would sometimes ride out to McLain Forest. The public were allowed to hike here and the scenery was breathtaking. Towering fir trees, lush grasses and ferns, meandering creeks and open green meadows all could be seen on a fifteen or twenty minute trek into the woods.

Walking these acres called to mind fun-filled days in my youth spent camping with my family. During summer vacation we would head into the Cascade Mountains, enjoying nature away from the city and the crowds. We hiked, fished, picked huckleberries, built campfires, and made memories that have lasted a lifetime.

One of the most enduring recollections I have of those childhood adventures is an encounter that helped spark my fascination with animals. One day in early June my family and I were fishing in the mountains on the South Fork of the Rogue River. At this high elevation the tributary usually ran small and meek, but spring rains and snow melt runoff had swollen its volume considerably. The icy cold water tumbled and churned with treacherous strength as it flowed toward the distant ocean. Its rocky path sliced through the dense forest that crowded the banks on both sides. The open strip of brilliant blue sky overhead was a perfect backdrop to the rich green of the pines and firs towering around us. The day was sunny and warm, but a pleasantly cool breeze wafted off the water wherever there was a patch of shade.

We were fishing for trout along the banks, working our way up-stream. Just ahead a fallen fir tree had made a natural bridge out to some flat boulders in the middle of the river. My mom had walked across the log and was fishing off the large rocks when she let out a yell. My dad and I looked up, alarmed, and we saw mom waving frantically for us to come to her.

Dad and I put down our fishing rods and ran upstream. We got to the fallen tree and walked rapidly across on the trunk, balancing as we traversed the rushing water just below our feet. When we got to the cluster of huge flat rocks out in midstream, my dad asked what the problem was. Mom pointed to the edge of the boulder on which she stood.

Something brown and wet was perched on the rock at the water's edge. At first I thought it was a small creature like a beaver, then I did a mental double take and realized that it was the head of a young deer. The animal's body was completely submerged in the freezing water, its chin and front feet perched precariously on the lip of the rock. It must have fallen in somewhere close by, and had tried to pull itself out of the churning river onto the flat expanse of stone. But it could not get a grip on the slippery wet surface, and now its struggles had weakened to the point where it could do nothing but hang on desperately. It was only a matter of time before it lost the battle with the river and drowned.

My dad decided to try to help the failing animal. He cautioned us to stay back, and bent down to grab the deer's forelimbs where they protruded from the river. It offered little struggle, and with a heave he hauled it clear out of the water and onto the flat rock beside him. Dad made sure we were off the log so that the deer could have a clear path to freedom should it decide to bolt. But it was in shock and too weak to move. It just stood there on trembling legs, staring at us. It was a young buck, with two velvety new antlers barely a finger-length in size, forked just at the ends. Dad patted its rear and coaxed it from the rock surface up onto the log. From here it was a straight shot to the bank of the river, but again the deer just shivered and made no attempt to leave.

"The poor little guy's cold and exhausted," dad said, standing to the front of the little animal. "I wonder if I have anything for him to eat." He fished around in his pockets, and came up with a butterscotch candy. When he unwrapped it and offered it to the deer, it sniffed and then eagerly snatched the treat, munching vigorously. Its shivering was gradually subsiding in the warm midday sun, and we began to feel like it was going to be okay.

Dad stood smiling, hands on his hips as he watched his candy being devoured. He said, "Well, he's obviously feeling better. It doesn't look like he's eager to move yet, but he's stable enough to leave him. He'll go to shore when he's ready."

With that, dad led us single-file back across the log to the river-bank. I was last in line, and I turned around at the shore to see the deer one last time. To my surprise it was right behind me! "Hey, look, he's following us!" I exclaimed.

My dad turned and said, "No, he's just heading for shore after we led the way. Get out of his path now so he can go."

We retrieved out fishing poles and resumed our trek upstream. The deer stood by the riverbank watching us go. As the trail led us into a thicket of trees I lost sight of him. We hiked onward a short distance, and then I heard a twig snap behind me. Looking around, I saw once again the deer following in my footsteps, only a few paces behind!

I called to my family ahead of me, "Mom, dad, look, he's still with us!" My dad looked back and his eyes widened in surprise. "Well, I'll be...," he exclaimed. "I've never seen a wild animal do anything like that before. He seems to have no fear of us at all. In fact, he's actively pursuing us!" He shook his head in disbelief. "This is wilderness country; there's no way that this little guy is ac-customed to people. He's totally wild and yet he's decided that we are okay. This is really extraordinary."

That word described the entire day. Everywhere we hiked and fished along the river the little deer followed us. He seemed to crave our companionship, staying as close as he could to one of us at all times. When we stopped for lunch in a small clearing, the deer sat with us, calmly chewing his cud. He allowed my brother and me to touch and pet him, not flinching from any contact. We caressed his incredibly soft, velvet-covered antlers, in awe at seeing him up close. My dad said that even tame deer usually wouldn't allow such contact, as the newly grown velvet was very sensitive.

While we ate we pondered how this shy animal had become in-stantly tamed. We concluded that it was a combination of things. At first the deer had been too weak to resist, then it had been helped out of the water and had gone unharmed by us, and possibly most im-portantly, my dad had given it a sweet candy. That series of positive events had completely wiped out the instinctive fear these animals had for humans. It was hard to believe, but we couldn't deny what we were seeing.

When we finished lunch and resumed fishing, the little buck stood and came along once again. He was amazingly agile and navigated the rough terrain with ease. The trail along the river was little more than a faint animal path, crisscrossed with fallen logs and overgrown with heavy brush. I and my family had to crawl over and under obstacles as we went. I was young and in shape but the little buck made me look lumbering and clumsy. He casually leaped over the logs and bushes, or ducked his head and squirted through amazingly small gaps in the brush. It was almost surreal seeing this wild forest creature, normally glimpsed only at a distance, trotting along happily beside us. It felt like having an exotic family pet on our outing.

The deer went to unexpected lengths to be near us. One time my dad jumped from the bank onto a small rock in the river to better reach a fishing hole. The footing was barely large enough for him to stand on, but suddenly he found himself straddling our new friend as well. The buck had jumped out onto the rock with him. It took some deft maneuvering with the deer between his legs for dad to turn around and jump back to shore.

When our fishing was done and the afternoon was stretching toward early evening, we headed back through the woods to where our truck was parked. The rear of the pickup had a canopy on it and a bench seat installed inside where my brother and I would sit. As we climbed in the back, the deer hovered near the door and looked like he was going to join us. My dad would have none of it, saying, "I'm not about to let him in there where he'll panic when the vehicle starts to move. He's got to stay behind." Sadly, we said goodbye to our new friend, then we got in the truck and drove slowly away. The last I saw of the little buck he was still standing at the roadside watching us go.

For years after that we wondered what had become of our wild companion. We all hoped that his trust in humans hadn't earned him an early death. Of course, we thought that we would never know the answer. But the best true stories have happy endings, and as fate would have it, we got the chance to hear the conclusion of this one.

My dad told the tale of our adventure with the deer many times over the years. He was an accomplished storyteller, and hearing him bring the events of that day to life in his words helped keep the memories vivid in my mind. Years later we were camping again in the same wilderness area, and while we were eating lunch at a picnic site, a Forest Service truck pulled up. The ranger was friendly and came over to say hello. In the course of chatting with him, my dad told the story of our implausible meeting with the deer.

The ranger's eyes widened and he said, "I wonder if that's the same buck I heard about."

My dad asked him what he meant, and the ranger replied, "Well there was a logger named Jim Swanson who was working in these woods years ago. He didn't like driving clear back to town between shifts, so he had a little trailer he hauled up here. He was camped by the side of the road not too far from the river, and one day into the clearing walks this little fork-horn buck. Right in broad daylight, and it walks straight up to the guy without batting an eye. Old Jim about fell out of his chair, to hear him tell it. The deer was as tame as could be, and Jim could pet it like a house dog.

"Well, he was worried that the animal would be shot come hunting season, as it had no fear at all. So he gets a big burlap bag and tackles the deer. After a struggle Jim manages to get it bundled up in the bag and loads it into his truck. Then he drives out to a friend he knows who has a lot of acreage, fenced and protected from hunting. The property owner was a real animal lover, I guess, and he had some other injured animals that lived out there. Jim released the buck on his friend's property and he said it was real happy staying there. No hunters to worry about, at least."

He paused and scratched his neck reflectively, then said, "I'll bet that was your little buck he found. We never could figure out how a deer up here could be so tame, and it was around the same time as when you had your adventure. I guess it all turned out well in the end."

One can never know with certainty, but I like to think that he was right, and that our forest friend lived a long and happy life.

CHAPTER SIXTEEN

In the classroom our work progressed as winter term neared its end. Gross anatomy continued to challenge us all, but I could see the usefulness in most of it. Learning major body structures, the organs, the primary blood vessels, the large muscle groups, all had relevance to the practicing veterinarian. The part I had the hardest time with was memorizing minutia that I might never use. If I really needed to know the anatomy of some obscure little structure ten years later, I could quickly pull out a textbook and see a good illustration of it. But for class we had to know it all.

One of the worst examples of this was learning the arteries and veins of the feet. Dogs and cats had four or five toes on each paw, and we studied the names of all the vessels supplying the feet and digits. I memorized the radial artery, the cranial superficial antebrachial artery, the digital arteries, and so forth. Once I finally had those straight in my head I breathed a sigh of relief, and then we began to study horse and cattle feet.

These animals had entirely different foot anatomy than a dog. The cloven-hoofed animals like cattle had two well-developed toes that made up the two hooves. Horses were even more extreme and walked on only one large toe, the middle finger. Because of these differences, the names of the blood vessels varied between species, but they were just similar enough to cause major confusion. Trying to keep them all straight for more than five minutes was the source of much wailing and gnashing of teeth among my classmates.

Stan Hulbert, the tall charismatic student I had met during my first interview, was one of those struggling to keep up. I would see his head bent over an anatomy specimen time and again, his thick black curls nearly motionless as he tried to commit the myriad details to memory. One day he came over and asked me, "How do you keep all this stuff straight? Like the damned arteries and nerves in the feet? It's so confusing, and I'll think I have it down, then when I wake up the next day it's all a jumble again."

He sounded so discouraged that I tried to cheer him up, saying, "Well, you're not alone! Just remember, we won't need to know most of the trivia after we graduate, and we'll have books to refer to when needed. Right?" He nodded, and I continued, "The important anatomy we'll see over and over again in classes like surgery. By the time we're veterinarians we'll have it burned into our brains."

He smiled at that, but then looked worried again, saying, "What about the exams? I don't want my grades to fall, and I don't seem to do well on Dr. Warner's tests."

I grinned at him, and replied, "Tell me Stan, are you getting passing grades?"

He shrugged and said, "Well yeah, but mostly B's, and maybe only a "C" in this course."

I told him, "Well, those are decent marks for this program. You don't need to pull A's here to be successful. I hear that some of the best practitioners were just average students. My advice is this: concentrate on learning the essentials, and then commit as much of the trivia to memory as you can. Do you want to know my secret?"

Stan nodded eagerly, and I said, "Well, little details like the vessels of the feet drive me crazy. Right before an exam I review that stuff so it's clear in my head. Then on the test I answer any questions involving those structures first, before I forget what I committed to short-term memory. After that I can do the rest of the test. If you asked me to tell you about the arteries of the feet two hours later I'd be in trouble. But for the exams I can get it right. Does that help?"

Stan smiled and thanked me, looking somewhat relieved. As he walked back to his desk I called after him, "Remember, a passing grade gets you a diploma."

A week later I passed by his desk and saw a small sign posted on the cabinet next to his desk. Inscribed on the white card in felt tip marker was the equation, "C = DVM." Apparently Stan had taken my advice to heart.

Soon after that we had our winter term final exams. When we got our grades Stan came to me and thanked me profusely. "Your little trick worked, Mark!" he said. "It almost feels like cheating, but I nailed the vessels and nerves of the feet. I scored a ninety-two on the written test! Of course I can't recall a lot of it now, but it sure feels good to have a high score." I laughed and assured him that he would remember the anatomy he needed to know, and told him to keep up the good work.

It was like that in our class all year long, and not just with Stan and me. The students took Dr. Lawson's opening day advice and helped each other whenever possible. The supportive atmosphere was a reflection of the solid character of my classmates. My entire veterinary school experience was much more enjoyable as a result.

There was no break after our final exams. When spring term commenced in early April, histology developed a new twist as the microscope gave way to gross pathology. In this portion of the course we visited the necropsy room and examined deceased animals, looking for abnormal lesions visible to the naked eye. The large scale of things was a drastic change from the tiny tissue slides we had scrutinized for months. It was a refreshing change, although gross pathology brought with it an unsavory aspect we hadn't encountered in histology: odor!

The rest of our courses offered less novelty, but there were some especially fun moments in class, none better than when we could have a good laugh at someone else's expense. One of the few times we worked with live animals as a group was when we practiced semen collection on dogs. The histology professors wanted fresh samples so we could see what live sperm looked like under the microscope.

One afternoon nine male dogs were paraded into the anatomy lab. One dog was allotted to each team of four students. Our task was to don gloves and manually stimulate the dogs to obtain semen samples. When my group obtained our dog, we all looked at each other for a moment. Blushing, the two girls told Mike and me, "You guys can do it. You have more experience at this!"

Not one to let an opportunity pass by, Mike immediately quipped, "Aw, c'mon Molly! You're married, so you should know what to do!" That turned her face an even deeper shade of red.

Finally Mike and I relented and agreed to do the honors. We stood our dog on the floor by the desks. He was a good natured Springer Spaniel mix. Mike crouched down and stroked the dog's penis for about a minute. Presto! There was our sample, which we dutifully collected in a small, preheated glass container. Warmth kept the sperm more viable so that they would exhibit strong movement.

We made semen smears on microscope slides and examined them. It was pretty impressive to see. The entire visual field was crowded with scores of tiny swimmers jostling for position.

After we each had a peek, I looked around to see how other tables were managing with their dogs. Some groups were examining samples with their microscopes, and others were still working to obtain semen. Those lucky few performing the "task at hand" were diligently concentrating with serious expressions on their faces. Some were working up quite a sweat in the process.

By contrast, those standing by and watching the proceedings were lightheartedly enjoying the show. Jokes and suggestions on improving technique abounded. In the end persistence paid off and eventually everyone got their samples. Everyone except the group that Stan Hulbert was in.

Stan was good-natured and popular, so predictably he had been nominated by his team to do the dirty work. By the time I saw that Stan's group was still going at it, a good half hour had passed since the lab had begun. I have no idea how long they had been polishing the dog's rocket, but Stan was beginning to look desperate. His brow was furrowed in concentration and his tongue stuck out a bit as he feverishly worked.

Finally he slumped in defeat, saying, "My arm is dead. Someone else give it a go." A second group member had at it, and then a third, frantically stroking away with their gloves. All the while the dog stared straight ahead bemusedly, tongue lolling and tail wagging as if he had no idea what was going on but was enjoying it nonetheless.

Finally Dr. Warner came over and said, "What seems to be the problem here?"

Stan shrugged, his hands on his hips, and replied, "I have no idea. We can't get him to ejaculate and we've tried everything."

Dr. Warner crouched down to examine the animal, and in a moment he gave a bark of laughter. It was the first time I had seen him show amusement all year. He stood up, his face incongruously split with a huge grin, and proclaimed, "Your dog has no testicles. He's been neutered! Didn't you notice? You'll be working a long time to get anything out of *that* boy!"

Stan just shook his head and stared down at his feet, chuckling sheepishly. Todd Taylor, the student who had most recently been on his knees working the dog, slowly stood up and threw his gloves down in disgust. He was usually a smug and cocky individual, and seeing him brought down to earth warmed my heart. The entire class was laughing, and the mood was decidedly jocular for the rest of the lab. As I passed by Stan, I clapped him on the back and said, "Hey that's OK. Better the dog than you, eh?" He had to agree with that one.

CHAPTER SEVENTEEN

One weekend in April my team-mate Molly Boyer had a party at her home. Her husband had taken their two small children to visit relatives, and she decided her house was too quiet. On the spur of the moment she asked a number of students if they would like to come over, and we all thought that was a great idea.

I asked Cindy if she wanted to go and she accepted enthusiastically. She was eager to meet some of my classmates and it was a good break from our routine. Molly's home resided in a quiet neighborhood on the west side of town. It resembled a cute cottage, painted pale yellow with white shutters and trim. The front yard was well maintained, with hydrangea bushes near the house and a yellow wooden fence around the lawn.

We parked on the narrow street and rang the doorbell. Molly answered the door with a smile and invited us in. As she took our coats I noted the family pictures on the wall, the knick knacks on the tables, and the kids' toys stuffed in one corner. Molly had definitely settled down. I realized that some day I wanted to have the same, perhaps with someone like Cindy.

The party was a casual affair, strictly jeans and T-shirt, and we did it potluck style with everyone contributing a dish or snack. Cindy and I brought cookies and tortilla chips. Molly had provided beer and soft drinks.

When we arrived, about fifteen people had already showed up. A basketball game was playing on the television. The stereo was cranked up as well, blasting out either rock or country music, depending on who was at the controls. Eight or ten people were sitting in the living room laughing and conversing, some on the floor, others lounging on chairs and sofas. Another half dozen stood in the kitchen holding plates and drinks.

A few people had spouses or significant others with them, but Cindy grabbed the eyes of the male students as soon as we walked in. I made the rounds introducing her to everyone. Among others I saw Mike Callahan and Amy Baker from my study group, "Special" Ed Martinelli, and Stan Hulbert. As I finished the introductions, Mike tossed me and Cindy a couple of beers from the kitchen. We grabbed plates and helped ourselves to some food. Then we headed into the main room where most everyone was. Cindy and I sat cross-legged on the floor and dived in to our food as we chatted with those around us. Cindy seemed right at home and quickly was involved in a conversation with several of my classmates.

It was entertaining seeing everyone in a social setting outside of the classroom. Ed was in his element and had downed three beers before I got halfway through my first. I doubt that he missed many parties. In one corner of the room Stan was telling off-color jokes, his deep voice holding the attention of four or five people around him. Every now and then a burst of laughter would erupt as he told a punch line.

Mike Callahan and a few other guys were watching the basketball game. Their conversation was occasionally punctuated by groans or cheers as the game unfolded on the screen.

The most fun I had the entire night was watching Molly. It turned out she had a knack for doing impressions, especially accents. She started with an Irish lilt, teasing Stan who had come to stand nearby. "Ay, there be a strappin' lad. I bet ye could turn many a bonny lass's head, no?"

Then she turned on Mike Callahan, switching to an Australian twang, "And who's this little thunder from down under? Not got a lady friend eh? Well, no worries, mate, a bloke's gotta keep tryin' till he's dyin'."

She pointed to Ed Martinelli, using a thick Cockney accent, "Now, 'ere's a right pretty sight. Bloody 'ell. Don't pay 'im no never mind, he's just sittin' on 'is lazy bum all day."

Hearing the different dialects spewing out of our prim proper classmate was enough to have us all rolling on the floor. I never would have guessed she had it in her. She was laughing herself, and watching her was like seeing the genie let out of the bottle.

I also remember Joe Wrobel getting pretty relaxed after a couple of beers and sharing hair-raising stories about his rodeo days. He was a small town boy from the rural sagebrush country of eastern Oregon. In his youth he had done some bronco riding before he had wised up and decided to go to college. Hearing his tales, I could understand why.

It started when someone asked him about his scar. Joe was sitting on the sofa with a can of beer, and whenever he raised it to drink, a large linear scar stood out prominently across the back of his hand. When Ed asked him about it, he rubbed it reflectively and said, "That's a rope scar. When you bronco ride, you wrap the saddle rope tightly around your hand several times to anchor you to the horse. It's held down against the saddle between your legs." He clenched his left hand into a fist and held it down between his knees. "The other hand stays free so you can wave your arm for balance as you ride." So saying, he waved his right hand in the air over his head.

"So how did you get your left hand so scarred up? Is that just from riding?" Ed prompted.

"Well if a horse throws you, you're supposed to fall clear and get out of the way," Joe said. "But if the rope doesn't come loose when you let go, then you can get dragged by your hand. That's what happened to me. The horse was bucking and I was flying around like a balloon on a string, and the rope cut into my hand pretty deep by the time I got free."

"Ouch!" Ed exclaimed, and his sentiments were echoed by several others who were listening.

Joe just laughed. "Oh, that was nothing. I've gotten hurt much worse, believe me."

He took another gulp of beer and shook his head.

"What's the worst injury you had bronco riding?" Stan's deep voice piped up from the easy chair where he sat.

"Well, I...." Joe hesitated, glancing at the women seated around him.

"Go on, spit it out," Stan encouraged.

"I got kicked in the family jewels by a horse once," Joe admitted with an embarrassed smile. A chorus of groans went up from the males in the room, and Joe nodded. "Yeah," he continued, "but that wasn't the worst of it."

"You mean it gets worse?" Ed asked incredulously.

"Well, yes, because the kick knocked both of my jewels back into my body."

"Owww!" erupted from multiple throats as the assembled students, both male and female, winced at that image. Ed appeared a bit green about the gills.

Joe was apparently quite amused with the reactions to his story. He just sat there grinning broadly and sipping his beer.

Ed's next words were so quiet that they were barely audible, as if dragged from him against his will: "So…what happened then?"

"Well I went to the doc, and he said we could wait to see if they came back down on their own. I waited two months and nothing happened."

"So, did they ever…?" Ed prodded, looking not at all certain that he wanted to know the answer.

Joe nodded emphatically as he gulped his beer. "Oh, yeah, not too long after that I got kicked again, this time in the stomach, and that popped 'em back out. I'm tellin' ya, *that* hurt worse than when they went in!"

"*Ewww!*" Ed exclaimed as he cringed and turned away, and the groans from the group were now mixed with laughter. I saw Stan Hulbert shaking his head, saying "That's just nasty" over and over. I began pondering if it were possible to stand sideways while performing procedures on horses.

Joe's stories generated much animated discussion and laughter as the evening unfolded. Everyone was loose and relaxed, chatting amiably and strengthening the bonds of emerging friendships. I thoroughly enjoyed myself and I got to know my classmates as real people with lives outside of school. Cindy had fun too, and having her there at my side made everything richer. I hoped that we would have many more opportunities to share good times like these as we went along.

CHAPTER EIGHTEEN

As spring term progressed it brought with it some nice perks. The rain lessened and the sun pushed its way through the clouds with increasing frequency. I received several delectable packages from home, along with notes telling me about life back in Medford and inquiring about my studies. I sent a couple of long letters back, thanking mom for baking the treats. In them I wrote about my classes and life in the dorm, and I also mentioned having met a wonderful girl named Cindy. I was serious enough about her that I thought I might as well break the news.

By this point in our freshman year my classmates and I possessed enough basic knowledge to begin helping out with hospitalized patients. On occasion we were called upon to assist the doctors and senior students while observing in the hospital ward.

I began to learn the fundamentals of handling and restraint for large animals. The cattle were relatively easy. They usually were submissive and their ability to bite and kick wasn't as well developed as in the horses. You could stand in front of a whole herd of cows, wave your arms and yell "bah!", and they would run before you like an African lion was after them. Their kicks were not terribly devastating, though oddly enough they preferred to jab out sideways instead of straight back.

The horses commanded more respect. Larger, quicker, and more temperamental, they could be dangerous patients to work with. One blow from a heavy hoof could send you to the hospital, no matter where it landed. Equines also could deal out a nasty bite. Their bulky bodies could crush you against the wall of the stall, knocking the wind out of you or cracking a few ribs in the process. Some were sweet, affectionate creatures, but others did not like being treated and had no compunction about telling you so.

Restraint methods varied depending on the nature of the beast and what procedures needed to be done. A halter and rope sufficed for physical examinations and for most minor treatments such as giving injections, oral medications, drawing blood, and so forth. For fractious horses a twitch might be applied.

Not having come from a farm background, I found the concept of a twitch fascinating. One would take a small loop of rope, often the same one attached to the halter, and encircle the horse's loose upper lip with it. Then you twisted the rope down to tighten the loop, pinching the trapped lip snugly. For some reason this had a remarkable calming effect on the horse, and often would allow the handlers to accomplish routine tasks without use of heavier restraint or chemical sedation.

For the most difficult patients or procedures the animal could be walked into a gated squeeze chute in the treatment room. An injected sedative could be administered in the chute as well.

I learned how to approach a horse or cow, from the front but a little off to the side. You didn't want to surprise or startle the animal from behind, but a head-on confrontation might seem a bit threatening. Once close, one needed to handle the patient firmly. A light touch might tickle or feel like a biting fly landing on the skin. We would rub or pat the skin with vigor so there was no doubt that the contact was human. A firm approach also implied confidence, and the more assertive animals could spot a tentative handler a mile away.

We always had to be careful of our position relative to the patient, especially with horses. When working around the rear quarters, you needed to stay very close (nearly touching) or very far back. Standing one or two paces from a horse's rear feet was a great way to receive a nasty kick. We needed to stand out of range or so close that a hoof couldn't gather momentum before striking us.

The stethoscopes we used in the hospital were very elongated. This allowed a person to put the end of the stethoscope well under the ribcage of a large patient, without having to bend over to listen. Keeping one's head up out of the path of flying hooves was an important safety precaution.

I picked up other little tricks as well. The glass thermometers the senior students used all had a long piece of flexible rubber tubing stuck on the back end. Looking closer I saw that the tubing led to a small alligator clip. When I asked a senior what that was for, he laughed and said, "I'll show you." He pulled up the tail of the heifer he was examining, and stuck the thermometer deep in her rectum. The glass end was barely protruding, but he took the alligator clip attached to the rubber extension and clipped it to the hair on the tail. "This keeps us from losing thermometers," he said, grinning. "Otherwise the animals tend to suck them up inside and we have to go fishing for them. Or they squirt them out and they break on the ground."

Being able to contribute in the hospital was a major boost to my morale. Much of the medicine was still beyond my understanding, but I could don my coveralls and help restrain patients or fetch equipment when needed. It made the first year of my education come alive in a way that classroom lessons could not.

Meanwhile, our anatomy lab marched forward in a never-ending succession of dissection and memorization. The horse and cow cadavers now stood completely hollowed out in the center of the room, some of their limbs detached and sitting on tables as students continued to explore their smaller anatomic features. The dog carcasses similarly were appearing more and more fragmented as our scalpels slowly disassembled them.

Paralleling the wear and tear on our specimens was the progressive soiling of our once pristine lab coats. Students now walked around cloaked in dingy grey garments spotted with formalin and nameless bodily fluids. Even laundering with bleach could not save the abused fabric and we eventually gave up trying. Instead, we decided the colors were a badge of accomplishment, like progressing from a white belt to a black belt in the martial arts. We didn't look any better but our self image improved.

A few diversions added some spice to the otherwise predictable lab sessions that quarter. On one occasion a recently deceased sheep donated a pair of lungs for us to inspect, and Dr. Warner attached an air hose to the trachea, inflating the lungs as we watched. The spongy organs swelled to several times their original size, then shrank again when he turned off the compressor. It was a great demonstration of the elasticity of the tissues and how they expanded and contracted during breathing. The doctor repeated the demonstration several times until he over-pressurized the stressed organs and blew a hole in one, spraying blood droplets over the students. A fun time was had by all.

Toward the last half of spring term we also noted some disturbing changes in the horse and cow cadavers. The specimens had been in the classroom daily for many weeks. Although they were stored in the cold room at night, they had begun to acquire a distinct odor over time. It seemed that the formalin preservative had not saturated all the tissues evenly. Maybe it was coincidence, but I noted that as the aroma grew, the numbers of students eating snacks in class shrank proportionately.

The ripe cadavers didn't repulse everyone. As the weather warmed outside, flies began to appear in the anatomy lab. They were large and black, nearly as big as bumblebees, and they buzzed ponderously around the classroom. When they landed they were so slow that you could catch one with a quick snatch of your hand. Despite their formidable size, I knew from my entomology background that they were harmless. I caught one or two to prove this point to my classmates. Then the fun began.

Staring at anatomy specimens for countless hours can warp even the most balanced minds. As the tedium wears you down, you find that any alternate activity, no matter how outlandish, begins to have amusement value. As a result, several students began to catch and examine the flies that landed on their desks. Soon someone got the bright idea of plucking long strands of hair from female students to make leashes for the tiny critters. Once the hair was carefully tied around the fly's torso, you could fasten the other end to your finger. Now you had a miniature pet who would buzz around at the end of its tether, then land back on your hand. This was good for hours of entertainment.

Eventually the investigational mindset kicked in, and students wanted to know if the insects could fly as a group. They took several fly leashes and tied them together, then tossed the group into the air. The flies all tried to go in different directions, and invariably landed in a chaotic heap on the floor. Apparently the lack of any real brain precluded cooperative aerobatics. The insects were amusing, but I had more fun watching the group of highly educated people animatedly pointing and debating the results of the experiment.

Eventually everyone had had their fill of fly behavioral studies, but we didn't want all our hard work to go to waste. It seemed only fitting that the insects should adorn the door of Dr. Warner's office. He had been out of the lab all day so he knew nothing of our endeavors. We took half a dozen flies and taped their tethers to his door. Whenever someone passed by they flew out and buzzed furiously in a small black cloud before landing once again. It was the oddest sight I had ever seen. What Dr. Warner thought when he encountered the bizarre display I have no idea; I suspect that even he might have cracked a grin despite himself.

Late spring was a time of personal fulfillment for me as well. Cindy and I continued to grow closer as our lives gradually became more intertwined. We enjoyed movies at the campus theater, ate meals together at the cafeteria, studied side by side in her dorm room, and went for walks when the weather was mild. Along the way we discovered the joy that comes with sharing oneself unconditionally, and in return being accepted without reservation by the one who knows you best. My memories of those exciting weeks are yet one more reason that spring remains my favorite time of year.

CHAPTER NINETEEN

As the school year neared its end and the weather waxed hot, it became harder to concentrate on class work. One of the diversions that the students cooked up to have fun was a friendly picnic and competition between the seniors and the freshmen.

The seniors organized the whole thing, and we gathered in a park not far from the vet school. Saturday afternoon was partly overcast but comfortably warm. We brought ice chests full of beer and pop, and the seniors provided the food. The park had picnic benches set in the shade of large maple trees. Near the benches were built-in barbeque grills, so we soon had hot dogs smoking over glowing charcoal.

Being outdoors enjoying good food with friends was a simple pleasure that never grew old. It was a meaningful gathering as well, being a last chance for the two classes to interact before graduation. The senior class would be the very first to receive doctorates from the program here. We all wished them the best in their careers as they headed out into the world of veterinary medicine.

The afternoon's contests had been devised by the seniors, and of course were rigged to favor their class. For example, one of the fourth-year students was skilled with a bow, so they had us pick a "champion" from our class who would represent the freshmen in a target competition against their archer. For safety's sake they used a plastic target and arrows tipped with suction cups. Predictably, we lost.

The same went for the syringe toss, wherein syringes were thrown at a target to see if you could impale the bull's eye with the needle. There was a trick to it, as the syringes wouldn't fly straight like a dart. Rather, you had to throw them end over end like a knife, timing the rotations so the needle hit the target straight on. The senior champion had obviously practiced this ahead of time but we had not. Again, we were beaten badly.

Then it was on to the hand scrubbing contest, wherein blindfolded contestants used a surgical scrub brush to remove black dye from their hands within sixty seconds. The seniors had been through surgery classes, so they knew how to scrub thoroughly even without looking. When the time was up and blindfolds came off, their hands were respectably clean, whereas the competitors from my class had missed large portions of the dye.

It went that way contest after contest, and we took it good-naturedly, knowing it was the seniors' last hurrah. At least until we came to the final contest, which was arm wrestling.

For this competition the seniors had set up a small card table on the grass, with two folding chairs pulled up to it. When I saw the senior contestant step forward, I was suitably impressed. He was built like a wrestler, with a thick torso and beefy arms packed with muscle. I remembered that his name was Mike O'Connor, and that he hailed from a farm in the mid-Willamette Valley. Looking at him, I envisioned that he would be perfectly suited for large animal work. He could probably heft a well-grown calf under each arm and not break a sweat. It was obvious the seniors figured they had this contest sewn up as well. Then we brought up Jerry Heinemann.

Jerry was one of those guys who looked average enough with coveralls on. Even in a loose shirt he hardly warranted a second glance. He wasn't tall of stature and he was well-proportioned, no single feature exaggerated. But he was a serious body builder, and when he wore a snug T-shirt, as he did now, he was an amazing specimen. His biceps bulged and rippled as they stretched the shirt fabric to its limits, and his chest was huge, his sculpted body a classic V-shape. Most of the seniors had no prior clue as to Jerry's physique, and I heard one of them exclaim softly, "Wow—look at that guy!" I grinned to myself; this would be very interesting indeed. We freshmen might be good sports, but we did have our pride as well. We would not go down in this last contest without a fight.

Jerry sat down opposite Mike O'Connor and they clasped hands in the classic arm wrestling stance. The two classes crowded behind each contestant, those in the rear straining to get a look. The students were hushed with expectation as the referee held up his hand and counted, "One, two, three, GO!"

He brought his hand down in a slashing motion and the contest was on. Jerry and Mike's arms unleashed their full strength against each other, their massive thews instantly becoming taut cords as they strained to gain the upper hand. Mike was a fraction quicker in his reaction time at the start, and had an initial advantage. He forced Jerry's hand down toward the table for fifteen or twenty seconds, and then Jerry began to make up ground, pushing Mike's arm slowly back up to vertical. The freshmen clapped and shouted, cheering him on.

The senior's efforts redoubled in a furious attempt to halt Jerry's progress. He succeeded, and for close to a solid minute they remained immobile, locked in a stalemate. Their arms shook with effort and the strain was evident in their faces. Perspiration beaded

Mike's forehead and Jerry was grunting with each breath, the veins of his arms standing out in bold relief. Both classes were going crazy, whooping and urging their champions to give everything they had.

Slowly, slowly, Jerry began to force Mike's hand down. This time the senior had no answer. He strained and grimaced, pain written across his visage as he watched his arm pushed inexorably toward the tabletop. Finally his knuckles touched the surface, and in a flash it was all over. Both men collapsed back into their chairs, their chests heaving as they gulped air. My classmates were cheering wildly and slapping Jerry on the back. It was our only victory of the afternoon, but it more than made up for all the losses.

After a moment Jerry offered his hand to Mike, this time in friendship, and the senior grinned and took it. They eyed each other with obvious respect and Mike said, "Nice match, man."

Jerry replied, "Thanks. You, too." Then he turned to his freshman classmates and raised his arms in victory. So ended the events of the first ever senior-freshman spring party at the School of Veterinary Medicine.

Of course, class work still required our attention despite the diversions. Though we all had spring fever to varying degrees, this was offset somewhat by the course materials becoming more interesting. In neurology class this took the form of interactive exams on live patients. Any hospitalized case with a lameness was subject to our poking and prodding as we did neuro testing on its limbs. It was both fun and educational as we got to apply what we had learned in lecture.

In anatomy class we were finally done with the horse and cow specimens, and now moved on to a variety of smaller animals. The time spent on each of these was relatively brief, mainly just highlighting the unique attributes of each species. We dissected sheep, pigs, and chickens. After that we spent a week on a handful of "pocket pets"—meaning rats, gerbils, hamsters, guinea pigs, and rabbits. For each there were only a select few anatomic structures that Dr. Warner wanted us to learn, so we made quick work of these. It was a refreshing change from the daily repetition we had become accustomed to. Gross anatomy had almost become—dare I say it?—fun.

The final exams for spring term would cover material from the entire school year. Over the three terms my class notebooks had acquired an imposing bulk, and I shuddered at the thought of committing all that information to memory. Fortunately, we were told that the anatomy and histology exams would emphasize material from the current term, with less coverage of previous notes. But we still had to review it all.

With exams bearing down on me in the final few weeks, I didn't have a lot of time for playing. Morning, noon, and night I was either studying in class or studying in the dorm. Cindy and I took a brief respite from work one weekend and made a quick jaunt to McLain Forest. It was only for a couple of hours, but it felt fantastic to get away and be together. We walked hand in hand down the sunny gravel road as I finally got to share with Cindy the natural beauty I had discovered there. She loved it just as I had. Our time was short, so we enjoyed each stolen moment to the fullest.

Another week of frenetic studying followed. That next Saturday I came dragging back to my dorm room in early evening after working for hours in the anatomy lab. I found Daryl inside, combing his hair in the mirror and slapping on cologne. When he saw me he flashed a smile and said, "Hey Mark, Trish and I are going out for dinner tonight. Just pizza, nothing fancy. Would you like to bring Cindy along, make it a double date? I'm heading out right now."

Just then that sounded like the best idea in the world, and my stomach rumbled at the thought. I told Daryl to wait right there. The prospect of fun gave me an unexpected burst of energy and I bolted up to Cindy's room, taking the stairs two at a time. My prayers were answered when she opened the door to my knock. "Oh, great, you're here!" I gasped, a little short of breath from my run.

"What's up?" she asked, looking surprised.

"Daryl and Trish are going out for pizza and they invited us to come," I answered. "They're heading out in a couple of minutes."

"Hey, that sounds great! I'm famished, and it's been awhile since Trish and I got together. Just let me brush my hair and get my purse. I'll only be a minute."

I stood by her door as she disappeared back inside, and true to her word she was in the hall ready to go in less than sixty seconds. I gave her a quick kiss and we headed back to my dorm room. Daryl was waiting in the doorway. We headed out to his car and Cindy and I got in the back. He drove us over to Trish's dorm which was only a block away. After parking the car, Daryl turned to us and said, "Be right back guys," and he got out and went into the building.

Left alone in the back seat of the car, Cindy and I looked at each other. She grinned slyly and gestured "come here" with her finger. I didn't need a second invitation. Undoing my seatbelt I scooted over to Cindy's side and we reached for each other. They say time flies when you are having fun, and it seemed like only a few seconds had passed when the car doors abruptly opened and Daryl and Trish hopped in.

Trish was laughing as she closed her door. "What are you two lovebirds up to back there?" she asked, looking around with a huge grin plastered on her face. "Oh, Cin, you're blushing! I never thought I'd see the day!" Then she giggled some more as Cindy denied all charges. Trish was obviously enjoying her friend's embarrassment. She looked at me playfully, saying, "Hi Mark. It's nice to see you again."

We had dinner at a pizza parlor in downtown Corvine. Daryl claimed it had the best pizza in town, and I had to agree it was pretty good. The slices were piled high with toppings, and beverages were served in huge glass mugs which had been frosted in the freezer. It was simple food, but as I bit into the hot cheese and followed it with a gulp if icy root beer, I sighed with contentment and found myself quoting my dad, "That hits the spot."

Cindy and Trish chatted away nonstop, catching up on what they had been doing in recent weeks. I don't remember what Daryl and I discussed, but it was probably man talk involving sports, power tools, the intricacies of gutting a fish, or something of the sort. Seeing the four of us together brought to mind the first time we had met, that fateful day when the girls had chanced to sit down across from Daryl and me in the cafeteria. So much had happened for all of us since then and still it was only the beginning.

The girls took a break from their conversation and Trish focused her attention on me, eyes glinting with mischief. "So Mark, you managed to capture this lady's heart," she said, nodding at Cindy. "You must be something pretty special. None of us thought we'd ever see this little wild thing settle down."

Cindy shook her head as she listened. "Hey, I'm not that bad!" she protested.

"Oh yes," Trish continued undaunted, winking at me. "This girl was certifiably single all these years. She was just too picky, I think. No guy was ever good enough. Either he was not cute enough, or not smart enough, or if he was good-looking *and* smart, then he was self-centered and egotistical. That's all we ever heard, one excuse after another. How did you catch her, Mark? You must be a genius with a huge…heart and a maestro's hands to boot."

"What the…?" Cindy snorted, putting on her most offended look. "Have you been smoking contraband or something?"

"Hmm, there may be another explanation," Trish mused, talking to me conspiratorially as if Cindy weren't right there listening. "I think Cindy's settling down because she's getting older and her biologic clock is ticking. Can you hear it? Tick, tick, tick, like a bomb waiting to detonate. It won't be long until she explodes and has a whole litter of kids crawling around her ankles."

"Trish!" Cindy exclaimed, blushing deeply.

"Ah, so I've hit closer to the mark with that one!" Trish ribbed her friend mercilessly. "What a lovely shade of pink you are!"

We were all laughing, even Cindy, but I felt sympathy for her, as she was obviously a bit self-conscious. I changed the subject after that and gave her a respite from Trish's wicked sense of humor.

Later that evening after we had all said our goodbyes, I stood with Cindy at her doorway and bid her goodnight. I leaned into her and kissed her softly, then I paused, frowning. I cupped my hand to my ear, saying, "What—what is that noise? Can you hear it?"

"Hear what?" Cindy asked, puzzled. "I don't hear anything. It's totally quiet up here."

"No, I can hear something. It's pretty faint, but...there it is again! I think it's coming from you! What is that? It sounds like 'tick, tick, tick....'"

Cindy's eyes widened and she exclaimed, "Oh, *you*!" There ensued a chase down the hallway as I tried to escape her wrath. My laughter proved my downfall as I could not suck enough air to run. She caught me before the elevator and punched me on the shoulder, then switched to tickling which was far more effective. She had me on the floor begging for mercy when she finally relented.

"That will teach you to mind your manners," she grinned with satisfaction, standing over me. "We don't need you picking up bad habits from Trish."

I held my hand out and she clasped it, pulling me to my feet. Once there I wrapped my arms around her and showed her how I truly felt. She quickly decided that I was worth the trouble after all.

CHAPTER TWENTY

Final exams arrived with a vengeance. The written portions were the longest I had ever taken, and I waded through page after page of questions that seemingly had no end. Some were multiple-choice, some required long answers. Histology wasn't too bad, mostly just identifying slides and regurgitating information from the spring term, plus some general questions on the older material. Physiology was also relatively straightforward.

It got more challenging from there. Gross anatomy was a long and strenuous exam, involving dog, horse, cow, and smaller animal specimens all laid out in the lab with structures to identify. The written test proved nasty as well, and I felt drained when I finally handed in the sheaf of papers and walked out of the room. I hadn't known all the answers; with Dr. Warner's exams I never did. But I had done the best I could and I was satisfied.

The neurology final was the most intriguing of all. It thoroughly tested our knowledge of the subject, but at the same time also managed to be pretty entertaining. In the lab portion we examined several live animals with various neurological problems. One I remember distinctly was a Shetland pony with a mild lameness. We watched it walking and I determined that the left forelimb was being favored slightly. After testing reflexes and looking for pinprick response over the lower leg, I found a small area that was numb on the left side of the foot. Only one small nerve branch had been damaged. I grinned as I wrote the answer on the test page; it was very satisfying to realize I now possessed the skills to make a diagnosis.

Other students felt the same way. Though the two-hour test left us dragging, I heard classmates afterward making comments such as, "That was a great exam!" or "What about that pony with the damaged lateral palmar digital nerve? Wasn't that great?"

In truth it really was. We felt like "Baby Docs" now, and we had made it through our first year with our so-called sanity intact.

After our exams were over, the sense of relief was indescribable. An almost manic rush of positive feeling swept over me as I headed upstairs to the anatomy lab to clean out my desk. There I found many of my classmates already doing the same, and everyone was smiling. These were precious moments we lived for as students, when the last work had been done, the final question answered, and nothing loomed on the horizon for a good long while.

My teammates Amy, Molly, and Mike showed up one by one while I collected my things. We bid each other goodbye in turn. Amy gave me a hug and wished me luck with Cindy. I thanked her and told her I'd see her in September. Molly smiled shyly as she said goodbye to the rest of us. Her husband Terry had come to the lab to help her with her things, so we finally got to meet him. His auburn hair was trimmed short and he dressed conservatively in slacks and a cardigan sweater. He had a quiet persona, seemingly a mirror image of Molly. I'd have bet that one could hear a mouse squeak over their dinner conversations...unless maybe she was hosting a party!

Mike Callahan was capering around as if he had just come off vacation. Watching him you would never guess we had just finished a grueling day of exams. He emptied his desk cabinet and chatted with everyone he saw, laughing and waving at people as they headed out the door. I bid him *adieu* and thanked him for his help in anatomy class. He just grinned and waved his hand dismissively, saying, "Aw, well, that was a team effort. You helped a lot and it was fun working with you! Have a great summer, Mark!"

I wished him the same and picked up my backpack. Looking around one last time I paused, realizing that I would probably never sit in this room again. It had been quite a year, all in all. But it was time to move on, and gladly so. I looked forward to summer break and the next stages of our education to follow.

As I headed out the anatomy room door for the final time, someone tapped me on the shoulder from behind. I turned to see Stan Hulbert's smiling face. He offered his hand and I shook it firmly. He said, "I wanted to thank you again for your help during the year. I guess I just needed someone else's perspective. You really made a difference in how I did on my tests, and I owe you one for that."

"You did all the hard work," I told him with a smile, "but I'm glad my input helped. I've enjoyed having you as a classmate this year."

We said goodbye then, and as I turned to leave Stan waved and said, "See you in Tullville!"

I walked down the stairs and out of McNairy Hall into the bright June sunshine. The afternoon air was warm on my skin and I leisurely strolled back to my dorm to begin packing my belongings. There was no rush, since I wasn't leaving town until the next day. I was riding back to Medford with my friend Daniel, and his exams weren't done until the following morning.

When I got to my dorm room Daryl wasn't there, but his closet was open and clothes were laid out on the bed next to his suitcase. The scene took me back to the first time I had entered this room. Nine months earlier I'd gazed at that same suitcase wondering what my roommate would be like. It felt like years had passed since then.

I opened the black travel trunk on the floor next to my bed. During the school year it had served as a table to set things on. I'd gotten used to thinking of it as part of the furniture. Now it would be put into service traveling once again. I opened my closet and pulled most of my shirts and pants from the hangers, laying them out neatly in the trunk. Some of my books and other odds and ends went in as well. I laid out one shirt and a pair of jeans on the bed for the next day and closed the trunk.

Just then the door opened and Daryl came in. He saw me and smiled, saying, "Ah, you're dressed." Then he turned his head to look out the doorway, saying, "It's OK, Trish, come on in."

Trish rounded the door and grinned at me, saying, "Hi there, Mark. Are you ready to head home?"

"Just about," I answered. "I'm not going until tomorrow, though; my ride isn't available until then."

"I see," she said. "We're heading out for Eugene this evening. Daryl lives there and I live in Springfield; we're practically next door neighbors! So he's going to drive me home and we'll be able to see each other all summer!"

"That's great! You'll get to visit Roseanne anytime you want," I teased.

Trish rolled her eyes and said, "Yeah, I sometimes think he loves that snake more than me."

Daryl replied, "That's because she gives me a lot less aggravation."

Trish poked him in the ribs and he laughed. With hands on her hips she declared, "Well, you're all mine, so you'd better tell Roseanne to move over." So saying, she snuggled up to Daryl and he grinned and winked at me; the two of them seemed really good together. I hoped they lasted for the long run, as I had a weak spot for happy endings.

That reminded me of my own source of happiness. "Hey you two, have a good summer, okay?" I said, heading for the door. "I've got to go see someone before she leaves town." Now it was my turn to wink at Daryl, and he laughed.

"Hold onto that lady," he said with a grin. "She's definitely a keeper."

"You be good to her, Mark," Trish added. "Otherwise I'll come after you!"

"Not to worry," I replied, laughing. "I know not to get you angry. Daryl's told me stories!"

Trish feigned shock and shook a fist at Daryl, and he protested, "Hey! Now see what you've started, Mark? I'll never hear the end of it, all the way to Eugene."

"Ah, a little trouble is good for you, toughens you up!" I called back over my shoulder as I left the room. I could hear them laughing behind me.

I took the elevator to the fourth floor and went to Cindy's room. I knocked twice, and my hand barely had drawn back for the third tap on the door when it flew open. Cindy grabbed my hand and pulled me into her room, shoving the door closed with her foot. I found myself wrapped in a steely grip by those velvet smooth arms, her soft lips pressed urgently against mine. I think she was happy to see me.

When I finally caught my breath, I grinned and said, "Nice to see you too." Looking into her eyes up close, I saw the swirl of emotions they contained. They were so expressive it was like peering straight into her heart, and I wanted to fall into those depths, losing myself there. Cindy must have seen something similar in me, because her expression softened and her smile grew.

We spent the rest of the day together. Both of us had finished our last exams, and we had nothing to do but enjoy each other's company until we traveled. We sat in her room and chatted for hours, knowing that it would be months before we could set eyes on each other again. What exactly we talked about is not important. What matters is that it was fun and funny, casual and intimate, and we loved every minute of it.

When afternoon stretched into evening, we went to dinner in the cafeteria for the last time. After we went through the chow line, I led the way to the far corner of the room. As we sat down next to each other I said to Cindy, "Do you recognize where we are sitting?"

She looked around blankly for a moment, and then it dawned on her, and a slow smile spread across her face. I had seated us at the same table where we had first said hello as strangers a lifetime ago.

We had a dinner of amorphous stew (affectionately known in the dorm as "mystery mush"), mashed potatoes with bland tasteless gravy (nicknamed "soggies"), tough bread rolls, and slightly wilted salad. It was absolutely wonderful because we shared it together. Later, as we put our trays in the dishware bin and headed out the door, Cindy said to me, "I'll always have a soft spot in my heart for this old cafeteria, because I met you here."

"Me, too," I replied with a smile. Then I laughed, adding, "It certainly couldn't be because of the food."

Together we walked back up to her room. There we sat on the bed and discussed our plans for the upcoming summer break. Cindy grabbed paper and we exchanged home phone numbers and addresses. We promised to write each other, and then the talk turned to what we would do come fall. I would be in Tullville for the school year, and Cindy would be here in Corvine finishing her degree. There would be long months apart, only connected via phone and letters. There was no Internet then, no way to instant message or chat via web cam. We would have to work hard to remain close.

We decided that I would stop in Corvine on my way north to Tullville in September, and also on my way home during the holidays. Beyond that we would need to play it by ear. With our plans made as best we could, we snuggled and talked late into the night. Eventually we fell asleep on the bed, Cindy's head nestled on my chest. I awoke around two A.M. and saw her face close by mine, her delicate features peaceful in slumber. That was a sight I longed to wake up to again and again. I promised myself that I would make it a reality someday, if I had any control over my destiny.

I knew I should head back to my room to keep tongues from wagging, but it was the end of the year and it felt like heaven holding Cindy close. Soon I fell back into a deep restful sleep. I didn't awaken again until daylight was stretching its glowing fingers through the window blinds.

Cindy began to stir as I yawned and stretched. Her eyes fluttered open, then her gaze focused on me and a smile lit her features. "Hi, baby," she murmured in a sleepy voice.

I leaned over and kissed her nose. "Good morning, Miss Webster," I replied, looking down at her.

She giggled and said, "So formal!"

"I guess I still respect you in the morning," I grinned. At that she laughed out loud, and I knew that I could never tire of that sound. "This was wonderful, waking up next to you," I said quietly as I ran my fingers slowly through her hair. "I could get used to this."

"Me too," she replied with a smile.

"I know we've not formally discussed it, really, but...." I paused and swallowed before continuing, "Umm, how do you feel about making this a long-term commitment?"

Cindy rose up on her elbows and gazed at me intently. "How long-term?" she asked, her eyes wide awake now. Her voice suddenly sounded very small, like a little girl's. "Do you mean really long-term?"

"Yes," I replied, meeting her eyes without flinching. "That is exactly what I mean."

Her mouth worked for a moment, but nothing came out. I was beginning to wonder if I had made a mistake when she abruptly threw her arms around me and hugged me for all she was worth. Her voice was close in my ear as she softly said, "Oh, yes, yes, I want that! I want you! I'll always want you." I closed my eyes and returned her embrace whole heartedly. We held each other like that, unmoving, for a few perfect moments. In the midst of my happiness the thought popped into my head that now I'd have some really interesting news for my parents.

CHAPTER TWENTY-ONE

Back in my dorm room, I finished packing; Daryl had left for home and the space looked empty and abandoned. His mattress was stripped of bedding, the closet hung open, and the desktop where Roseanne's cage had sat all year was vacant. I made one last sweep to be sure I hadn't missed anything. Satisfied, I grabbed my suitcase and trunk and left the room for the last time. As I exited, I turned and briefly looked back, remembering the nine months I had passed here. Then I closed and locked the door and headed downstairs.

Cindy and I had said goodbye, so I had no reason to linger. I turned in my key at the front desk and went outside into the morning sun to wait for my old friend Daniel. Eventually his familiar car pulled up to the curb and we crammed my belongings on board, with my bike roped onto his roof rack. When we were done, I hopped in the front seat and looked over at my long-time companion. It had been months since we had seen each other. He grinned back and hit the gas, and we drove off into the brilliant day that was the start of summer vacation.

The next few weeks were a time for catching up with old acquaintances. In Medford I visited with Daniel as well as a few high school friends. My mom and dad were fascinated and more than a little amused by some of the stories I carried with me from my first year in school. As would be expected, they also were very interested in Cindy. I had a small, wallet-sized picture that she had given me, so my family could see what she looked like. Dad's eyebrows shot up appreciatively when he took a peek, and mom said, "Oh, she looks sweet. What a nice smile." I told them that Cindy and I were getting pretty serious, and left it at that. Exactly *how* serious was something that could come out over time, once they'd gotten used to the idea of her.

Of course I had to visit Drs. Strom and Thurman at the veterinary clinic. Both seemed thrilled to see me and welcomed me back enthusiastically. Doug Strom was curious about what they were currently teaching in veterinary schools. He asked a lot of questions regarding the curriculum. I don't think my answers were very satisfying. As I had only gone through the entry-level subjects, I couldn't really comment on the latest and greatest medical advances which were probably his main interest.

Throughout my summer break I kept in contact with Cindy. We wrote to each other nearly every week, occasionally talking on the phone as well. My parents wanted to keep the long distance bills to a minimum, so the calls were far apart and far too brief. Cindy and I both cherished the occasions when we could hear each other's voice. The letters she wrote were sweet and heartfelt, sharing a mix of everyday events in her life, plus a helping of intimate thoughts and feelings. Though I could not see or touch her, those handwritten words on paper kept our relationship real and alive for me.

By late August I found my thoughts turning more and more to my fiancée. I would get to be with her soon when I headed back to school. It was only a couple of weeks in the future, so close and yet so frustratingly far away. I could do nothing but count the days and wait. In all my years of school I had never been so eager for summer break to come to an end.

YEAR TWO

CHAPTER TWENTY-TWO

Of course time did pass, and the day eventually arrived when I traveled north to Corvine. I would stop over for a weekend there, visiting Cindy, and then proceed on to Tullville, Washington the following Monday. My parents drove me to the bus station where I bought my tickets. After my luggage was stowed in the cargo bay of the bus, I bid mom and dad a fond farewell, giving each a heartfelt hug. Then I climbed aboard and settled in for the duration of the trip.

With the approach of fall term a lot of young people were traveling. By the time we pulled out of Medford around one P.M. the bus was full. I had a window seat next to an older gentleman who was maybe in his sixties. About my height, he had a solid build that had grown soft around the middle. His dark hair was graying at the temples and thinning on top; a devilish corner of my brain wondered which process would win the race. He wore a plain ensemble of faded blue jeans and a darker blue cotton shirt, and his hands looked rough and calloused. I surmised that he was no stranger to hard work.

My riding companion proved friendly and talkative and we soon struck up a conversation. His name was Mel, and it turned out he was a retired linesman for an electrical utility company. He entertained me with tales about his work for a couple of hours. I learned about power grids, high tension electrical lines, substations, and more.

As we traversed the mountains north of the Rogue Valley, Mel pointed to a string of towers which crossed the freeway and headed straight up a forested hillside, eventually disappearing over the crest. "Those were a real pain to build," he commented. "Rough terrain, and we had to clear a fifty-meter swath in the trees all the way up, to put the towers and lines in. It was dangerous work, and one of my buddies was killed on that project."

We also talked about my studies in school. Of course, when Mel heard of my career choice, I got to listen to several stories about his beloved Chihuahua, Ned. One of the hazards of my profession is being a captive audience while pet owners expound on the unique and wonderful attributes of their animals. It's the verbal equivalent of watching a neighbor's home movies or sitting through slide shows of Uncle Herman's trip to Europe. But I smiled and listened graciously, laughing at all the right times as was part of my calling, and Mel was happy being able to talk to someone who understood his love for little Ned.

The last portion of the trip seemed to drag on forever. I dozed lightly off and on while watching the scenery sliding by. With stops along the way, we rolled in to Corvine nearly five and a half hours after we had left Medford. I felt my pulse quickening with anticipation when I saw the familiar streets of the town. Cindy had my itinerary and I knew she was expecting me.

Once the bus parked, we all got up and began to shuffle out. I turned to Mel and wished him well, and he smiled warmly and shook my hand. Then we separated in the crowd of departing humanity and never saw each other again. Many years have passed since that day, and I am sure that Mel lives now only in my thoughts. I wonder how many people's lives I might have similarly touched over the years, and who then might recall me, even if it were only in passing, after I am gone. It does make you think.

The inside of the Corvine bus station was cramped and dingy, looking as worn as my suitcase. But I had no eyes for that. My gaze was captivated by the lovely lady standing alone off to the left. Cindy was wearing a yellow summer dress which highlighted the tan of her arms and legs. When she saw me her face broke into a radiant smile, and with a cry of delight she came running. I dropped my luggage and met her halfway. As we came together I wrapped her in a tight embrace and picked her off her feet. Holding her warm and close in my arms, the sense of incompleteness that had haunted my days and nights the past three months was swept away. For a minute I just stood there, my face buried in her soft fragrant hair, basking in the reality of being together again.

After a moment we reluctantly pulled apart and just drank each other in, grinning. I told her, "C'mon, let's get out of this place," and grabbed my travel bags. She led the way out the door and to her car, and we piled the luggage and ourselves inside.

We drove slowly through the streets of Corvine. Seeing the sleepy little town brought back memories of my first year here. It was nice to be back, but much of the drive I spent simply looking at Cindy. She was so beautiful with her skin browned from the summer sun, her long dark hair cascading over her bare shoulders.

While we drove we caught up on each other's lives. She and I were both keyed up and the conversation ran lively and animated. We spoke of our summers and the upcoming school year, and neither of us could stop smiling all the way to her apartment. I ran my fingers through her hair and she sighed and leaned her head back into my hand.

We reached her place in less than ten minutes and parked. Cindy's apartment was actually a converted second floor of a small house. A built-on staircase allowed direct access to the upper level from the outside. We hauled my suitcase up the long flight of stairs and Cindy unlocked the door. Inside the place was spacious, with a nice kitchen and living area and two decent bedrooms. After giving me a quick tour, Cindy grabbed my hand and walked me to a big overstuffed loveseat in one corner of the living room. She dropped into the seat and pulled me down alongside her. Winking, she said, "How about some snuggling, my boy?"

I grinned broadly. "Oh, you speak my language," I replied as I reached for her, and then I paused. "Where's your roommate?"

Cindy waved her hand dismissively. "Oh, Stacy's not going to be back for at least an hour. We'll hear her coming up the stairs when she does."

"Good enough for me!" I answered. And while I always loved how we could talk heart to heart, Cindy reminded me once again how much I appreciated her skill at nonverbal communication.

We spent two glorious days talking, romancing, walking the town and driving the countryside. The weather was warm and sun-drenched, perfect for enjoying the sights. Cindy also introduced me to her roommate Stacy, a short and spunky pony-tailed redhead who was studying performing arts.

The weekend passed in a flash, and neither of us was happy when I had to board the bus for Tullville. The ride to the station was much more subdued than my arrival had been. Cindy drove with her left hand on the wheel, her right clasping mine tightly the entire way.

When we got to the bus depot and I had checked in, we sat in the waiting area and talked quietly. "I'm going to miss you so much," Cindy said plaintively. "This was way too short a visit, Mark. When will we be able to see each other again?"

I sighed as I considered my options. I had learned that with Cindy it was best to be bluntly truthful rather than sugar-coating the situation. "I'm afraid I won't be able to leave Tullville until Thanksgiving break," I finally answered. "Until then I'm stuck in school. But nothing is going to stop me from seeing you when I travel to Medford. I promise I'll find time to stay over in Corvine whenever I travel south. You can count on it."

"What about the long term?" she asked, unappeased. "We're going to be living far apart for so long. It takes time spent together to keep a relationship strong. I really worry about us over the next couple of years."

In truth I shared her concerns, but it wrenched my heart to hear the anxiety in her voice. I squeezed her hand and said, "We'll be fine, Cindy. I know we will. My parents were apart for long stretches when my dad served in the Air Force, and they are still happily married decades later. What we have isn't going to vanish, not if we want it badly enough. And I do want this with you, more than you can know," I concluded emphatically.

That at least got a smile from her, and she kissed my cheek gratefully, wiping away a tear or two as she did so. Thankfully, the mood of the conversation lightened from there. We continued to discuss the future, but instead of hand-wringing we tackled the logistical problems facing us with an eye to problem solving. We even discussed marriage plans frankly for the first time.

"We're going to be apart for at least the next year and a half, until I get back to Corvine as a junior," I began. "It should get better after that. You'll be graduating next spring, so you'll have to move to wherever you find work. That's not going to be in Corvine, but hopefully when I return, we'll live close enough to see each other every week."

"Well, I'm going to keep my job search within Oregon and maybe southern Washington," Cindy offered. "Portland and Eugene are good-sized cities with decent prospects; I'm pretty sure I can land something in the Willamette Valley."

I considered that pleasant scenario for a moment, smiling. Then I took a deep breath and said, "Have you given any thought to when you would like to get married?"

The transformation those simple words produced was really quite remarkable. Apparently a discussion of matrimony was a more effective antidepressant than any prescription medication. Cindy's face lit up, and you would never have guessed that a few minutes earlier she had been so glum. Suddenly excited and animated, she was full of ideas, and we discussed our options seemingly without a worry in the world.

Fortunately, we were of like mind when it came to this subject as well. Cindy was smart and practical, and she agreed that we would need at least one steady income when starting our life together. First she needed to graduate and find work. Any nuptial plans would almost certainly have to wait until then. These were heavy subjects we were tackling, but it felt good to talk openly and to have a least a general timeline for our lives. It made our parting a little easier to bear, knowing that our futures would remain intertwined.

The public address system announced my bus and it was time to go. We stood and shared a lingering embrace and one last kiss. Then I grabbed my luggage and headed through the door to where the bus awaited. After seeing my bags safely into the cargo bin, I turned for a parting look at Cindy. She was just inside the doorway, and she smiled and waved as I blew her a kiss. Then I climbed aboard the bus and she was lost to my sight.

Because I had waited as long as possible to board, there were few seats remaining. I ended up near the back of the bus. Once I was settled I didn't have long to wait before the doors closed and we began to move. The bus pulled out of the depot a few minutes after ten A.M. and we were on our way.

Initially the driver headed north on Interstate 5 toward Portland. Traffic was moderate and we cruised up the Willamette Valley past crop fields of corn and grass. The corn stalks were tall and mature this time of year, their green ranks standing proudly in endless rows as we passed. By contrast the grasses were mostly grown for hay production and had been harvested already. The once lush acres were now fallow, dotted here and there with hay bales, both the square and rolled varieties. The exposed soil lay dry and dusty as it awaited the rejuvenating rains of winter.

We reached Portland around 12:30 P.M. The city center was a concrete maze of elevated highways, towering skyscrapers, and bustling avenues. The landscape felt strange and foreign compared to the quiet towns of my youth. After winding through the downtown streets, we made a stop at the large modern bus terminal where passengers disembarked and boarded. From there our path turned east. Crossing the picturesque Willamette River in the heart of the city, the driver took us out of town on Highway 84 toward the Columbia River Gorge.

Just east of the Portland area the Cascade Mountain range runs north to south. The Columbia River flows west toward the ocean.

Where the two intersect, something has to give. Because the Cascades are relatively young volcanic peaks, the river predates them. As the mountains formed and grew upward, the erosion of the moving water kept the river bed from elevating, thus cutting a trough into the gradually rising land. Eventually a deep canyon had resulted, with basalt cliffs hundreds of feet high on both the Washington and Oregon sides of the river.

Our bus headed east into the heart of the gorge as the freeway hugged the south side of the Columbia. Close at our right rose majestic tree-covered mountains. Their angled slopes abruptly ended in sheer black cliffs facing the river, as if an axe blade had cleaved them from top to bottom to expose the raw stone hearts within. Mountain streams poured off these precipices here and there, creating long feathery waterfalls down the rock faces. The grandest of these was Multnomah Falls, which plummeted over six hundred feet (nearly two hundred meters) off the cliffs of Larch Mountain to the floor of the gorge. It was the second highest year-around waterfall in the United States, and I craned my neck to catch a glimpse of it as we drove past. Though its volume was shrunken this late in the dry season, the white ribbon of water was starkly beautiful against the dark basalt of the cliff face. It was only visible for a few seconds before the speed of the bus had carried us onward, and trees again blocked the view.

To my left the Columbia was impressive in its own right. Separating Oregon from Washington, the waterway was easily the largest in the Northwest. Historically a powerful river that had once cascaded over boulders and waterfalls, it had been transformed through a series of dams, so that it currently resembled a long flowing lake. The river was so wide that the other side seemed remotely distant, and so deep that only the largest prominences still reared above water level as small islands. No rocks broke the glassy surface of the river, no rapids or falls interrupted the smooth flow of the water to the ocean. The dams had provided flood control and irrigation opportunities, and generated electric power for cities and towns. But the Columbia as Lewis and Clark had known it existed no longer, and some of the natural beauty of the original gorge had been lost in the process.

As we headed through the rift in the mountains and out the east side, the landscape began to change before my eyes. Tall peaks faded into rolling hills which gradually tapered off into flatlands stretching to the horizon. The thick forests of firs and pines were also left behind. Oregon's rainy reputation applied mainly to the

Willamette Valley; east of the Cascades the land became a vast high desert extending for hundreds of miles.

I watched as we rolled out into a bleak landscape of rocky lava flats and grey-green sagebrush. Trees were few and stunted even at the river's edge. We came to The Dalles, the last community of significant size for hundreds of miles, and took the long bridge across the Columbia into Washington. Continuing east on the north side of the river, we passed through mile after mile of dry tumbled terrain. Outside our air-conditioned vehicle the relentless sun baked the parched ground. Here the landscape was broken by small outcrops of columnar basalt, clusters of vertical black pillars resembling odd forms of abstract art scattered among the brush.

Now and again we would encounter a small slumbering town with a few miles of cultivated farm land around it. Fields of watermelon and cantaloupe thrived in the hot sun, nourished by water taken from the river. Within a few miles we would pass through these islands of life and out into the barren countryside once again.

Eventually we turned northeast and left the river behind. Across the plains of eastern Washington on winding, two-lane roads we crawled, and as we neared Tullville the landscape began to rise and fall like a rollercoaster. We had finally entered Palouse country.

The Palouse is an extensive area of gentle rolling hills with a few higher bluffs here and there. Once covered in prairie grasses, this was now a major wheat producing region. By early September the crop had been harvested, and the undulating land was covered only with wheat stubble and dry soil. I frowned as I took in the view. The untamed landscape of the high desert had at least embodied a stark beauty, but these barren fields had little appeal. They simply rolled on, mile after monotonous mile, as the small highway twisted and climbed and dropped with the terrain.

The sun was lowering in the sky and the hills cast long shadows by the time the buildings of Tullville showed in our front windows. The wheat fields fell away as we entered the outskirts of town and passed tracts of square wooden houses set on the low hillsides. Many were two-story dwellings with steep roofs and large front porches, and looked to be built in the earlier parts of the twentieth century. Large shade trees lined the streets in the residential areas.

Our bus headed up the main road into the heart of the little town. Nearly six and a half hours after leaving Portland we pulled into a tiny depot and disembarked. Heading indoors I found a pay phone on the wall, and called for a taxi to take me and my luggage to the dorm. I had requested graduate student housing, and had been assigned a room in Goldstein Hall. Beyond that I knew close to nothing about my accommodations.

The taxi arrived in about twenty minutes and with my luggage stowed in the trunk, I got in the back. I told the driver which building to take me to and he nodded. We headed up what appeared to be the primary street through town and I gazed around curiously as we went.

Tullville conformed to the undulating landscape it was built upon. Whereas Corvine had been situated on a flat valley floor, everything here seemed to be either rising or falling. The main downtown area was situated on lower ground. Up ahead to my left I could see the large concrete and glass buildings of the university perched on a hillside, peering down over the smaller houses and businesses. We passed a few restaurants and a movie theater, and some steep residential side streets which came down off the neighboring hills.

After a few blocks the driver turned left onto a large avenue that climbed up into the campus proper. We passed by several multistory dormitories with white concrete faces and rows of small windows on each floor. The cab stopped in front of one of them. I squinted out the dirty window of the car and saw that the name over the building's entrance said "Goldstein Hall."

I thanked the driver and paid him, and then grabbed my luggage, heading for the front door. Inside I found a desk where I checked in and got my room key. My room was on the fourth floor; I was sharing it with Keith Dolman. I learned he was also the floor monitor for that part of the dorm, which meant that he could handle any questions or problems I had. This sounded good to me, so I nodded and smiled and headed upstairs.

When I got off the elevator I was immediately hit with a blast of noise. The hallway I stepped into had multiple dorm room doors along its length, and many of these were wide open. Loud rock music blared from at least two of them, and several young guys were kicking a soccer ball up and down the hall. Hauling my luggage I walked down toward the other end, squeezing past the soccer players, looking for the room I had been assigned.

As I proceeded I glanced into several of the open doorways. The spaces within were invariably strewn with clothing and books, and the walls held posters which seemed to focus on two major themes: professional athletes and scantily clad girls. Everyone I saw looked barely old enough to shave; the pervading ambience was that of a high school gym locker room.

I finally found my room and went in. More of the same here: clothes thrown carelessly on one bed, presumably that of my roommate, and sports equipment piled in one corner. When I closed the door I came face to face with a life-sized photo of a semi-nude blonde model stuck on the door's back; she was standing wearing only a bikini bottom, her ample breasts partly hidden in her cupped hands. I rolled my eyes and sat wearily down on the open bed. *"Well, Mark,"* I thought, *"At least you're here, and so is your luggage. Welcome to Tullville."*

CHAPTER TWENTY-THREE

Despite the pounding drum and bass rhythms vibrating the walls, I was tired enough that I laid back on the bed and eventually fell asleep. My slumber ended when the door was thrown open and several young "kids" (that was the only way that I could think of them) came crowding in, talking animatedly about—what else—baseball playoffs. As I sat up fuzzily, one of them said, "Oh, hello! You must be Mark."

I focused on the speaker as he extended his hand. He was tall and athletic-looking, with a boyish face and disheveled blond hair. In keeping with the Goldstein Hall dress code he wore gym shorts and a stained T-shirt. His smooth cheeks were trying desperately to sprout a five o'clock shadow, but the effect more resembled a few scattered dirt smudges—or maybe a mild case of mange. Perhaps I would have interpreted his pelage more charitably if my slumber had not been abruptly interrupted.

I put on what I hoped was a convincing smile and stood to shake his hand. His grip was surprisingly limp for someone with his muscular physique. "Are you Keith?" I inquired as we stepped back and sized each other up.

"Yeah,, that's me," he asserted, nodding emphatically and giving me a thumb's-up sign. His buddies laughed and gave him a few friendly pokes and jabs, then piled back out of the room to leave Keith and me to chat alone. I could hear them hooting and joking as they made their way down the hall.

"Quite the circus here, it seems," I commented, rubbing my eyes.

"Oh, yeah, it never gets dull," Keith replied. "That's what I like about dorm life: something's always happening."

"Is this a graduate student dorm?" I inquired, puzzled. "Everyone seems very young to me."

Keith laughed as if the suggestion was hilarious. "Oh, no! This is strictly an undergraduate dorm, mostly freshmen and sophomores on this floor. Graduate student housing is in little buildings that look like condos, down the hill at the edge of campus."

"That's odd. I'm a vet student and requested grad housing. I need plenty of quiet time to study. I don't know why they put me here." I shook my head, not happy with the situation.

Keith looked suitably sympathetic. "Hey, man, I don't know. If I were you, I'd check with Student Housing. They'd be the ones to help if anyone can."

"Great! Do you know where are they located?"

"In the Tower of Power," he replied without missing a beat.

"The what?"

"The Administration Building," Keith clarified.

"Thanks, I'll walk over there in the morning." I nodded and smiled, and then a thought struck me. "Where do we eat around here?"

Keith looked relieved to be fielding a question he knew the answer to. "That's easy. This dorm has its own cafeteria. Just go down to the main floor and toward the back end of the building. It's simple to find."

I thanked him again and went to grab some food. When I came back, I chatted with Keith as I unpacked my things. We talked for maybe an hour, and during that time there were at least three interruptions as students came calling. "Hey Keith!" a freckled youth with fiery red hair exclaimed as he peered in through the partly open doorway. "Where are the cues for the pool table kept?" Keith answered his question, and he scampered off with a hurried "Thanks, man!" flung back over his shoulder.

Just a short time later another resident put his head in the doorway, and asked what the hours were for the exercise room. Keith shot off a quick response and the questioner disappeared.

After that two guys showed up together, asking Keith to help organize a tug of war contest between the two wings of our floor. Keith laughed and told them he'd get together with them later to discuss it further. As the procession continued into the evening I began to suspect that being the roommate of the floor monitor might be more a curse than a gift.

The following morning I awoke early, showered and ate. It was Tuesday, and nothing was scheduled at the vet school until orientation and a welcoming party later in the week. Formal classes didn't start until the following Monday. I had some time to look into alternate housing, so I headed for the Administration Building. My campus map showed it located just a bit further up the road that passed in front of my dorm.

When I reached the towering gray concrete structure, I headed inside and found the appropriate office. A matronly lady sat at the desk wearing a formal business suit and a serious expression. She looked over her glasses at me and asked me what I needed.

I composed my thoughts and began, "Well, I'm a veterinary student, and I requested graduate student housing. I have a heavy course load and require a lot of quiet time to study. But you've got me stuck in a freshman dorm, and it's constant partying and noise. There's simply no way I can work there. I need to find something else."

She frowned and looked in a notebook. "Well, the graduate student housing is nearly full as it is. There are students already on a waiting list wanting rooms."

"Why didn't you put me there to start with?" I asked, feeling myself becoming exasperated. "I had requested it when I enrolled months ago."

The desk clerk adjusted her glasses and said, "What program are you in again?"

"The veterinary school," I replied. "I'm up from Oregon for my sophomore and junior years."

"Oh, well, that explains it," she said with a nod. "Out-of-state students don't qualify for graduate housing. We reserve those for in-state students only, as spaces are limited."

"Oh, great," I exclaimed in dismay. "So I can't get anything but a freshman dorm? I've got to go somewhere other than that! I don't have much choice."

She lost a bit of her professional detachment then, and smiled sympathetically. "Well, I think we can cancel your dorm contract so you don't have to pay for housing you'll not be using. We can't offer you grad student facilities, but you are welcome to check out our postings for housing off-campus. Lots of people rent space in their homes or want to share an apartment. You can probably find something that way."

So saying, she gave me a copy of an off-campus housing list she had in her files, as well as a recent edition of the city newspaper, the *Tullville Review*, so I could check the want ads. She also started paperwork to get my dorm housing deposit refunded. I thanked her profusely for all her help, and left the admin building much happier than when I had entered.

Now that I had freed myself from the dormitory, I needed to pursue leads for other housing. I had a flash of inspiration and stopped by the vet school as I walked down the hill. The College of Veterinary Medicine was a larger, older program here than at Northern Oregon University, and there were several substantial buildings that belonged to the teaching hospital. The main lecture rooms and administration offices were in Goltz Hall, and I headed there to check for veterinary student postings for housing. I struck gold.

A receptionist directed me to a bulletin board along one wall of the main hallway. There I found several ads posted by vet students saying "roommate wanted." I copied the information on all that I could find and hurried back to the dormitory to phone them. The main dorm office had a phone that was available to residents for local calls. I pulled out the folded piece of paper from my pocket and began dialing numbers.

The first two I tried yielded no results: one didn't answer, and when I called the second number, the student told me that the vacancy had already been filled. I was down to two ads. One was posted by a female student; I wasn't sure she'd want a male housemate, but figured I'd call anyway. No matter; the phone rang interminably until I relented and hung up.

I dialed the final number with some trepidation. I really wanted to room with someone in the veterinary program; he/she would understand my need for study time and would be fun to chat with as well. It would be a great situation, but it seemed I was getting a late start and the choices were dwindling. I was relieved when a male voice answered the phone, and my hopes soared when he said that yes, he still was looking for a roommate. I introduced myself and asked if I could come out and see his place. He said his name was Jake Levitt. He was a Washington University student and was in the sophomore veterinary class as I was. We talked for a few minutes, and he gave me directions to the trailer park where he lived. I promised to come out that afternoon to see him.

When I hung up the phone my heart was racing with excitement. This might be the break I had needed. My entire school experience in Tullville could be heavily colored by my housing situation. I ate a quick lunch and headed out for the long walk to the trailer park. Tullville was a small town, but my destination was at the very outskirts, a good couple of miles from my dorm.

I exited the dormitory and squinted in the brightness of the midday sun. As I turned left to follow the road down the hill, I took a deep breath and savored the warmth of the gentle breeze in my face. Having spent part of my childhood in Spokane, I remembered how cold Eastern Washington could get. It wouldn't be long before the Indian summer would be a thing of the past. But for now the heat seemed reluctant to relinquish its grip.

While I walked, I noticed that there were metal grates in the sidewalk at intervals. What drew my attention were the little wisps of vapor that came rising out of them on occasion. Peering through the grates, I could see large pipes running close to the surface, and what looked like a sizable passageway below. I wondered what purpose such a tunnel would serve. When I reached the edge of the campus at the hill's bottom, the sidewalk grillwork ceased as well.

I turned right and followed the main street back through town, past old neighborhoods with elm-shaded streets on my right, and the businesses of the downtown area on my left. Three bars, a couple of gas stations and a movie theater later, I had passed through the center of Tullville and turned left onto Grant Avenue, which headed south and out of town. I hiked onward past a few outlying buildings and into the barren countryside.

Once I left the city streets behind, the rolling hills were smooth and featureless, covered with wheat chaff and straggling weeds remaining after the crop harvest. The arid terrain was different from anything I had known west of the mountains. Though it lacked the lush beauty of the forests I had grown up with, the novelty of it all held my interest.

Finally I saw the landmark that Jake had told me to watch for. Ahead on the right arose a large solitary concrete structure with the logo of the United States Postal Service emblazoned on its clean grey walls. Directly behind the Post Office I spotted rows of trailer homes rising in tiers up the side of a low hill. The road to the trailer park was just past the postal building, leading off to the right and up a steep incline. I found myself puffing a little as I hiked the narrow pavement toward the summit. On the way I passed four driveways on my right, each leading off between rows of trailers. Jim had said that his residence was on the top row near the far end.

At last I reached the crest of the hill where a fifth driveway angled off along the flattened summit. I caught my breath for a moment, turning around to gaze out over the surrounding countryside. Far off to my left I could see the trees and buildings of the outskirts of Tullville. To my right the barren hills rolled on endlessly like ocean waves until I lost them in the distance. The sky overhead was a brilliant Robin's egg blue, the air warm and dry, every distant detail standing out crystal clear in the bright sunlight. I concluded then that whether or not I found housing here, the walk had been worth the effort.

Turning back, I headed down the final driveway, following its winding course past residences with cars parked in front, until finally I came around a turn and spotted the trailer I was seeking. It was a small mobile home, white and weather-beaten, standing on concrete blocks which elevated it a couple of feet off the ground. Someone had added a small platform with three wooden steps which led from the ground up to the single door in the trailer's side. I approached the little dwelling and was about to climb the steps when I heard a masculine voice above me say, "Are you Mark?"

Startled, I looked up and saw a man's youthful face framed by light brown hair peering over the edge of the roof. I shielded my eyes from the sun and smiled up at him. "Hi," I replied. "You must be Jake, I guess."

"The one and only," he chuckled. He held a wide paintbrush in one hand, and now he gestured behind himself with it. "I'm up here patching the roof, and my hands are covered with tar. Let me grab a rag and clean up, and I'll be right down." I noticed he had a few black smears on his T-shirt and cheeks, and I encouraged him to take his time. I figured the cleaner he was before he shook my hand, the better.

Soon Jake climbed down the ladder he had propped against the back of the trailer, and he came over so we could introduce ourselves. After the formalities were over, he invited me in to see his place. I followed him up the steps and through the trailer's narrow door.

The interior layout was simple, a necessity since the floor space was smaller than most apartments. We entered what passed for the main living room, which merged on the right with a tiny dining nook and kitchen. Though cluttered, the place didn't seem to be excessively dirty, and the furniture was decent. We headed left down a hallway which led to the bedrooms and bathroom. The room for rent was on the right of the hallway, and I peered in the open door.

The space was miniscule, barely enough to accommodate the single bed which sat in the corner. One wall held a narrow closet and a built-in bureau with a few small drawers. A tiny, dirt-streaked window over the head of the bed let in the afternoon light. I pursed my lips as I assessed the situation. The cramped quarters left much to be desired, but it was private, and there were no loud dorm students partying around me, so it seemed a vast improvement over my current situation.

"Well, what do you think?" Jake asked me as we stood in the doorway.

"It looks good to me," I replied, nodding.

"Great! Let's head back to the living room and we can go over the details."

Once there I spotted some familiar veterinary texts stacked on the small coffee table, and we began chatting about school and our experiences in the programs at Washington versus Oregon. Sharing tales from our freshman year, we quickly relaxed and became comfortable with each other.

Eventually the talk turned to the business at hand. "Your ad said you wanted $75.00 a month. Is that correct?" I asked him.

"Yes, that's right," he confirmed.

"That's reasonable. I'll take the room if you're okay with the arrangement," I offered. Part of me worried that he would find some reason to say no, but we had hit it off pretty well so far, and after only a moment's hesitation he grinned and told me that he'd like to have me as a housemate. I tried to hide my elation as we shook hands to seal the deal; this was a major burden off my back.

A short while later I headed for the door, eager to get back to the dorm and pack my things. I paused in the doorway as a thought struck me. "I'll have to get a taxi to bring my stuff out here, so I'm not sure when exactly I'll be back," I said to Jake. "I'd like to get out of the dorm tonight."

Jake pondered a moment, hands on his hips, and said, "Well, if you don't mind waiting until tomorrow, I could give you a ride in my car. I need to finish this roofing while it's warm or I'd help you today."

"Wow, that would be great if it's not too big an imposition," I replied.

"Not at all," he said. "I'm going to be on campus tomorrow anyway, buying some books and taking my ad off the wall at the school. I'll pick you up after I finish my errands." So it was arranged.

My walk home was energized by my good fortune. I got back to the dorm in great time and packed everything I could in preparation for the move. When Keith came in, he asked what was up and I filled him in on the day's events. He congratulated me and wished me luck in my studies.

I was humming a lively tune as I worked. Even the music pounding through the wall and the constant knocks on our door couldn't spoil my mood. It's amazing how tolerable everything becomes when one isn't facing the prospect of nine more months of the same. I went to sleep that night with a feeling of optimism about my second year in school.

CHAPTER TWENTY-FOUR

The following day I bid Goldstein Hall an enthusiastic goodbye and moved into the trailer park. Jake gave me a ride as promised. By noon I was comfortably settled in to my new quarters (comfort is, after all, a relative term.) I unpacked my suitcase and trunk, storing my clothes in the closet and bureau, and threw my extra belongings under my bed. I asked Jake where he did his food shopping, and he mentioned a supermarket on Grant Avenue toward town. I remembered passing it on my hike the day before. It was only a quarter-mile or so from the trailer park. I told Jake I'd walk down for groceries, and he said he might be out when I got back. He fished around in a kitchen drawer and found a spare key for me. I thanked him and said I'd catch up with him later.

Jake was indeed gone when I returned, and after I put away my groceries I took the opportunity to inspect the trailer further. The hallway off the living room led to three doors. One was to my bedroom, the second was the bathroom door, and the one at the hall's end led to Jake's room.

The bathroom was small but clean, and had a full bathtub and shower. While I was inspecting it, I heard a peep like a bird chirping. At first I thought it came from outside the bathroom window, but when the sound came again, it seemed to originate from Jake's room. Curious, I walked to the door at the end of the hall and turned the knob to peek inside.

A deafening cacophony of screeches and whistles burst forth as the portal swung open. I stood frozen with my hand on the door, staring at the scene before me. The entire room was lined with bird cages, floor to ceiling, on every wall. There was a gap in the menagerie where the closet door was located, and a small area in the center of the room where a mattress lay on the floor. Other than that there was no space left unoccupied. My ears weren't the only sensory organs taking a beating; the aroma in the cramped space was pungent and powerful.

Birds of every size, shape and color populated the cages. Parrots, cockatoos, cockatiels, and others I couldn't identify fluttered and squawked from their vantage points on the walls. Directly ahead a green parrot with a yellow crown fixed an unblinking eye on me as he bobbed his head furiously up and down. To my left a large African Grey Parrot used his powerful beak to hoist himself up and down the sides of his enclosure, every so often letting out a raucous screech at my intrusion. I shook my head in amazement. Jake had mentioned that he had an interest in avian medicine, but this was a bit extreme. The noise continued unabated as the agitated birds protested the invasion of their space by a stranger. With one last look, around I eased the door shut, glad that I had my room all to myself.

I walked out to the living room and turned on the television, in part to drown out the din still emanating from Jake's bedroom. After awhile the trailer became quiet and I began to nod off.

I was suddenly jolted awake when a furry white projectile flew up from the floor and landed in my lap. I stared down to see a long-haired Persian cat looking up at me with large green eyes. A glittering collar encircled its neck, and a small nametag proclaimed the feline's name to be Delores.

The cat looked young, and a loud purr emanated from her throat as I stroked her head. "How are you, Delores?" I asked her. "Do you like living in a house with a hundred feathered friends to play with? I'll bet Jake doesn't let you in his bedroom, does he? Oh, the birds would love to meet you, I'm sure." Delores just purred louder and settled down to warm my lap.

We stayed that way until the front door rattled and opened, and Jake entered. "Hi Mark!" he greeted me with a grin. "Ah, I see you've met Delores."

"Yeah, I didn't see her when I came yesterday," I replied, stroking the cat's back.

"She's a little shy when there's any commotion or visitors. If you settle down and hold still awhile she's very friendly," Jake explained as he unloaded some books on the dining room table.

"I noticed," I said with a wry grin. "I practically dropped a load when she landed on me the first time."

We both had a good chuckle at that, and we talked for awhile about our interests in unusual pets. I wanted to practice on small animals such as ferrets, rabbits, rodents, and reptiles, in addition to the usual fare of dogs and cats. Jake's interest in birds was obvious. We seemed to have a lot in common; both of us were considered oddballs by our classmates due to our fascination with exotic species.

I took this opportunity to pick my roommate's brain regarding Tullville, the campus, and vet school. The talk turned to weather and Jake confirmed my suspicions. "Yes, it does get pretty cold here in winter," he said. "You'll want a warm coat. Oh, and these old trailers have almost no insulation, so a heating blanket would come in handy as well."

I made a mental note to acquire one, and I asked him about snow. He nodded. "Oh, we get that, usually not a lot of depth, but any snow we have stays around quite awhile. Say, did you notice the sidewalks on campus? They're steam-heated."

A little bell went off in my head as the grates with the pipes and wisps of vapor suddenly made sense. "Yes, I saw what looked like steam rising from metal grates today," I replied. "I wondered what that was about."

"Well, it's too early for the sidewalks to need heating," said Jake. "They're probably just testing the system so it's ready for winter."

Now I wondered exactly how severe the weather would be in a few months. Heated sidewalks, for Pete's sake! And me living in a flimsy trailer on the top of a hill, fully exposed to the wind and elements. It sounded like loads of fun.

Later that night I snuggled into the narrow bed and fell asleep reveling in the peace and quiet. My alarm was set for eight o'clock the next morning, since I needed to buy books and go to an orientation meeting at the vet school. It would be a busy day.

It turned out that I didn't need my clock. At about five A.M. I was dragged from the warm depths of slumber by a shrill note. It sounded like someone putting his fingers in his mouth and giving a short, high-pitched whistle to hail a taxi. And it felt like it was right in my room. Blearily I looked around, but I could see nothing. That wasn't surprising, since it was still pitch black. For a moment I wondered if maybe I had dreamed the sound. Then I heard it again and realized with a sinking feeling that it originated from Jake's room. The paper thin walls might as well not have been there at all; the noise pierced both my room and my eardrums with startling clarity. It was soon joined by another voice, slightly different in pitch but essentially the same call. They continued whistling every thirty seconds or so, and eventually I heard the squawks of the other birds as they awakened.

I looked at the clock and my heart sank. It wasn't even dawn yet. Peering outside, I could make out a faint glimmer of light on the horizon, but no one besides a vampire would glorify the event by calling it daybreak. Apparently the birds thought otherwise.

I later found out from Jake that the early risers were in fact a pair of Lovebirds. These were smallish green birds in the parrot family, rather pretty to look at. They were so named because of their tendency to bond closely with a mate, but I can tell you they tended to induce the opposite emotion in humans who were forced to wake up with them. Jake seemed totally immune, sleeping soundly right there in the midst of the cages, but then he was a bit eccentric when it came to his birds.

Every morning that week I was awakened in the predawn hours by the charming sounds of the little angels singing. During this time I discovered that chronic sleep deprivation can warp your frame of mind. I like songbirds, but as I grew more desperate day after day, I began to develop a sinister alter ego. I would lie awake in bed, teeth gritted, contemplating various ways that little birds might disappear. Maybe the cat would accidentally get into Jake's room and learn how to unlatch their cage door. Perhaps one of the bonded pair would trip and fall, injuring its vocal apparatus. Its partner would then be devastated by the silence and choose to sing no more. As the days wore on, I began to wonder whether Lovebirds had enough meat on them to make worthwhile rotisserie items.

Well, I am happy to say that no ill befell the birds. In the end a cheap set of foam earplugs worked quite well in place of more dire solutions. I could still hear my alarm clock come morning, but the chirps and whistles faded thankfully into the distance and I finally lost the shadows under my eyes.

That first week the vet school had a meet-and-greet at Goltz Hall. I entered the building and followed the map included in my school paperwork, eventually finding the lecture auditorium. The door to the room was located at the back, exactly opposite from the arrangement at Northern Oregon.

As I walked in I was struck by how much larger this lecture hall was than the one I was accustomed to. The facility looked fairly modern and well appointed, but the walls, floors, and desks all had a well-used feel to them. The glossy newness I had grown accustomed to in my freshman year had long since worn off the fixtures here.

There were also a lot more students in class this year, judging by the size of the crowd milling around inside the room. Our Oregon class held thirty-six individuals, but I had heard the Washington group was twice that size. Our sophomore class was not going to be as small and intimate as in the previous year.

Among the many strangers I picked out some familiar faces. Stan Hulbert's ebony mane towered above most of the people around him, and I caught his eye and waved. He grinned and waved back. Eventually I tracked down Mike Callahan and Amy Baker standing together in a corner. Mike was as energetic as ever, dressed in shorts, sandals, and a garishly-striped shirt. Amy sported a deep tan from working on her father's farm over the summer break, her blonde hair bleached even lighter by the hot sun. She wore it pulled back in a tight ponytail. The three of us joked and caught up on each other's lives since last we had last met. We also traded stories about our quests for housing in Tullville, and for some reason Mike and Amy seemed to find my dorm experience quite amusing.

After awhile a professor came in and made his way up to the front podium, and on cue the students took seats in the auditorium. The doctor in question was grey bearded and distinguished, with a mass of short silver curls atop his head, dressed in a nicely tailored suit. I leaned toward Mike and murmured, "He must be one of the senior staff members here."

Mike smirked and replied, "Gee, what gave you that idea? Anyone much older would need a séance to talk to us."

The speaker cleared his throat and spoke in a gravelly voice. "Hello and welcome to both the Washington and Oregon classes. I'm Dr. Otterman, and I'm available to answer any questions as we get started this year. We are very pleased to have you here, one and all. In addition we sincerely hope you find the educational experiences of the next couple years to be of the highest quality. It's always a challenge integrating two programs and two groups of students midway through their studies. I ask that you all embrace the opportunity to make new friends and to help each other in any way you can.

"You should all have your class schedules and facility maps. While you are here today, you may wish to tour this building and find the rooms you will be in next week. Most of the lectures are held in this auditorium, but some will be in smaller rooms, and the labs are scattered around as well. We'll have a formal tour of both the main buildings once classes begin.

"In the meantime, take this opportunity to begin getting to know your new classmates, and we'll see you Monday morning!" With that the old professor waved his hand and smiled, stepping down off the podium and slowly making his way up the central aisle toward the door at the back. Along the way he was accosted by a group of Washington students and he stopped and chatted with them awhile.

I spent most of my time that day getting reacquainted with my Oregon classmates, and touring the building to find where I needed to be the following week. I met a number of Washington students, but other than Jake their faces were a blur to me. I noted that the Oregon and Washington classes tended to band together in separate groups, which was not surprising since at this point we were total strangers. I hoped the two programs would merge harmoniously as the year progressed.

The following weekend passed lazily, life deceptively calm as the last days of summer vacation wound down. I rested and walked around town a bit. Exploring the campus occupied most of one afternoon as I tried to learn my way around. The overall size and student population of Washington University was remarkably similar to that of Northern Oregon, but there the similarities ended. The surrounding community was much smaller than Corvine, with open fields only a mile or two away from any spot in town. As far as I could tell, Tullville offered few diversions, which was perfect if you lived only to study. The undulating terrain also took some getting used to, and the steep streets reminded me of a miniature San Francisco. This seemed really an odd place to locate a university, unless one considered that it was an agricultural college situated in the heart of Washington's wheat farming region.

On Sunday I phoned my parents in Medford to let them know all was well, and I also called Cindy in Corvine. She was excited to hear from me and we talked for a long while, sharing stories about our new roommates, class schedules, and housing. Cindy was fascinated with my descriptions of the campus and the landscape, so different from what we had known in the Willamette Valley. Listening to her distant voice in my ear made me happy and sad at the same time. It was going to be very difficult being so far from her in the upcoming months, but knowing that she was mine filled me with joy.

When I hung up the phone I felt reenergized, centered again, knowing I had ties with people who cared, who were thinking of me and waiting for my return. That last night before my classes began, I slept more soundly than I had since my arrival.

CHAPTER TWENTY-FIVE

Monday morning I crawled out of bed to face my first day of classes in the Palouse. Jake and I attended the same morning courses, so he gave me a ride to school. Unfortunately, this wouldn't be an every day occurrence. Jake sometimes ran errands before class and left the trailer very early. On those days I would need to walk or utilize another option for transportation.

Since arriving, I had fretted over the prospect of long treks through snow come winter. Without a car my choices were limited, and the creative side of my brain had eventually cramped and given up thinking of solutions. Then, just a day before classes began, an answer to my quandary had literally come knocking.

As chance would have it, two other Washington vet students, Todd and Shannon Hagel, lived in the trailer park on the level directly below ours. They knew Jake well and had paid us a friendly visit one afternoon. After chatting awhile, they had unexpectedly offered to carpool with Jake and me to save gas. What a piece of good old-fashioned luck! Chance had favored the impaired mind, and now I could catch a ride nearly every morning.

But as I said, Jake was my chauffeur on the first day of school, and upon arriving at Goltz Hall we entered the rear of the auditorium together. I found a seat and watched as students wandered in singly and in small groups until the place was packed nearly to capacity. It felt like a huge crowd compared to the freshman class size back in Corvine. I rubbed my eyes and yawned, trying to fight off the summer break hangover.

Suddenly out of nowhere Mike Callahan landed in the chair to my right. He grinned at me as I glanced upward to see if perhaps there was a trapdoor in the ceiling that might explain his entry. Even at this hour Mike looked as energized as ever, smiling and practically bouncing out of his seat. Maybe he had an IV line pumping caffeine into his veins while he slept. I had to fight not to look at his arms for signs of venipuncture. He clapped me on the back and gave me a hearty "Good morning!" I humorously growled something about how those two words did not, in my opinion, belong together.

A young professor stepped up to the podium and began the now familiar introduction routine for the class. He went over general rules, the hours that the building was unlocked, and so forth. Once general announcements had been covered, Dr. Hill took us on a tour of the facilities, starting with Goltz Hall. This building housed the lecture auditoriums, and some laboratories and administrative offices were located here as well. After seeing the main features, we were taken out the door at the end of the building and down the slope to Aimsley Hall.

Aimsley looked older than Goltz, and in fact was the first veterinary building on campus. We entered the arched doors under the ivy-covered brick walls, and toured the main floor. After passing by reception, we entered the small animal hospital, where client-owned patients were treated. There were half a dozen examination rooms, a large treatment room area, and surgery suites where state of the art procedures were performed. Some cases were brought in by local pet owners, but Tullville lacked a big population base, so a fair number of patients were referrals from places like Spokane. Those cases typically needed expertise that only the teaching hospital could provide.

Further back in the building were extensive kennels housing mostly dogs and cats. One room off the main hallway was home to scores of birds, from small parakeets to large parrots and even raptors such as hawks and owls. Dr. Hill explained that some of these were wildlife that had been injured and could not be released back to the wild. We saw a large, regal-looking Red-tailed Hawk that had permanent damage to his left wing and could not fly. In the next enclosure a petite Screech Owl stared out at us with one good eye and one blind eye; he would never be able to effectively hunt.

Our last stop on the tour was a cavernous room with numerous surgery tables. We were informed that this was the infamous small animal surgery classroom, where we would someday cut our teeth learning to cut our patients. I looked around at the gleaming steel tables, the banks of surgery lights, and the numerous anesthetic machines. It dawned on me that I was inching closer to the day when I would be performing procedures rather than reading about them.

For now, though, it was more classroom lectures and lab work. We barely had time to settle in to our surroundings before we were hit with a full load of study materials. The Washington school was on a two-semester system, rather than the three terms per year at Northern Oregon. Our new courses still provided generous helpings of note-taking and rote memorization, the two activities best capturing the sweatshop charm of learning medicine. However, the subjects were inching closer to being clinically relevant, something we had been hoping for since starting vet school.

Microbiology was typical of this transition to practical knowledge. We sat in the lecture hall and took down endless pages of data about microbes, the good and the bad, the beneficial and the disease-causing. There were minutiae galore, yet much of the material applied to clinical practice, such as learning which bacteria are normal to find on skin, or in the bowel, or in an ear canal. Those that could cause disease especially drew our attention; here at last we were beginning to acquire pieces of the arcane wisdom associated with being a doctor.

We learned about nasty organisms like Clostridium bacteria, which could cause swollen, putrefying infections in the feet or limbs of farm animals. The ailments they produced came with dire-sounding names hailing from the olden days of veterinary medicine, such as Blackleg, Big Head, and Black Disease. We also learned about other bacteria with commonly-recognized names like Staph, Strep, and E. coli. I was surprised to find that some Staph and Strep can cause harmful infections, whereas others are meek and mild. The Staph bacteria found on normal skin are actually beneficial.

They compete for space and nutrients on the body surface, and help deter less friendly organisms from taking root. Without the normal bacterial flora on our skin, we might all be battling constant fungal infections or worse.

Much of this information was worthwhile, but try as I might, I could not see the usefulness in learning trivia such as the length (in microns) of all the different species of bacteria. As I poured nightly over my notebooks, filled with page after page of must-know material, I would not have been surprised to see my cerebral cortex start to bleed onto the white sheets in front of my blurry eyes.

Despite the workload, our second year classes rekindled our excitement for veterinary medicine. Parasitology was one of the most entertaining subjects we would encounter in our curriculum. Animal parasites held a revolting fascination for us, and Dr. Dick Wesley brought his subject to life in a fun and humorous way that had us actually looking forward to lectures. He was in his fifties, with a broad face and ruddy complexion that called to mind a country farmer. His full head of auburn hair belied his age, and the laugh lines around his eyes gave testimony to his ever-active sense of humor.

Dr. Wesley knew parasitology inside and out, literally, and could discuss internal parasites such as worms, or external parasites such as fleas, ticks, and lice with consummate ease. But he often did so with a tongue-in-cheek approach which made us grin as we jotted down notes. He might refer to a particularly nasty tapeworm species as "this cute little feller," or suddenly sidetrack into a joke that came to him during his lecture. Never mind that the punch lines were usually groaners; his fun approach was a breath of fresh air.

The lecture notebook also added to the charm of the class. A former student with some artistic talent had seen the need for pictorial summaries as a learning aid. He had created cute, hand-drawn caricatures of the parasites and their life cycles to help us keep the complex lives of worms and other critters straight in our heads. Smiling-faced nematodes followed little arrow pathways from egg to larva to adult, through whichever hosts they inhabited, all graphically and humorously summarized in the cartoons.

The lab portion of the class proved interesting as well. We got to see preserved specimens of worms, ticks, and other parasites, some quite large and pickled in jars of formalin, others very miniscule and preserved on microscope slides for us to peer at.

Throughout the term Dr. Wesley's subject matter certainly kept our attention. Add in the professor's good-natured banter, and it made for a memorable experience in the midst of our strenuous curriculum.

CHAPTER TWENTY-SIX

Despite the alienation of being thrown into a strange program, I found the Washington students to be quite approachable. Our new classmates tended to band together, but many were outgoing and made efforts to bridge the gap between our two schools.

One event that I'll always fondly recall happened just a week or two after school began. We were in microbiology lab, staining and viewing bacterial samples under the microscope. The Oregon students and some of the Washington group were in the early afternoon section. We were working away diligently at our tables when the door of the lab burst open and a small group of men and women filed in.

Each of them carried a musical instrument. Three had guitars, one had a fiddle, and one a flute. They arranged themselves in a loose circle in the center of the room and one of the male musicians cleared his throat and said, "We'd like to welcome the Oregon students here today. We're from the senior class here at Washington. To my left is Linda," he continued, gesturing toward a slender woman with long brown hair. The rest are Steve, John, and Stacy, and I'm Mike." Each member nodded or smiled in turn, and Mike said, "We know how difficult it is coming up here, leaving family and friends behind, not to mention tackling the curriculum! So we thought we'd entertain you with some music this afternoon. We know you're busy, so we won't take much of your time, just a few little numbers."

With that he grinned and turned to his companions, saying, "Okay, here we go, one, two, three...." They launched into a lively little folk tune that capered and jumped, and it soon had our feet tapping in time with the instruments. The flute and fiddle played the main melody with the guitars providing background chords, reminiscent of Irish folk music. When the song ended, the seniors followed it with a couple of others, and our entire class sat and smiled, the microscopes and culture plates momentarily forgotten. It was one of those uplifting moments that we all remembered long after it had passed, and that little gesture of goodwill did indeed make us feel welcomed.

During my first few weeks in Tullville, the fading heat of late summer transitioned to the cool but dry weather of autumn in the Palouse. Days dawned bright and crisp, requiring a light jacket in the morning, with temperatures becoming pleasantly warm by mid-afternoon. The sky remained a clear pale blue dotted by a few cottony white clouds. Cottonwood, elm, and aspen trees lining the town's streets became resplendent in reds, oranges, and yellows as they began to withdraw nutrients from their leaves in preparation for the winter ahead.

As time allowed I took opportunities to learn a bit more about the veterinary facilities at Washington. Between classes I wandered through the buildings, looking at hospitalized dogs and cats, reading their case histories and treatment plans. I peered into the avian room on occasion, mostly attracted by the large raptors with their intent eyes, hooked beaks and sharp talons. It was a thrill to see these regal birds of prey up close.

Once a staff veterinarian was there checking on the animals, and he let me hold one of the hawks. "Here, put this piece of leather over your arm first, so his talons don't dig holes in your skin," he advised, and I did as he suggested. The bird's grip was powerful, squeezing my forearm tightly as it balanced its considerable weight on my outstretched arm.

The vet gestured at the hawk and said, "His feet are his main weapons. He'll dive and hit his prey with them, usually killing it just from the force of the impact. His mouth is relatively harmless; he has a sharp beak for tearing flesh, but it's not very powerful. It really can't do much damage once you get beyond that pointed tip. Watch this." The vet tapped the bird on its face and it opened its mouth in irritation. Quickly he slid his finger in between the upper and lower beaks, just behind that wicked-looking hook. The hawk clamped down, but couldn't do more than gently squeeze the vet's finger. It tried to spit out the offending appendage after biting down several times, and the doctor relented and removed his finger. "Don't try that with a parrot or cockatoo!" he advised me with a stern look. "You'd pull back a stump. Those birds have beaks designed to crack hard tropical nuts, and they have incredible crushing power."

I thanked him for the information and for letting me handle the hawk. Though I haven't pursued avian medicine in my career, I enjoyed having the opportunity to touch such exotic creatures while in school.

Another room that held a fascination for me was the museum filled with preserved organs and other animal parts. There I found entire dried limbs of horses and cattle, dissected to various depths to show off different aspects of anatomy. Even more bizarre were the preserved cow stomachs. Cattle have four stomachs to assist them in digesting their high-fiber diet of grasses, hay, and tough weedy plants. Someone had managed to lacquer and preserve these organs with their connections to each other intact. The result was a great three dimensional model which aided students' understanding of the flow of food through the bovine gut. The tissues were shiny orange-brown and felt brittle when I ran my fingertips over them, like a giant eggshell. A sign warned viewers to handle the display with care due to its fragility.

My walks home after school were enjoyable during those September days of sunshine and balmy breezes. Once I left town, the route was quiet and peaceful. There was little traffic and often no sound but the wind rustling through the dry grasses along the road. Walking here gave me ample opportunity to think of those that were far from me. Faces I knew well swam before my mind's eye: my parents, my brothers, my friend Daniel, and most of all Cindy.

I also found an oasis in the undulating desert of brown hills. During my walks home I had noticed a large grove of trees off the road opposite the trailer park. A small paved lane led toward the grove and one day I decided to follow it. Maybe twenty meters in I encountered an ancient-looking wrought iron sign hung beneath the branches of a weeping willow, which carried the words "Tullville City Cemetery."

I hiked a bit further in and soon discovered a treasure of wonderfully manicured lawns set under the shade of old pines, oaks, and maples. Inside the grounds the road turned to gravel which crunched beneath my feet. Curious to see more, I strolled leisurely up into the heart of the cemetery.

Soon I wandered off the road and across the grass, looking at the weathered gravestones and enjoying the cool relief from the heat outside. The inscriptions on the markers often spoke of times long past, and I felt a profound sense of history walking alone in that silent place. After awhile a touch of melancholy began to take hold despite the warmth and brightness of the day, and I made my way slowly back down the road toward the cemetery entrance.

When I got near the gate, I sat on the ground at the edge of the shade, gazing out at the bright afternoon sun slanting across the hill beyond the cemetery. A small movement off to my right caught my eye. I glanced over to see a small reddish brown head peering at me from the grass. I sat motionless for a moment and the little creature came further out of the hole it was hiding in. It sat up on its haunches like a prairie dog, and I realized it was a brown and grey ground squirrel. Its stocky, well-fed body was cloaked in thick fur. The shiny black eyes gazed at me intently before it raced across the lawn to another large burrow and disappeared inside.

I got up and went over to look. The burrows were scattered over the dry grass at the cemetery's edge, and I could see more in the weeds and brush outside the gate where the land was uncultivated. Watching for a few minutes, I saw other individuals popping up and scampering here and there, like busy denizens of an underground city. I grinned and spent quite awhile observing the little animals' antics.

As the afternoon lengthened I finally called it a day and headed home. I felt totally relaxed and restored. The cemetery had been a worthwhile discovery, the closest thing to a scenic park that I had seen in Tullville. I would visit there again several times that fall, sometimes bringing my camera to photograph the hills, the cemetery grounds, and the busy little squirrels. The images captured in my photo album still take me back to that time and place where I found peace and a respite from the harried life of a vet student.

CHAPTER TWENTY-SEVEN

I squinted at the radiograph, trying desperately to see what the instructor had talked about. The thoracic X-ray hung on a light box on the wall which illuminated it from behind. It showed the chest of a large breed dog viewed from the side. Readily visible were the ribs, spinal vertebrae, and bones of the forelimbs which had been pulled forward so that they would not overlap the lung fields. Also easy to recognize was the prominent heart, roughly egg-shaped, that sat in the lower mid portion of the chest.

I recalled my lecture notes about pulmonary lesions and radiography, and tried to make sense of what I was seeing. Lungs normally showed black on X-ray images, due to being filled with air. On this film the lung fields had been infiltrated by a hazy pale gray, which indicated fluid had moved into them. That much I understood. But the pattern of gray was supposed to tell us whether the alveoli (microscopic air sacs) of the lungs were filling with fluid, or whether the serum was accumulating in the tissues outside of the airways. It was no use; my untrained eyes saw nothing but a hazy gray and black pattern, just like the prior X-ray which supposedly had showed different lung pathology. I turned to Amy Baker who stood next to me and said, "Can you tell the difference between an interstitial fluid pattern and an alveolar pattern? I'm stumped!"

Amy shook her head and brushed her blond hair back, saying, "It beats me, I can't really see much to distinguish them. There's supposed to be a difference in the fluid distribution, and also whether or not the airways are visible."

I examined the films for awhile longer and then shook my head in frustration. "I guess I'll have to get one of the profs to come explain what we're looking at—again."

Such was my introduction to the mysteries of radiology. This was a class that included some theory but was mostly clinical; we had to know how to take and interpret radiographs if we were going to be competent practitioners. It was just the sort of thing we had been wishing for, since it was genuine doctor knowledge. It was also genuinely difficult.

The lecture portion taught us how an X-ray machine worked, using a high-powered cathode to beam radiation down onto the table in a targeted area. As the X-rays passed through the patient, some of the beam made it through to the film, and some was absorbed by the body structures. This created the lighter and darker patterns seen on the film, which became a picture of the animal. Size really does matter with some things, and a large dog's body absorbed more of the X-ray beam than a toy poodle would. The machine's settings had to be adjusted both for the thickness and type of tissues we wanted to look at, so the film would not be overexposed, resulting in a picture that was all black, or underexposed, making the film turn out too white and hazy.

Once we understood the theory and method of taking pictures, we also had to learn to develop the X-rays in a darkroom. Nowadays automatic processors handle this chore in a few minutes, yielding fast and consistent results. But this was the early 1980s, and the radiology department utilized manual developing tanks. This meant that we had to hand-dip the films in developer and fixer, and then dry them on hanging racks. This wasn't as easy as it sounds.

A typical developing session might proceed as follows. After taking an X-ray, a couple of students would go off to the darkroom. There we were reduced to using our sense of touch to find our way around. The room had a dim red safe light which was supposed to allow us to see without damaging the film. It was about as useful as the glow from a single star in the sky. You could look up and tell that it was on, but seeing your hand in front of your face was wishful thinking.

We would try to memorize the locations of the tank lids and other necessary landmarks before closing the darkroom door. Once that portal clicked shut, we might as well have been entombed in the bowels of the earth. Immediately losing our bearings, we would stumble and fumble our way around inside like a couple of stooges. Being educated individuals, we would of course discuss the matter intelligently while we did so.

"Can you see?"

"No."

"Hmmm…me neither. Where are you?"

"Here."

"Where is here?"

"Umm…I dunno. Where are you?"

"Here."

"Oh."

"Well, try to find the developing tank. I thought it was here, but apparently I missed it. Maybe it's there."

"Okay, let me move over this way."

"Ouch! Watch the elbows!"

"Sorry, was that you?"

"No, it was one of the other hundred people in here. Of course it was me!"

"Sorry. Wait a minute, I'm finding something…"

CLANK.

"What was that?"

"Hey, I've found the tank lid!"

"Which one, the developer or the fixer?"

"Umm…dunno."

"Come on, this is taking forever!"

"Really? How much time has passed?"

"Hmmm…I dunno. This is ridiculous! People are going to think we died in here. It couldn't get any worse."

"Yes it could."

"How?"

A long pause.

"Well?"

"Please don't fart in here."

"*What*? Why did you bring that up? When have I ever…?"

"Never mind. I was stating a preference, not making an accusation."

"Oh. Well, that goes for me, too." Another long pause. "I guess that *would* be worse."

"Yes."

"So, what next?"

"I've got the tank open. Give me that film already!"

"Here you go."

"*Ouch!*"

"Sorry."

When miraculously the task was somehow completed, we would lurch out into the blinding light of a normally lit room, eyes squinted and faces flushed from heat and stress. Our feeling of accomplishment would be instantly wiped away when a glance at the clock showed that twenty or more minutes had passed. Invariably the radiology professor would say something helpful like, "What took you so long? We thought you had fallen in the developing tank!" In such situations I thought it best to bite my lip and not tell him what he could do with his tanks.

But for all the challenges of mastering X-ray techniques and film developing, those came easy compared to making sense of the final product. Reading a radiograph wasn't something one could memorize. The abnormalities shown on a film were often subtle and easily missed. I soon realized the biggest obstacle was trying to learn what normal looked like.

Each individual is unique—in shape, size, exact organ positions, and so forth. Therefore, each animal's X-ray is unique as well. One has to know what is simply individual variation and what is beyond the norm. This takes a long time to get a feel for, with hundreds or even thousands of images being viewed before your mind can see pathology with confidence.

Even when we did recognize something as abnormal, we often didn't know what it was. Dealing with multiple types of animals, with their vast variations in anatomy and diseases, multiplied our headaches exponentially. As one Washington student said forlornly while she stared uncomprehendingly at a radiograph, "Oh, it's just no use; I'll never develop X-ray eyes."

Dr. Parry and Dr. Barton were the senior radiology professors at Washington University, and they bore a striking resemblance to each other. Both were big, stocky men, with dark hair that was thinning on top, and they rolled a bit from side to side when they walked. The students dubbed them "the penguins."

It was obvious these two were experts in their field, although the sophomore class had a difficult time following what the doctors were pointing out on the films. Dr. Barton in particular delighted in seeing what we could not. We'd be inspecting a horse radiograph that showed an enlarged heart and hazy lung fields, and he would casually walk by and say, "Oh yes, this patient has chronic obstructive lung disease with secondary cor pulmonale and cardiac enlargement." (This meant the heart was having a hard time pumping blood through the diseased lungs, and had become enlarged as a result.)

So the next time we saw a big heart with hazy lungs on an X-ray, we'd make the same diagnosis and the professor would say, "No, no, no…this patient has chronic heart disease and is in congestive heart failure, which is causing the lungs to fill with fluid." It was exasperating! Trying to figure out which came first, the pathology in the heart or in the lungs, made my skull want to fill with fluid as well. The class referred to such undecipherable films as Dr. Barton's Imaginographs.

With time and experience I came to realize that it wasn't always easy even for the veterans. In class they made it seem like child's play, but when we saw them discussing films from current hospital cases, it was a different story. More than once I saw Dr. Parry and Dr. Barton disagreeing on the diagnosis, sometimes even wagering a bet on what the eventual answer would be. When the referring internist or surgeon showed up to see what the radiologists had uncovered, he or she would sometimes offer another diagnosis as well. If the patient went to surgery and a definitive answer was found, it would invariably vindicate one doctor's opinion. Then he or she would strut about the halls preening for a few days, occasionally toting a bottle of wine that came with winning a wager. It all made me feel a little better about my own inadequacies in radiology. On the other hand, it was depressing to learn that I might never be entirely certain what an X-ray meant no matter how long I practiced.

While our attention was focused indoors, the weather in Tullville gradually began to deteriorate. Restless winds drove clouds helter-skelter across the sky, foretelling harsher storms to come, but as yet little precipitation spilled on the parched ground. When the nights were clear, temperatures dropped and a bright haze of frost whitened the hills when I awoke, sparkling like fairy snow in the morning sun.

As the weather cooled, I discovered that the thin walls of the old trailer had no detectable insulating properties. On some mornings I could have sworn the air inside the trailer was in fact colder than outdoors. Jake was reluctant to turn on the heat unless ice was forming on the water faucets, citing the need to conserve dollars.

I'm usually a sluggish person in the morning, but when I crawled out of the warm cocoon of my heating blanket I was spurred into frantic action by the kiss of the frigid air and an icy cold floor. I had always set my alarm as late as possible to squeeze every iota of sleep from the night. Then I would rely on a streamlined shave/shower/eat routine to get out the door quickly. Over the years I thought I had refined the whole process to be as fast as humanly possible. Now I found that risk of frostbite could inspire unimagined gains in speed and efficiency. The only thing that slowed me at all was learning how to shave while shivering.

CHAPTER TWENTY-EIGHT

There were also some amusing aspects to the classes that semester. Not all of these were positives, but we could smile wryly at them nonetheless. A prime example was pharmacology lecture. On paper this was another subject we had been eagerly awaiting, a chance to learn material that would critically impact our lives as doctors. Unfortunately, we had to endure the presentations of Dr. Borland.

The pharmacology professor was a smallish man in his mid fifties, bald but for a grayish fringe around the sides of his head. He typically wore a clean white, full-length lab coat to lectures. While speaking he stood nearly motionless at the podium, hands gripping both sides of the wood surface as he stared alternately at his notes, then at an undetermined spot well above the heads of the students.

We all entered the class excited to learn the intricacies of drugs and therapeutics. Dr. Borland took the podium the first day, consulted his pages, and began his lecture. He discussed the overall organization of the course, how we would learn different classes of medications, from antibiotics to narcotic pain relievers and everything in between. Drug uses and contraindications, toxicities and overdoses, all of the important aspects of pharmaceuticals would be touched upon. Later in the year, during spring term, we would cover anesthetic drugs and the basics of anesthesiology.

This was material that should have riveted our attention. But even on day one of class, with a new group of students hanging on his every word, Dr. Borland ponderously ground out his lecture without the slightest inflection or emotion. His voice droned along in a dry monotone that would have made a hypnotist drool with envy. I could have read the ingredients off the back of a cereal box with more enthusiasm.

The effect was amazingly potent and rapid. Within minutes I found myself fighting the Special Ed syndrome and yawning repeatedly, my eyelids growing heavy as I struggled to take down notes.

Amy Baker was sitting to my left in the lecture hall, and Mike Callahan to my right, in a near recreation of our first year group. Both of them had caustic senses of humor. As Dr. Borland's spell numbed our brains, Amy leaned over to me and whispered, "Who needs to learn about anesthetic drugs? He could knock out any animal by just talking to it." She mimed nodding off to sleep and I nodded in agreement.

A few minutes later Mike rubbed his eyes and shook his head, then summarized his thoughts with, "This guy's about as interesting as a rectal polyp." I suppressed a chuckle and told him that his comment was rather insulting—to the polyp.

Of course the sophomore class was merciless in its assessment of pharmacology lecture. "Dr. Borland" was quickly mutated to "Dr. Bore-land," or alternatively "Dr. Snore-land." But I must give credit where it is due, and the information he presented was well organized and pertinent. Despite the challenge of remaining focused in class, I did manage to learn the basics of pharmacology. The core material of that course served as the foundation for my knowledge of medicines thereafter.

By contrast, parasitology class continued to entertain as well as educate. Dr. Wesley's presentation made all the difference. One afternoon he was discussing Trichinosis, an illness caused by a vicious little parasite found in pigs named *Trichinella spiralis*. The worms formed cysts in the pig's muscle tissues where they lay dormant until eaten. People who consumed undercooked pork meat could then become infested.

Once ingested, the worms awoke and burrowed into the intestinal lining of the unfortunate person. The resulting digestive upset would soon pass, but then the worms would produce hundreds to thousands of tiny larvae that migrated out of the bowel and into the person's muscles. They formed new cysts there with coiled worms inside. This caused pain and cramping, scarring of the muscles, and in severe cases could even be debilitating. It was a decidedly unpleasant experience, and was by itself a strong argument for fully cooking meat before consuming it.

After covering the worm's life cycle and health implications, Dr. Wesley paused thoughtfully. Then a huge grin split his face as he recounted a tale from the grand old days of parasitology. He began, "In times past they didn't know how Trichinosis was spread, how a person became ill with it. They had identified a parasitic worm as the probable culprit producing the symptoms. No one knew how the worms got there however. And that's where things became really fun.

"At a national veterinary conference two of the preeminent parasitologists of the day, Dr. Thomas Merril and Dr. Aaron Stormberg, debated the conundrum of Trichinosis. Dr. Merril had become convinced, via careful history-taking of affected patients and examination of human and pig muscle tissues, that the disease could be contracted by eating undercooked pork meat. A common source back then was sausages which were often smoked or cured but not thoroughly cooked. Dr. Merril had an example of such a product on the podium beside him, a large piece of juicy-looking pork sausage, and he would pick it up and gesture with it as he made his case for this being the source of the disease.

"Dr. Stormberg, on the other hand, thought this was hogwash. The debate raged on for nearly an hour, with tempers flaring and voices rising. Eventually Dr. Stormberg had had enough. He slammed his hands down on his podium and bellowed out, 'There is no way that sausages cause Trichinosis! I'd stake my reputation on it! And that's final!'

"Dr. Merril, also at his wit's end, pointed at the pork sausage and retorted, 'Well if you are so certain, take a bite of that sausage! I dare you!'

"The audience of veterinarians listening to the debate had been getting louder and more boisterous as the speakers' level of agitation had risen. Now as Dr. Stormberg hesitated, the crowd began chanting, '*Eat it, eat it, eat it!*'

"Dr. Merril stood with his hands on his hips, looking from Dr. Stormberg to the sausage and back again, silently challenging his opponent. Finally with a scowl Dr. Stormberg grabbed the sausage, tore off a large bite with his teeth, and threw the remainder back down on the podium. He then stomped off the stage to wild applause and cheers from the audience."

Laughter erupted throughout the class as Dr. Wesley finished his story. He spread his hands wide and proclaimed, "Now, *that* was a fun time to be a parasitologist! They don't have seminars like that anymore!" Maybe not, but our professor made his course lectures as entertaining as anyone ever did during my four years in veterinary school.

The fall term naturally came with its quota of exams along the way. Luckily the Washington program was a bit friendlier to us than at Northern Oregon. During our first year the exams had always been clustered, making for high anxiety levels as we prepared for multiple tests at once. Now the sophomore courses deliberately separated their tests to facilitate our studies.

Between the easier exam schedules and the lack of diversions in Tullville, I pulled the best grades of my veterinary education during that time, getting straight A's during one semester. It wasn't important to have perfect marks in vet school, but I could look back with some pride and say that I had done it. In any event, studying helped keep me from going stir crazy that year.

As the weather grew ever colder I contemplated ways to protect my face from the freezing winds, especially on long walks to school when I had no ride. Ever since my undergraduate days I had toyed with the idea of growing a beard. Cindy and I discussed the matter, and she wanted to see what I would look like with one. As the semester steamrolled into an early winter, the idea sounded more appealing than ever.

Cultivating a beard is an exercise in patience, and it helps to not be self-conscious. For the first month or so it really looks like you've gotten lazy about personal hygiene or lost your razor. The patchy, moss-like growth in the early stages was a far cry from the solid dark covering I had envisioned. I tried to dress in my nicer clothes so I wouldn't be mistaken for a derelict. After about five weeks of this I finally began to see the end product, and I liked the look. It's one I've kept all these years since then.

Between all my classes and adjusting to life in the Palouse, I kept in contact with Cindy regularly. We shared handwritten letters nearly every week. Long-distance phone conversations were a luxury to students trying to make ends meet, but we indulged when we could. One evening shortly before Thanksgiving that year, I spent close to an hour on the phone with Cindy. Hearing her voice instantly melted away the months and miles that separated us. When I closed my eyes, I was once again there by her side, enjoying the warmth of her embrace, the taste of her lips, the whisper of her words uttered softly in my ear. I felt such longing for her right then that it was a physical ache.

Cindy was missing me as well. When we got to discussing Thanksgiving break, she said, "You can come visit me in Corvine over the holiday, can't you? I really need to see you then. Please?"

Even from far away the warmth of her affection washed over me, and I was smiling as I told her, "Nothing will keep me away, Cindy. The only problem is that classes don't finish until two days before the holiday. I'll be taking the bus the day before Thanksgiving and it's an all-day ride to Medford. I will have to go straight there to be able to spend the holiday with my family. I already promised them I would."

"Oh, no! Then I won't get to see you on the way down! I'm planning to stay in Corvine during the break to just rest and catch up, so I'll not be with my family on Thanksgiving. My roommate will be out of town too and I'll pretty much be alone. I was hoping for a little company."

The disappointment was evident in her voice and my spirits sagged. Before I could say anything Cindy continued, "I understand, though; how about we meet after the holiday on your way back up?"

I started to agree and then a wonderful thought struck me. "Cindy, what do you think about coming to Medford with me for Thanksgiving? The bus stops in Corvine, so if you got a ticket you could jump on there and we could ride together! It really would be nice if my parents got to meet you before we formally announce our engagement. Only my younger brother and I will be at home, so there will be plenty of room. Mom's a good cook and you'd love her, she's a lot of fun. You two will have all sorts of things to talk about, I'm sure."

Once I had broached the idea I found myself racing on excitedly, leaving little room for Cindy to get a word in edgewise. Finally she started laughing and said, "Mark, slow down, take a breath! The answer is yes, I'd love to come with you. I guess it's about time I met your family. Oh wow, I'll get to spend several days with you too. This is going to be a lot of fun!"

I certainly shared that sentiment, but there were some hurdles to jump before then. The week before Thanksgiving I had a radiology exam, so I spent much of my time studying in preparation. I reviewed radiation safety protocols, positioning of patients for X-ray studies, calculations for proper film exposures, and so forth. All that was fairly easy for me; the hard part was pouring over the example radiographs and trying to see what they supposedly illustrated. My X-ray eyes were still in need of corrective lenses.

When the exam finally came, it was much as I expected. The written portion was straightforward enough, and I attacked it confidently. After answering the last question, I felt good about my mastery of the theoretical side of the course. Evaluating the radiographs tacked up on the light boxes was not going to be so easy.

Deep in the radiology section of the teaching hospital was a long hallway with multiple viewing stations on the walls. X-rays of all types were hanging there with questions attached to them on small white note cards. Some asked us to identify a particular anatomic structure, highlighted on the film with a small arrow. However, most questions dealt with abnormalities illustrated on the pictures.

The question might relate to a specific lesion pointed out to us, or might be more general, such as "Identify all pathology seen in this patient." Some were tricky, as the patient we were looking at could be totally normal. Dogs, cats, horses, cattle, and sheep were pictured, challenging our knowledge of anatomy and radiographic interpretation. The two professors circulated among the students, making themselves available in case any of the questions needed clarification.

I found some radiographs to be fairly easy. A good example was the canine leg X-ray showing a spiral fracture of the femur. The two bone fragments were minimally displaced and overlapped each other, so the fracture wasn't visible on the lateral (side) view. However the A-P (front to back) view showed a thin line running obliquely across the shaft of the bone. This was a great demonstration of why two views are essential on any radiograph—it is the only way to achieve a good feel for the three-dimensional anatomy of the patient.

There were X-rays showing degenerative arthritis in the ankle of a horse, congestive heart failure in a cat (yes, I did get that one right!), rocks in a dog's stomach, and on and on. Nearly forty radiographs in total were included in the exam. By the time it was over, I once again felt the sense of total fatigue that seemed an integral part of the testing experience.

There were a few films on the exam that I just could not figure out no matter how long I stared at them. One that stood out was a study of a horse ankle and foot, which showed no degenerative changes, no rough or thickened bones or joints, no soft tissue swelling, nothing abnormal that I could see. The question was, "Describe any abnormalities demonstrated by this patient." I wasn't at all sure, but I finally had to jot down "Normal" on my exam form.

When the test was over and students were milling in the hall outside of the radiology department, I heard Stan Hulbert asking Mike Callahan about that film. My ears immediately perked up and I listened in as Mike answered with enthusiasm, "Oh yes, wasn't that a cool film? The horse was totally lacking P-2, the second bone in the foot. He only had P-1 and P-3. What a weird birth defect!" My heart sank as I realized that here was one question, at least, where I had missed the answer totally. Stan must have done the same, because he grimaced and shook his head before slowly walking away.

But overall I felt good about my performance in radiology, and I certainly did as well as most of my classmates. With the exam no longer hanging over our heads, the last few days before the holiday were relaxed. After lectures on the final day of school, I bid my friends good bye and left the building to hike home. That afternoon the air had a sharp cold bite to it, a west wind blowing strong in my face. I hunched over and zipped my coat up as high as it would go, warming my hands in my pockets to keep my fingers from going numb. The long walk to the trailer was becoming less entertaining with each passing week.

The following day I prepared to leave town and head home. I packed just one suitcase to travel light, and got a ride from Jake to the bus station downtown. I was fidgeting with excitement and eager to be on my way; this would be my first trip out of Tullville since I had arrived. It looked like I was leaving just in time. Forecasts had predicted winter conditions and the sky brooded with impending weather as I boarded the silver-and-white bus for Portland and beyond.

CHAPTER TWENTY-NINE

My ride to Portland was relatively uneventful, despite heavy rain squalls that periodically lashed against the bus windows and slicked the roads. After a stopover in the city, we headed south on Interstate 5 through the Willamette Valley. In about two hours we arrived in Corvine and pulled into the small bus depot. I waited in my seat, wanting to hold it so that Cindy and I could sit together. Some passengers unloaded and then boarding commenced. A number of men and women filed in, but I didn't see Cindy among them as they shuffled slowly down the aisle of the bus. I began to worry that she had not made the terminal in time. A young man asked to sit next to me and I told him that I was waiting for someone. Just then a wonderfully familiar face came into view at the front of the bus. Cindy looked even better than I remembered, dressed in jeans and a heavy blue winter jacket, her dark glossy hair spilling down her back.

I waved frantically to catch her attention as her eyes searched down the length of the bus. Her gaze passed over me at least once and I suspected she didn't recognize me with a full beard. When at last she saw me her face came alive, and she impatiently waited for the line in front of her to move. Our eyes hardly left each other as she slowly drew closer. Finally she slid into the seat beside me, all flushed with the cold and excitement.

We gazed intently into each other's eyes, drinking in what we had missed for so long, and then I wrapped her in a close embrace. For a good long moment we remained like that, simply enjoying being able to touch once again. I could feel Cindy quivering against me, and I didn't think it was from the cold. Within my encircling arms her body felt warm and supple even through the heavy winter clothing. I eventually pulled back and saw a couple of people across the aisle smiling knowingly. My face felt suddenly flushed and I looked away.

Cindy wanted to know all about my classes and the town of Tullville, the weather, the countryside, my roommate, and anything else she could think of to ask. In turn I inquired about how her studies in organic chemistry were going, and how apartment life was treating her. We also talked about where she might find work in June when she graduated. Her career would begin much sooner than my own, and she had already begun to explore job options. Most of the good opportunities in Oregon were in the Portland area. She suspected that the city was where she would end up come summer.

This was also Cindy's first look at my facial makeover, and her eyes squinted appraisingly as she ran her fingers lightly down my cheek. "It's grown in pretty well, baby," she murmured as she smiled at me. "I like the way you look in a neatly trimmed beard; it's scholarly and masculine at the same time. If you want my opinion, I'd say keep it." That response was good enough for me, and I've not been clean-shaven since.

Just being together made the time fly, and for a change the trip to Medford seemed almost too short. The bus pulled into our destination at 7:30 P.M., nearly twelve hours after I had boarded the bus in Tullville. Even then I didn't feel tired, only elated that I was home and Cindy was with me.

My parents and younger brother Ted were awaiting our arrival at the terminal. As I descended the steps off the bus, I could see mom smiling and nearly hopping with excitement. She was eager to meet my girlfriend, I could tell. Oh, and maybe she was just a little bit happy to see her son too.

Cindy followed close beside me as we made our way through the crowd of people to where my family stood. She smiled tentatively at my parents, and after I got a hug and a handshake from my mom and dad respectively, I made formal introductions all around. My mom was her usual bubbly self, and she gave Cindy a hug and told her, "It's so nice to finally meet you, dear, after all the wonderful things Mark has told us about you."

Cindy blushed and murmured a quiet greeting in return, but by the time we had piled into the car she and mom were chatting away like old friends. I had expected that they would get along well, since each had an outgoing disposition that people warmed to quickly.

When we arrived at my parents' home I saw Cindy's eyes darting around curiously, as she saw for the first time the place where I had spent much of my youth. It was not a large or impressive dwelling, but my family maintained the yard fastidiously, and the ranch-style house sported a fresh coat of white paint.

"So this is where you grew up?" Cindy asked.

"From the age of twelve onward, yes," I answered.

She said, "It's a cute place! It reminds me of my home in Bend when I was a kid. I still love seeing that house; it always brings back memories. I'll bet you enjoyed your childhood here." I smiled and told her that I certainly had.

It was evening and dinner was already mostly prepared. As mom went to put the finishing touches on the food, the smells wafting from the kitchen made my mouth water. I paused for a moment when I saw the dining room table set for five. It was hard to believe that my girl would be sitting here having dinner with the family. It made our relationship seem official somehow.

Dad showed Cindy to the guest room, while I put my luggage in the bedroom which I had called mine before moving away to school. Many of my things were still there, and someday soon I would have to come collect my belongings when I had found my own place to live.

Later at the dinner table, my parents asked Cindy about her family and where she had grown up. Mom was also curious about how we had met. I let Cindy tell most of the tale of our first encounter and also our subsequent dinner together in the dining hall. She had a humorous manner of storytelling, so the meal was replete with a fair share of laughter, some of it at my expense. "He was so shy I thought I'd have to spill my drink on him to get him to say something," Cindy giggled.

"Mark always was the consummate lady's man," Ted chortled.

I waved my hand dismissively, saying, "I refuse to comment on the basis that whatever I say may be used to incriminate me." In truth it was a bit embarrassing having my initial tentativeness with Cindy exposed, but I didn't really mind. It sure beat being single, and whenever Cindy poked gentle fun at something I had said or done, she looked at me smiling, and the affection was evident in her eyes.

After dinner I helped clean up the table and then Cindy and mom shooed the men out. "I'd love to have your help, but this tiny kitchen barely fits two people at a time," mom declared. "You guys go watch television and get out of here."

Suitably cowed, we retreated into the family room and dad turned on a football game. As we watched, I could hear the women chatting busily in the kitchen, with occasional laughter punctuating their conversation. I couldn't make out what they were saying, but I would have loved to be a fly on the kitchen wall just then.

For our part, dad and I spent time quietly enjoying each other's company and watching the game. Ted had left to visit some friends in town after dinner, so we had the family room to ourselves. As we each sat in our accustomed easy chairs, it seemed like I had never been away.

During commercial breaks we would chat, and at one point dad spoke approvingly of Cindy. "She's got a good head on her shoulders and a lot of moxie. She also seems very sweet. You made a good choice there, son." Then he winked at me and added, "She's a nice-looking girl, too. She reminds me of your mother when we first met. Makes me wish we were twenty-five again."

We laughed, and I told him that I hoped I could make it last as long with Cindy as he and mom had achieved. He looked thoughtful for a minute, watching the game as it resumed. Then he looked over at me and asked, "Do you two have any timetable for when you plan to get married?"

Cindy and I hadn't officially announced our engagement to either family yet, but dad didn't miss much, and I guess he could tell where things were headed. I shifted uncomfortably in my chair, and said, "Well, we've talked about it, but we're not sure yet. A lot depends on when and where Cindy finds work. We definitely want to wait until one of us has steady employment and can make ends meet. That could be a year or more from now. I just don't know."

Dad nodded and said, "Well, at least you're approaching things sensibly. There's no rush when it comes to these decisions. You've got a lot of time." I agreed with his assessment, relieved that he approved of Cindy and of our plans. Then a big play drew our attention back to the game and the discussion turned to other subjects.

Thanksgiving Day was slow and lazy, with no one getting up early. When I arrived at the table for breakfast, mom and dad were already having coffee. Cindy appeared soon after, smiling demurely as she sat down in the seat next to mine. Ted arose from the dead when we got tired of waiting and dad thumped on his bedroom door. Then we shared a hearty breakfast, with dad making his signature pancakes, one of those few culinary items that mom insisted he did better than her. Afterward we sat and talked awhile, and then I borrowed mom's car and took Cindy out for a drive around the Rogue Valley, showing her the sights. We ended up in Jacksonville, a tiny historic town just southwest of Medford.

During the holiday season the town was decorated charmingly, the main street hung with lights, tinsel, and other touches that made it seem like a page from a nineteenth-century Christmas tale. The old brick and wood buildings that once had housed essential goods and services during the Gold Rush era now featured restaurants, art and curio shops, and upscale clothing outlets.

Cindy and I browsed slowly along the sidewalks, peering into shop windows, sometimes venturing in to check out their wares. We held hands, walked, talked, and made the most of our time alone together. It had been far too long since we had been able to share this simple pleasure. We reveled in the moment, both aware of how painfully brief our time was.

After walking for an hour in the cold November air, we both felt twinges of hunger. It wasn't long before a little corner café beckoned to us. Its antique windows were hung with strands of festive holiday lights, and looking inside, I saw chocolate nut clusters on display in a glass case near the front. A tiny silver bell over the door jingled delicately as we entered to the warm aromas of cinnamon and spices. I soon discovered that the scent originated from hot apple cider that patrons were sipping at a nearby table. Just then the idea sounded marvelous, and we both ordered spiced ciders. Mindful of the Thanksgiving dinner we would be tackling that afternoon, we abstained from lunch, but did sample a couple of cashew clusters smothered in dark chocolate. The warm cider washed those down most delightfully.

We didn't want to leave mom to prepare dinner without help, so with the winter chill successfully driven from our bodies, we headed back to Medford. Once there, we got busy helping out in the kitchen. With two of her sons home and a guest as well, mom was bustling with enthusiasm as she moved from oven to stovetop to refrigerator and back again, preparing various dishes for the afternoon feast. The dining table was set with china dishes and crystal goblets, atop the white lace tablecloth that was only brought out for the holidays.

When the turkey was golden brown on the outside and juicy on the inside, I was once again given the honors of carving the bird. I approached the task with more confidence and aplomb than on the previous Thanksgiving, deftly slicing off thin, even cuts of meat, and separating the wings and legs neatly. Cindy watched with appreciation, saying, "You're handy with that knife. I think you'll make a good surgeon, sweetie."

I chuckled and replied, "Well, I don't have to worry here if I mess up. A live patient will be a different story."

She squeezed my shoulder and said softly, "I know you'll be great." Just then my mom asked Cindy to help her move dishes to the table. I smiled to myself as I returned to my carving. Simply knowing that Cindy had faith in me made it easier to trust in my own abilities. Seeing myself through her eyes, I could believe that one day I might in fact be an accomplished practitioner.

Dinner was impressive, both in quality and quantity. The large turkey was tender and savory; along with it came stuffing, cranberry sauce, mashed potatoes with gravy, soft buttered dinner rolls, a tossed green salad, and fruit salad. The conversation around the table fell mostly silent for awhile as everyone dug in and concentrated on the feast set before them. Gradually as hunger was pushed back a bit, we began talking and jesting. Ted and I sat across from each other, and partway through dinner he looked at me smirking and said, "So, Mark, is that a beard, or did you glue a dead rat on your face?"

I paused, eyebrows raised, then grinned evilly and replied, "At least I've got enough testosterone to generate facial hair."

Ted regarded me thoughtfully over a bite of turkey and came back with, "I doubt it. It looks like you had it transplanted from your back."

That was a good one, I had to admit. I countered, "Well at least I didn't have to comb out my nose hairs to make that stringy mustache." That got a chuckle out of him. And so we continued a long-standing tradition, exchanging good-natured insults and barbs back and forth, each seeing if he could outdo the other in a verbal thrust-and-parry.

Cindy's eyes were wide, her fork frozen halfway to her mouth, looking from Ted to me as the exchange ricocheted between us. My mom laughed at her expression and reassured her, "Oh don't worry dear. The boys are just having fun. They don't mean any of it! You should hear it when all four of them get together, oh my!"

Cindy looked relieved then and laughed, shaking her finger as if to scold me while I grinned back at her. Shortly thereafter she was animatedly talking with mom and dad as if she had sat at this table for years. I felt a sense of relief, since I knew how nervous she'd been about meeting my family.

Between conversations we managed to plow through the mountains of food crowding the table. As if the generous portions were not enough, on the heels of dinner came freshly-baked pumpkin pie and whipped cream. A hefty slice of the warm pie was enough to obliterate any space remaining in my stomach. I practically rolled out of my chair when I got up to leave the table. I waddled into the kitchen to help clean up, feeling as stuffed as the turkey.

Cindy insisted on helping as well, and Ted brought dishware from the table so we could begin washing. I scrubbed and Cindy dried. When you are with someone special, even the most mundane of tasks becomes enjoyable. I was acutely conscious of Cindy's proximity, and of our bodies touching at hip and shoulder as we worked. She was humming happily as the pile of dishes shrank. While working, I occasionally used my pinky finger to flick a little water Cindy's way. It took three or four times before she realized it was deliberate, and then I got smacked with the towel.

Late that evening Cindy and I went out for a walk around the neighborhood. We were dressed in heavy jackets, but we walked close together, hands clasped tight as the white streamers of our breaths trailed behind us in the chill night air. The clear sky overhead had brought a rapid drop in temperature come sundown, but the brilliant stars made up for it in stark beauty as they shone against the velvet backdrop of the heavens.

Strolling the sidewalks along the quiet streets, we talked about my family, and Cindy told me how much she liked my parents. I let her know that they liked her too, at which she smiled gratefully. We paused beneath a street lamp, bathed in the yellow glow where it pushed back the darkness. Nearby the skeletal branches of a leafless tree reared blackly into the sky, the dew-coated surfaces glistening as they caught the light. We stood and talked and watched the stars, pressed close together to combine our warmth, enjoying the silent magic of the night. Cindy's presence made a simple walk a thing to be remembered forever.

The rest of our stay flew by as good times always do, and soon we were at the bus station saying goodbye to my parents and Ted. My younger brother was attending college in nearby Ashland, as I had done, so he lived at home. My mom hugged me and told me to study hard, and she gave Cindy a hug as well, saying how happy she was to have met her at last. Cindy blushed and smiled, replying, "Thank you for your wonderful hospitality, Mrs. Bridges. I really enjoyed getting to meet all of you. Mark always says such nice things about his family life growing up. You raised a good son, I think."

Mom looked me up and down and offered, "Yes, I think he turned out all right, more or less." We laughed and then mom admonished Cindy, "Call me Jane, my dear, not Mrs. Bridges. You'll make me feel old talking like that!" Cindy promised not to forget, and soon after we said goodbye amid wishes for a safe journey.

As Cindy and I approached the open door of the bus I glanced back one last time. Mom looked ready to cry as she watched us go, but dad just stood and smiled broadly. With a final wave we stepped inside the bus. Amidst the line of boarding passengers, we moved slowly down the center aisle until we found two seats open where we could sit together.

We spent most of the trip north talking about everything that came to mind—our families, schedules, school, the next chance to meet during Christmas break—as we tried to cram a month's worth of conversation into those last few hours together. When the bus arrived at the Corvine station several hours later, we hugged and said goodbye, Cindy pulling me to her with a desperate strength. "I'm going to miss you so much," she breathed as she nestled her head on my shoulder. "You be safe, and come to me next month, promise." I told her that I wouldn't miss it for the world, and she laughed a little then kissed me. As she grabbed her purse I saw her eyes glistening with tears and she wiped at them self-consciously. "I told myself I wouldn't do this," she fretted. "It's embarrassing."

"It's very sweet," I told her. "I love knowing how you feel, because I'll miss you just as much."

For some reason that made her cry more. She smiled through the tears and punched me on the arm, and told me to stop saying nice things or her makeup would run down her face. Sometimes a guy just can't win.

She gave me a final hug, and her hand lingered on my arm a moment before she pulled away and walked down the aisle. At the front of the bus she looked back and smiled, then vanished down the steps and out.

With a sigh I settled back in my seat and waited for the remainder of the trip to be over. Now that Cindy had gone, the romance and charm of the journey vanished too, and it was just a long, tiring bus ride to Tullville that awaited me.

CHAPTER THIRTY

After Thanksgiving the weather in Tullville turned downright cantankerous. There were times when I could not get rides from my classmates and had to walk to college in the morning. Always entertaining when half-awake, now the long trek brought the added joys of freezing winds, driving rain, and sleet.

I encountered an interesting phenomenon in the Palouse. Precipitation didn't obey the law of gravity as in the normal universe. Instead it insisted on falling sideways most of the time, whipped by strong gusts into a skin-soaking force that an umbrella was powerless to repel. It also seemed that no matter which direction I was walking, the wind always blew against me, driving the moisture it carried straight into my face. I adopted the ludicrous-looking stance of holding my umbrella out in front of me rather than overhead, peeking around it to see where I was going. I'm sure that onlookers found the amusement factor enhanced by the wind periodically flipping the umbrella inside out, leaving me frantically trying to restore it to working order while being pelted and buffeted by the weather.

Our classes continued to evolve as the semester progressed. Pharmacology now shifted from studying beneficial drugs into toxicology. There were plenty of poisonings to learn about, including overdoses of medications (both animal and human varieties), accidental exposure to pesticides, ingestion of toxic plants, and so forth. Dr. Borland plodded his way relentlessly through each of these, reciting the clinical signs, diagnostic methods for confirming the type of poison, and remedies. His lifeless treatment of the subject elicited about the same level of interest as watching a fungus spread. Occasionally I would experience a flutter of excitement when the professor's face twitched or he raised an eyebrow. Unfortunately those highlights were few and far between.

In microbiology we took a break from studying bacteria and focused for awhile on virology. Viruses were important disease-producing organisms both in animals and humans. The problem was that we had fewer weapons against them than with bacteria. Sadly, with the severe diseases the end recommendation was often isolation and euthanasia. This was especially true with herd management in cattle and sheep. A virulent contagion in a group of animals could spread like wildfire and kill thousands of livestock, wreaking financial ruin on the unfortunate farmers and untold misery on the affected animals.

Back at home, I found that my health and comfort were increasingly tied to the heating blanket on my bed. It was the one source of true warmth in the trailer. I would wrap its thick folds around me as I huddled on the bed pouring over my books, and when it came time to sleep, I buried myself under its protection all the way up to my eyes. Rolling out of that cozy haven each morning was not for the faint of heart. The ancient oil furnace creaked and groaned most of the night, but its efforts were inadequate in the face of the plummeting temperatures outside.

About two weeks after Thanksgiving the first real snowstorm hit Tullville. Overnight it dumped about four inches on the ground, and I awoke to find the hills transformed into a brilliant white fairyland. Visually it was a vast improvement from the bare dirt fields I had been gazing at for months.

While in school that day I periodically glanced outside between classes, and noted that snow was still falling off and on throughout the afternoon. Parasitology lab was my last class of the day. There I spent an hour peering through the microscope at mites, ticks, and lice found on various species of animals. I became intimately familiar with the mouthparts, genitalia, and other structures used to identify each diminutive parasite.

Species identification of ticks often involved close examination of their anal anatomy. Midway through this exercise it occurred to me that I had traveled far and spent considerable money to enjoy this privilege. I pointed this fact out to Stan Hulbert who sat at a nearby microscope, and he grimaced and replied, "Only in vet school could this be considered normal behavior." I raised an eyebrow at this insightful observation, then shrugged and peered back into my scope. The things one will do to earn a degree.

By the time I returned the specimen slides to their boxes and put away the microscope, it was nearly 4:30 P.M. I rubbed my weary eyes and grabbed my coat and backpack, making for the door to head home.

A blast of frigid air hit me as I exited the building. I tucked my collar tight around my neck and hugged my arms close to my sides, hunkering down against the cold. Snow was falling heavily, the large flakes swirling and dancing as they wove their silent paths to the ground. Having grown up in a climate where snowfall came briefly only once or twice a year, I was always struck by the beauty of it.

Once on my way I descended the vet school hill without difficulty. The sidewalks were wet but free of ice thanks to the heated pipes beneath them. Steam billowed out of the grates set into the concrete, white plumes rising eerily to hover ghost-like above the ground. The snow blanketing the roads had reduced traffic to a fraction of normal, so that an uncharacteristic hush lay over the land.

When I reached level ground at the bottom of the hill, I also reached the edge of campus. One moment I was strolling along confidently, and the next step I was pin-wheeling my arms for balance as my feet hit ice and I lost all traction. In a split second my backside was planted in the snow. Of course I did what any mature adult would do in that situation, scrambling to my feet quickly and looking around to see if anyone had noticed. Once I regained my balance and my dignity, I baby-walked gingerly the rest of the way home.

The new ground cover made for interesting drives as well. Todd and Shannon, the two vet students in our trailer park who gave me rides to school, had an old Dodge sedan which demonstrated winter traction characteristics similar to that of a bobsled. It didn't help that Todd showed utter disdain for his car's lower gears. Driving down off the hill in the morning seemed to me more of a controlled slide than a powered descent. The narrow road had no retaining barrier, and the drop-off to our left loomed precariously close as we slewed around the curves. Our return in the afternoon consisted of Todd gunning the engine at the bottom of the slope, trying to gain enough momentum to carry us to the top while the wheels spun and the rear of the car fishtailed back and forth.

It was hard to decide which direction was worse for my blood pressure. On some days I'm certain that my fingers left permanent imprints in the seat upholstery, but beggars couldn't be choosers. When we arrived, I'd thank Todd for his white knuckle taxi service, and totter off shakily to my trailer to find a bottle of Scotch.

Since I'm telling this tale, it stands to reason that I survived all my commutes. The few weeks between Thanksgiving and Christmas passed in a flurry of class work, and suddenly it was time for the winter break. We had ten days off over Christmas and New Year's, but the students' excitement was tempered by one sobering fact: semester final exams were immediately after the holiday. This meant taking home class notes and spending at least part of vacation absorbing the course materials we had accumulated. It was not a great way to enjoy a holiday, but such was life in the veterinary program.

I talked to Cindy on the phone just before the break. We would not be able to see each other for Christmas, since I was heading to Medford and she to Bend, each to spend time with our families. But we decided to meet in Bend after the holiday, so that I could see her and meet her parents before returning to school. Any formal announcement of our engagement would only happen after introductions had been made with both families.

Another winter storm had hit Oregon and Washington, and it showed no sign of letting up. I worried about this impacting my travel plans, but the bus was in the Tullville depot on schedule and I was told the route was open. As I boarded, I saw that the large vehicle was rigged for snow, the double tires at the rear outfitted with heavy chains.

The countryside was adorned in white and snow flurries fell sporadically during the drive to Portland. The black lava of the high desert showed starkly through gaps in the winter cover, like a charcoal sketch of a wilderness scene. Thankfully, the roads were passable. The main effect of the weather was in slowing the always drawn-out bus ride even further.

We hit the Columbia Gorge an hour behind schedule but right then I didn't care. I was too busy staring out the windows of the bus, taking in the stately ranks of tall conifers resplendent in their white gowns, and the towering cliffs with ice and snow clinging to their ramparts high above us. The waterfalls tumbling off those heights were now festooned with long graceful ice formations resembling still-life sculptures. I had my camera with me and I took pictures through the windows as best I could. As breathtaking as the gorge was during the warm season, winter brought a unique beauty to this area that I had never before seen.

After that, however, the weather became simply unpleasant. As luck would have it, this was one of those rare instances where the snow fell nonstop even west of the mountains. As a result, the pace of the ride was agonizingly slow, and we rode all day and into the night. By the time we reached the Rogue Valley my watch read eleven P.M., and over fourteen hours had passed since I had boarded the bus in Tullville. The tiny Medford depot wasn't even open at that hour; the bus simply pulled up to the curb in front of the locked building to unload its passengers. The streets were dark and silent, the only illumination coming from the pale glow of the streetlamps filtered through the falling snow. My energy flagging, I gathered my luggage as it was unloaded from the bin in the side of the bus, thanked the driver, and looked around to find my parents.

In a moment I spotted them walking toward me from their car, which was parked just down the street. Mom looked as grateful to see me as I was to have finally made it to the Rogue Valley. We hugged and made our greetings on the sidewalk, and then I hopped in the car for a warm and relatively brief ride home.

Once there mom made a grilled tuna sandwich and chocolate milkshake for me while I unpacked. It was the best midnight snack I'd had in a long time. We sat at the kitchen table and talked about school and travel and winter weather until my eyelids grew too heavy to hold open. Then I staggered off to the warmth of my old familiar bed and slept like the dead until nearly noon the next day. There's nothing like the beginning of a long vacation.

CHAPTER THIRTY-ONE

Christmas that year was a fun family affair. My older brother Stan, he of bumper sticker fame, visited from California with his wife and kids. With Ted and I also there, mom had three of her four sons home for the holidays, and she was ecstatic.

On Christmas morning we arranged ourselves around the Noble Fir in the family room, sitting either on the floor or in chairs. Dad played Santa and crawled around the tree, handing out the gifts one or two at a time so we could all see what was unwrapped. The room was filled with smiles, laughter and heartfelt thanks.

The other memorable event during that visit was when I bought Cindy's engagement ring. The rest of her gifts, plus a couple of small things for her parents, had been purchased and wrapped weeks before. This last item was all that remained to be found.

The ring I chose was gold sculpted into a delicate swirl with a center diamond and tiny baguette sapphires arranged around it. It was absolutely beautiful, which I thought made it perfect for Cindy. I had the store gift wrap the small box, and after parting with a nice chunk of my savings I made off with my prize. I was so excited I didn't remember the drive home; suddenly I was in my parents' driveway with no real sense of time having elapsed.

My vacation was split between Medford and Bend that year, so after only a few days with my family I was at the bus station saying goodbye to my folks. The trip north thankfully lacked any major drama. Our bus stopped at Salem and then headed east over the Santiam Pass toward Bend. Crossing the snowbound mountains in broad daylight gave us all a glimpse of the raw splendor of winter in the wilderness. As we climbed the winding way up the side of a peak, the land dropped away from us in a stunning vista of sculpted rock, trees and snow that filled our sight in all directions.

It was a harsh environment caught in the grip of midwinter, not a place to be lost without the amenities of heat, food and shelter. For the wildlife here it was a struggle just to survive until springtime. For humans who ventured into this untamed territory to enjoy winter activities such as cross-country skiing or mountain climbing, a careless step or lack of preparation could be disastrous. Every year several people became lost in the Cascades while challenging the wilderness, and sometimes their bodies were not found until the spring thaw when the snow pack receded.

As the bus descended the east slope of the mountains, I felt my anticipation building with each passing mile. It was not far to the city of Bend once we cleared the foothills and hit the high desert plateau. Here the weather was clear and sunny, with wispy clouds streaking an ice blue sky. A light coating of powdery dry snow lay upon the land around us. The passage of our bus kicked up the frozen precipitation on the shoulder into a miniature blizzard of dancing crystals that sparkled in the sun.

The landscape here was appealing and quite different from other areas I had seen east of the Cascades. Instead of endless sage flats, the terrain was broken by low hills and sprinkled with stands of mint green juniper trees. Their gnarled trunks and windswept limbs reminded me of giant bonsai specimens, and the dusting of white on their branches enhanced their rugged beauty.

We reached Bend less than an hour after leaving the mountains. The small bus depot was clean and modern-looking, and I noted that most of the town I had seen en route had that same fresh new feel to it. Bend was booming, fast becoming a popular vacation destination due to the numerous recreational opportunities nearby. Visitors could fish or raft several sizable rivers, hike and horseback ride the numerous wilderness trails, and, of course, head to the mountains for the ski resorts in the winter and campgrounds in the summer.

I waited impatiently for the bus to park and begin unloading, and it seemed that the line of passengers ahead of me took forever to move down the aisle and out the door. Finally I exited and retrieved my bags from the handlers. I followed the stream of travelers across the frozen parking lot toward the grey, single-story terminal. It was late afternoon and the sun had dropped low toward the mountains in the west, its ruddy light staining the packed snow beneath our feet. The chill air burned my throat as I toted my luggage carefully across the slippery surface.

I entered the building and looked around randomly for a moment, unsure of where to go. After a moment I heard my name being called by a voice I knew well and loved. I turned to behold Cindy in jeans, coat, and scarf, her eyes wide and hand waving as she tried to get my attention. She was standing across the room along with two other people who I realized must be her parents. I saw the older woman say something to Cindy and gesture toward me, apparently encouraging her daughter to come ahead and greet me. Cindy eagerly accepted the opportunity and crossed the distance between us in a flash. As we came together I dropped my luggage and gave her a huge hug. Conscious of her parents' scrutiny, we pulled apart after only a moment, and I contented myself with a brief peck on her cheek.

Cindy excitedly led me over to where her parents waited. I was relieved to see that they were smiling broadly as we approached. Her mother was a comely woman in her fifties, slender and fit-looking, and she wore a blue tailored pant suit topped by a stylish wool jacket. Her dark brunette hair, so like Cindy's, was lightly streaked with grey along the temples. Cindy's father was tall and angular, with a thick shock of wavy hair that was also deep brown. His matching beard gave him a scholarly look, and he bore a striking resemblance to our sixteenth president. I half expected his name to be Abe. Cindy looked up at me smiling and said, "Mom, dad, this is Mark."

Cindy's mom gave me her hand and said, "Hi Mark, I'm Nancy. We're so happy to finally meet you! We've heard quite a lot about you, as you can probably imagine." She was grinning as she said it, but I felt my ears burning anyway. I managed to say that I hoped they had heard good things, and then turned my attention to her father.

Her dad stepped up and offered me his strong grip in a handshake, and said, "Great to meet you, Mark. It's nice that you could come visit us here in the middle of winter. I know it's not the most convenient time to cross the mountains. I'm Evan, by the way. Let me help you with your luggage."

So saying, he grabbed one of the two cardboard boxes that I had packed with Christmas presents, and Cindy took the other. I thanked Evan for his help, and clutching my suitcase, I followed the others out to where their car was parked. We piled into a vintage sedan that was large enough to hold about half of the passengers on the bus. Then we drove toward the outskirts of town where Cindy's family home resided.

The appearance of the old car led me to think that her family had to watch their pennies carefully. Thus I was totally unprepared for the imposing, two-story white colonial perched atop its own hill on several acres of juniper-covered property. When Cindy pointed it out from the main road, I just stared, and she giggled, "Oh, it's not as big as it looks from here, being on top of the rise makes it seem grander somehow."

We left the highway and followed a private gravel driveway up the side of the hill. The view across the surrounding countryside as we climbed was spectacular. We reached the hilltop and the land leveled out. Their property was sizable, and the road snaked around through junipers and desert sage for awhile longer before the house loomed ahead.

Cindy was only partially right; the house did seem not quite so massive viewed up close, but compared to my parents' home it was still impressive. We pulled into a circular driveway in front of the main entrance. As we exited the car and grabbed luggage, I took in the stately dwelling with its four white pillars and formal lines. Beyond the driveway and a tidy lawn the terrain resembled a gigantic rock garden, with small boulders and native plants providing low-maintenance landscaping. The overall feel was of living in a natural setting.

We entered the house through large double doors. Cindy's mom led me up a broad curved flight of stairs to the guest bedroom I would be staying in. It was directly across the hall from Cindy's room. We deposited my things on the floor, and I looked around appreciatively at the tasteful décor, the polished hardwood floor covered by an oriental rug, the walnut nightstand and chest of drawers, the queen-sized bed with plush pillows and soft floral comforter, the intriguing art hung on the walls. Their old beater car notwithstanding, it appeared that the family led a quite comfortable lifestyle.

Cindy had one sibling, a younger brother who was away at college in Boston. She had celebrated Christmas with her parents already, but as we toured the spacious home together I noted there were some unopened gifts under the large tree in the living room. Cindy smiled and told me that those were for me. I mentioned the gifts I had brought with me, and her eyes lit up. "Oh, put them under the tree here, that would be great," she bubbled. "That was so thoughtful of you to get something for my parents too. I think they're going to love you. I know I do." And with that, she took advantage of our temporary solitude to wrap her arms around my neck and give me a proper holiday greeting.

Dinner that night was in a spacious dining room at a table that could have seated a score of guests. As we ate, Cindy's parents asked me about my school experiences and complimented me on my choice of profession. They had quite a few pets themselves, with three large dogs in a concrete run out back and about a dozen cats, mostly strays that had wandered onto the property and had benefited from the charity of the family. Cindy's dad had built a multistory outdoor condo for the felines. He grinned conspiratorially at me and said, "We call it the 'cat house'." His wife clucked disapprovingly and shook her head while Cindy and I laughed.

As the evening progressed, it quickly became evident that Cindy's father ("Please, call me Evan") had quite a sense of humor. He delighted in recounting stories of mischief that Cindy had gotten into as a child. "When she was little, she was a feisty thing, and when something didn't go her way, she could pitch an absolute tantrum. It was hilarious! She would throw herself down on the floor and pound the rug with her fists and feet. I would sit in my chair and laugh until my eyes ran, and the more I laughed, the madder she would get. I'll never forget that as long as I live."

Cindy looked at me ruefully and said, "Yes, that's what I'm afraid of."

Her father winked at me and remarked, "Don't worry; she's grown out of that phase. She hasn't pitched a fit like that in, oh, two or three years now."

"Dad!" Cindy growled, brows furrowed and eyes glinting menacingly even as her lips curved in a grin. It was obvious that she shared a close bond with her father, and I smiled to see it.

Later we all gathered in the living room to open the gifts under the tree, and afterward Evan and Nancy bid us good night and retired for the evening. Cindy and I stayed up awhile chatting until we caught ourselves yawning and finally called it a day. Alone in my room, I was preparing to sleep when I remembered the engagement ring. A sense of urgency hit me; I had to find the right moment to give it to Cindy before I returned to school. Soon, very soon. So thinking, I fell into the soft embrace of the plush guest bed and faded quickly into oblivion.

CHAPTER THIRTY-TWO

Late the following morning I was awakened by a tentative knock at my door. I rolled over groggily and looked at my watch. My eyes popped further open when I saw that it was nearly 11 A.M. "Yes," I groaned as another knock came tapping. "I'm awake."

Cindy's voice came through the door. "Are you decent? Can I come in?"

The day was starting off well. I smiled and replied, "Yes! Please do."

The door cracked open and Cindy's face peeked around the edge. Her hair was slightly disheveled and she had no makeup on. She had never looked better. I gestured for her to come in and she grinned and entered the room, closing the door behind her. She was wearing yellow flannel pajamas with hearts scattered over them. I thanked my lucky stars that I had become a part of her life to the extent that I could get to see her so casually garbed.

She came and sat on the edge of the bed, and then leaned over and kissed me good morning, her long hair falling about my face like a shroud. Now fully awake, I sat up and propped a pillow behind my back. Cindy snuggled against me and I held her close as we talked quietly for awhile. She informed me that breakfast was cooked and waiting downstairs. As if on cue I caught a whiff of bacon that made my mouth begin to water.

I ignored the demands of my stomach for the moment as I had something else on my mind. Being here with Cindy in an intimate setting, I felt this was the opportunity I had been waiting for. I reached over the side of the bed and into my open suitcase. After rummaging around for a moment I wrapped my hand around a small square object. When I turned back to Cindy, I held out the handsomely wrapped gift box that held the ring.

Her eyes widened as she said, "Mark, what is this? You already gave me lovely gifts. You shouldn't have…."

"Oh, I think you'll like this one more than the others," I grinned, and said, "Go on, open it already!"

Her expression quizzical but excited, she tore off the ribbon and paper to reveal the small velvet jewelry box. "Oh, my," she whispered. "Is this what I think it is?"

"Well, there's only one way to find out, isn't there?" I answered, gesturing at the box.

She opened the small case slowly, almost fearfully, and gasped as she saw the ring within. "Oh wow," she breathed, her eyes wide. "It's...it's...." She was utterly still for a few moments, just staring into that little box. Then her eyes came back to me, and I was struck by just how much can be communicated in a single look from a woman in love.

Before I knew it she had launched herself at me and I was bowled over onto my back. An instant later I found myself pinned to the bed as Cindy covered my face in about a dozen kisses. It was the most enjoyable "thank you" I could imagine.

The remainder of my stay was a wonderful mix of day trips into Bend to explore the diversions the city had to offer, tasty relaxed dinners with the family in the evenings, and time spent alone with Cindy whenever we could manage it. I found that I liked Cindy's parents a lot. Evan and Nancy were well-educated and well-traveled, having lived in various cities back east before settling down in Bend. Like the house they resided in, they seemed oddly out of place in this placid rural community.

Over dinner one evening, I asked them what had caused them to relocate here, and Nancy spoke up first, "Well, Evan and I had vacationed in Oregon soon after we married, and we loved the look of the area. Evan's a nature lover and a bit of a rock hound, and the geology here is fascinating."

Cindy's father added, "Sometimes Nancy misses the city, because of the museums and shows. We do go back east about once a year or so, to allow her to get her dose of culture."

Nancy smiled and said, "I'm also involved in the local art scene; Bend has a burgeoning artist community, believe it or not. There are no Picassos here, but some of the talent is surprising for such a small area. I have fun helping organize art shows and such." As I listened to Evan and Nancy talk about their hobbies and interests, I began to understand that they weren't entirely misfits in central Oregon after all.

The days slipped by, and the return of school loomed ever closer. With Cindy near I found it hard to study for final exams, but I summoned what discipline I could and spent an hour each evening enjoying quality time with a notebook. The prospect of long and strenuous tests just around the corner was enough to make me act like a student, at least for brief periods.

The day before I returned to school, Cindy and I took a walk on the family property. The day was crisp and clear, with the sun rising bright in the azure dome of the sky. We both wore jeans and heavy winter jackets, and her gloved hand clasped mine tightly as we started our way down the winding dirt road from the house. The chill air briskly caressed our exposed faces and the light layer of powdery snow on the road crunched under our feet. I felt invigorated, every sense acutely alive.

Seen at a walking pace, the details of the landscape could now be fully appreciated. The intricate branches of sage and rabbit brush sported frozen white highlights that traced each small twig. Many bushes were festooned with tiny icicles that dangled like glittering jewels in the sun. The larger twisted shapes of juniper trees dotted the terrain, their evergreen foliage adding the vibrant color of life to the otherwise stark landscape. Even the lava rocks and boulders scattered over the ground had a rugged esthetic that many a gardener has struggled to replicate.

As Cindy and I made our way slowly along the meandering track, we spoke of our families and our love for each other. Sometimes we didn't talk at all, comfortable in each other's presence and content to share the stillness that the countryside offered. Soon we came to the edge of the plateau the house stood upon. From there we followed the road down the side of the hill until it led out onto the flatlands below.

At one point we crossed a little wooden bridge that spanned a small creek. The frigid clear water tumbled and bubbled as it meandered darkly between snow-covered rocks. Where moisture splashed onto stone or stream bank, it had formed sheets of glittering ice. These brilliantly reflected the winter sun and made us squint to look at them. Cindy and I stood close together and watched the contrasts of snow and stream, light and shadow, still sculpture and fluid motion. It was an artistic display wrought without intent by Mother Nature herself.

We hiked awhile longer, eventually retracing our steps and ascending the hillside. Bundled up against the weather, I found myself growing warm on the upward climb. I unzipped my coat, enjoying the cooling touch of the brisk air against my shirt. Cindy saw this and playfully scolded me, saying that I would get sick if I became too chilled. I replied that real men didn't need coats and stuck my tongue out at her. An impromptu chase and snowball fight quickly ensued, with Cindy doing the chasing and most of the snow throwing. I can't imagine what inspired such behavior on her part. Despite her energetic attack, I did manage a few well-placed hits in return, eliciting some offended shrieks when the icy projectiles found their mark. Once when she bent over to pick up ammunition, I planted a hard thrown snowball right on her rump where the jeans fit snugly. She straightened up in a flash and exclaimed, "Ouch! That stung!"

I grinned and said, "Good!" at which she redoubled her attack.

When it all was over we were panting and laughing, our disheveled hair speckled with snow and our breath clouds mingling over our heads. At that moment I felt completely happy and totally in love, without a care in the world. If I had to choose a few precious experiences from my life to live over again, that winter walk would be one of them.

That was my last day with Cindy before leaving for school, and we stayed up well into the evening, neither of us wanting it to end. Finally we headed up to our rooms, since I had a long trip ahead of me and needed a decent night's sleep. We bid each other good night with a kiss, and her hand clasped mine for a moment. Her smile couldn't quite hide the sadness in her eyes as she pulled away. I reluctantly closed my door and went about the business of packing my things.

The following morning Cindy and her parents saw me off at the bus depot in Bend. When my ride arrived, Cindy's mom hugged me and wished me well, and I thanked her for all her hospitality. Her dad grinned and shook my hand firmly, saying "Good luck in school, young man." As I walked to the exit door at Gate Five, Cindy was close beside me, and we stopped just short of the gate. She wrapped her arms around my waist and stepped in close. Her dark eyes were bright and shiny, her voice barely more than a whisper as she said, "I'll miss you more than I can say. Have a safe trip and call me when you get there so I know you are all right!"

Then she looked around at her parents who were standing a short ways off, smiling at us. She turned back to me and shrugged, saying, "What the hell, they can watch if they want!" So saying, she kissed me full on the lips, grabbing the back of my head and holding me in a long, deliberate embrace. I could feel my face flush hot, but I didn't resist. It would be a long while before we would touch again. I glanced over Cindy's shoulder, and noted with relief and amusement that her mom and dad were diligently inspecting a rack of post cards that had suddenly captured their interest.

We held each other for a moment longer, then the moment passed and I was walking away while Cindy waved to me. I exited the building alone into the cold January air. Once outside I crossed the slippery pavement as quickly as I could and boarded the waiting bus which would carry me back to my other life.

CHAPTER THIRTY-THREE

On returning to school I found myself buried under an avalanche of class work and preparing for the fall term final exams. Radiology, parasitology, pharmacology, and microbiology all demanded my attention. It made the previous school year look easy by comparison, and I wouldn't have considered that possible twelve months earlier. At such times one's day-to-day existence can seem to be an endless run of thankless toil. Even then, life has a funny way of spicing things up, whether you wish it or not.

I remember one particularly bizarre day during the exams that semester. On the morning of my parasitology final, I had awakened early, since I wanted to get to the lab and review specimens before the test. As I shut off the alarm clock, I noted the glowing dial face showed the time to be 5:30 A.M. It was mid-January and the trailer was dark and cold, the long winter night still gripping the Palouse in its icy fingers.

My sneakers were not readily at hand by my bed, so I leapt out of the covers and attempted the ridiculously impossible exercise of running to the bathroom without my feet touching the frozen floor. I must have looked like an idiot, high stepping at breakneck pace with my knees nearly hitting my chin.

Once in the bathroom there ensued a super quick shower in the tundra-like environment, followed by a drying-and-dressing routine that would have been the envy of any bona fide hyperactive person. After downing a quick breakfast I grabbed my backpack with all of my class notes in it. Then I headed out the door into the winter darkness for the long walk to school.

Outside the predawn air was at its coldest and almost immediately I could feel my breath freezing on my face. The stars shone brilliant in the cloudless sky overhead as I walked down the hill. Once on the main road into town I was struck by the utter quiet around me. The roads were devoid of traffic, the air deathly still, and it seemed the entire world slept except for me. I trudged numbly along, pushing the pace to try to stay warm and to make my trip as fast as possible.

I had only walked a few blocks when a faint noise reached my ears. It came from behind me and grew steadily into the growl of a lone engine winding up the road. I turned to look and saw a motorcycle coming up the near lane. Due to the slippery conditions the rider was proceeding at a cautious pace, following a strip of clear pavement created by the passage of numerous tires. This was in the era before mandatory helmet laws and the intrepid soul was riding bareheaded. He slowed as he pulled abreast of me, and I saw that his long brown hair and full beard were frosted with snow and ice. He came to a stop and called out, "Hey there, do you need a lift?"

Somewhat taken aback, I took a closer look at this unexpected apparition. The rider was adorned in biker's leathers, including black snug-fitting pants and heavy boots. He wore gloves and his jacket was suitably thick for the frigid weather. His ride was a large, heavy-bodied machine whose engine chugged out a deep-throated growl as it idled. There was no one else on the road so I walked out to talk to the rider. As I approached I said, "I need to go to the college campus. Which way are you headed?"

He grinned and said, "I'm going there myself. I'm majoring in anthropology. How about you?"

I tried not to laugh at the image of this rough-looking gent sitting primly in anthropology class taking notes, and I replied straight faced, "I'm attending veterinary school."

"Oh, that's a cool line of work!" he said with another flash of teeth. "I know where the vet building is. Hop on and I'll drop you off there."

The seat of the big bike was plenty large enough to hold two, but as I moved around behind the vehicle I hesitated a moment. On the back of his leather jacket was a garish emblem featuring a stylized motorcycle with flames erupting from the rear, ridden by a wild eyed demonic creature. Crimson words below the picture proclaimed, *"Death on Two Wheels."* The perfect sentiment when riding on an icy road without a helmet. But there was the allure of a quick and effortless trip to school, with the bonus of thirty extra minutes to study before the test. Convenience won out over caution, and I "hopped on" as he suggested.

Straddling the large seat with my backpack slung over my shoulders, I grabbed the rider around the waist and he revved the engine. The bike lurched forward beneath me and I held on tighter. We headed down the road at a moderate pace, but it felt like traveling at light speed compared to walking. Our velocity turned the still air into a freezing gale that whipped my face, and I tucked my head in behind the driver to shield it as best I could.

The powerful engine vibrated and rumbled steadily between my legs as the motorcycle rapidly ate up the distance to the school. Landmarks that I laboriously trudged by every day went flying past in a heartbeat, and in only a few minutes we pulled up in front of the veterinary buildings. Just from that brief ride my face felt like it was frozen solid. Hoping that no part of my visage would crack and fall off, I grinned broadly as I dismounted and thanked the rider. He simply waved and rode off down the street.

I shook my head chuckling as I headed into the vet building. People are amazing, and they can surprise you when you least anticipate it. I never knew the biker's name, but I appreciated his unexpected charity on that cold midwinter's morning in the Palouse.

The day had yet more strangeness in store. A short while later I sat in the laboratory on the second floor of Goltz Hall, peering at slides of parasites through a microscope. No one else was in the building, and I was concentrating hard on an image in the scope when something intruded.

At first I was only peripherally aware of it, a sort of rumbling vibration of the building around me. The vet school had forced air heating that rattled the walls as it ran, and I remember thinking distractedly that they must have had the blower turned up high that day. That thought vanished a moment later when the entire room lurched sideways under me, shoving me to my left and nearly throwing me off my chair. I looked up startled from my microscope thinking, "What on Earth was that?!"

There were television monitors mounted high on the walls, and as I looked around I saw that these were swaying wildly back and forth in their mountings. The shaking continued strongly for another five or ten seconds, then faded away. I sat there bemused for a few moments, thinking to myself, "That felt like an earthquake!" I had never been in one before, but it was just as I would have imagined it. Then I thought, "No, silly, this isn't California."

So I shrugged and resumed my test preparations. I might not have given it another thought except that students began filing in an hour later, and the first thing out of each person's mouth was, "Did you feel that quake?" It turned out that in fact it had been a real earthquake, and it had originated in Idaho. The temblor was a powerful one, registering 6.8 on the Richter scale, and my being on the second story of the vet school had helped magnify the effects. The net result was that I got quite a ride from the disturbance, though no damage was done to the building. I can't remember a thing about the test I took that day, but I'll never forget feeling the earth move for the first time.

When it was all over, I did manage to get good marks on my examinations. As I mentioned before, being isolated in the Palouse with no family, no car, and no Cindy left me with few distractions. Studying was easy because, frankly, there was little else to do.

The fall semester ended on a blustery Friday afternoon in mid-January. Spring term began promptly on the following Monday; there was no time off in between because the holidays had just passed. That weekend was a brief blessed interval wherein I had absolutely nothing to study. The other students were similarly free, and of course that meant it was party time.

Both the Oregon and Washington contingents in our class had events planned, and I went to a party Saturday night that included students from both schools. Beer and wine flowed, snack foods abounded, and as is typical of the medical professions at social gatherings, the unhealthiness of the cuisine mattered not one iota. Here, for once, no one worried about the following day or how late we stayed up. It was quite liberating to be truly free for an evening.

Despite our efforts to avoid school topics, once or twice the talk did turn to the upcoming curriculum. The new courses generated a buzz of excitement among the students. Pharmacology class would now focus on anesthesiology in preparation for our forays into the operatory next year. In addition we would be taking a new course, "Intro to Surgery." We could hardly wait to see what it had to offer.

After staying out late, I slept in on Sunday. Around midday I took a stroll over to the cemetery across the highway. The sun was out and the hills were still covered in a white mantle. Snow blanketed most of the cemetery grounds as well, though dark bare patches of moist grass were visible under the dense foliage of the evergreen trees. The ground squirrels I had seen in September had long since hidden away to sleep for the winter.

As I walked the gravel road the crisp green smell of the pines brought to mind the time spent at Cindy's home near Bend. But here there was no laughter, no playful companion, just the pervasive silence all around. A pang of loneliness hit me and I fervently wished she were here at my side. Acutely aware of how far I was from those closest to me, I turned back toward the trailer park and made my way down the cold empty road to home.

CHAPTER THIRTY-FOUR

As we had hoped, spring term brought significant changes. Pharmacology class finally began to unveil the mysteries of anesthesia, from the old-time methods to the most modern. We learned of the oral, injectable, and inhaled substances that could induce sedation, muscle relaxation, unconsciousness, or block perception of pain. For most of these lectures we had Dr. Cavanaugh. He was a bald, wizened little man who was near retirement but still lectured on a limited basis; his main area of interest was anesthesiology, or as he put it, "gas-passing."

Despite his advanced years he was a lively soul who never tired of telling stories from his long decades in veterinary medicine. Many of Dr. Cavanaugh's recollections were of drugs that had long since fallen out of favor. It was evident that he had an incredible first-hand knowledge of the subject of pharmacology. Listening to him, I knew that I never would learn everything he had stored in his head, no matter how long I practiced.

The old doctor also cautioned us against falling victim to our own medications. He recalled colleagues who had been injured in the line of work and had later become dependent on pain killers or other substances. In some cases their careers and personal lives had been ruined by their addictions. The doctor sternly cautioned us to take care of ourselves physically and emotionally, and to be aware of the risks of any medication we might use.

His strong words made me wonder if some of his conviction came from personal experience. The way he described the effects of certain drugs, how they made one feel, sounded…firsthand. I never asked of course, but I always wondered if he had been one of those unfortunates who had, at least briefly, carried the proverbial monkey on his back.

Other students voiced the same thoughts when the subject of Dr. Cavanaugh was discussed. None of us knew if it was true, but if the old doctor really had battled addiction in the past, I was very thankful that he had managed to recover and continue teaching. His sharp mind held a vast treasure of knowledge and wisdom that needed to be shared.

I recall one episode in Dr. Cavanaugh's class with particular amusement. As part of our introductory lectures we were learning the different phases of anesthesia a patient goes through. This especially applied to gas anesthetics where the effect was more gradual than with an injection. To further our understanding of this subject, we were treated one day to an old anesthesiology film. The movie was in black and white, and looked like it was made when Dr. Cavanaugh was in diapers. It was purported to be a classic treatise on "stages of anesthesia." Perhaps it was, but the film was memorable for entirely different reasons.

For one thing, the archaic medications and equipment seemed outlandish compared to what we were currently experiencing. Holy cow, they were using *ether* to anesthetize patients! That substance had been abandoned long ago due to its low safety margin: a small dose could prevent the patient from moving, but a little too much would stop the patient's movement permanently. Ether also had the aggravating tendency to cause explosions if it leaked into the room air. This could be slightly inconvenient.

Besides the primitive methodology in the film, the subjects used were also quite riveting to second year veterinary students. You see, the movie came from the human medicine field. This meant that the patients illustrated were good old-fashioned *Homo sapiens*. It's widely understood that medical students become inured to the sights of blood, feces, organs, and other aspects of bodily functions and anatomy. What's not as well known is that the immunity we build to such things does not translate to all species.

The movie began, and at first our class had a good time laughing at the ancient equipment and old-style doctor smocks. The formal dry speech mannerisms of the lecturer, straight from the 1940s, lent to the perceived silliness of the film. When the patient was anesthetized with a cumbersome-looking mask over his face, more hoots and giggles ensued. At one point the movie commentator remarked, "During the early phases of anesthesia, nausea may occur with ether." Right on cue, the anesthetist pulled the mask off the patient, who immediately vomited over the side of the bed onto the floor. This elicited a mixture of laughs and groans from our class.

The mood abruptly changed a few moments later. When the patient in the film was deemed to have reached surgical anesthetic depth, the view changed to that of a bare torso scrubbed with iodine, and a scalpel incision was made down the man's midline from chest to navel. As blood welled up from the cut, the entire class suddenly went quiet, and I glanced around to see my classmates wide-eyed as they stared silently at the screen. You could almost hear the collective gulp.

I too was taken aback. I had become accustomed to seeing the insides of our animal patients, but I discovered that my veterinary experience hadn't prepared me for watching another human being opened up. It was fundamentally different somehow.

I still look back on that day and laugh, since it's the only time I can recall my entire class of boisterous individuals being silenced. I've had physicians tell me the same thing in reverse; they have no problem seeing a human surgery, but are squeamish when it comes to animals being operated upon. It's funny how the mind works. People are quite adaptable, and we learn to take for granted whatever we are familiar with.

Of course, other classes also occupied my attention during spring term. Radiology continued to be a mind-bending experience, with students squinting to see what could not be seen and filling in the gaps with creative speculation. There was cause for hope, however. Our X-ray filming techniques slowly improved, so fewer pictures came out jet black or pure white, and clear images of animals actually showed up when the films were developed. Darkroom forays no longer required a tent and provisions for an overnight stay. We could now stare at an X-ray for less than a week before offering up a tentative diagnosis, and even more astounding was the discovery that sometimes we were correct! Somewhere along the way, somehow, we began to transform into reasonably competent radiologists.

That spring also brought us two entirely new courses: "Small Animal Medicine" and "Introduction to Surgery." Just the mention of the words medicine and surgery was enough to quicken our pulses. At last we would be initiated into the essential art and science of veterinary practice, the knowledge we had been primed for in all the courses leading up to this moment.

Imagine, then, our disappointment when we discovered that "Intro to Surgery" was mostly a dry recital of general principles. The class completely lacked any practical descriptions of surgeries. Instead, we were treated to vague catch phrases such as "avoid aimless puttering" and "economy of hand movements." Most of the theory taught here was common sense, and probably could have been covered in ten minutes of lecture time.

The class also required us to learn a myriad of different surgical instruments. There were tissue forceps, hemostats, clamps, retractors, scalpels, and all sorts of fun toys for surgical girls and boys. Here the students paid attention. Even though it amounted to rote memorization, there was no denying the importance of this information. We absolutely had to know the names and uses of the instruments we would soon be called upon to wield.

We discovered that the suture materials utilized could literally make or break a surgery. As we reviewed the various types of surgical sutures, it amazed me that there could be such a large volume of information to learn about silly little threads. There were monofilament varieties, basically single smooth strands like fishing line. Other types were braided from multiple smaller strands, more like a string or rope is formed. Braiding made suture softer, more flexible and easier to tie, but also could cause the material to behave like a wick, drawing fluid and bacteria into the flesh. The latter trait made braided sutures undesirable for use in non-sterile areas such as on skin or in a bowel incision.

Some sutures were nylon, some polyester, and yet others were synthetics I had never heard of. There was even one called "cat gut," made of sheep intestinal lining, if you can believe that. Many sutures self-dissolved after awhile, whereas other types had to be removed when the wound was healed.

Sutures also came in different sizes, based on the thickness of the strand. Some were so fine as to resemble a wisp of hair, whereas the heaviest gauges began to resemble twine rather than something one would use in a live patient. The needles attached to the finest sutures were themselves feats of engineering, miniature curved blades that had been hand-honed to be razor sharp.

Hand-honed? That was cause to stop and think. I couldn't conceive what type of person it would take to sit all day sharpening needles a few millimeters in length, but such an individual would likely have a disturbed personality. If not when hired, then certainly by the time he or she had been on the job for a few months. My career choice was looking much better by comparison.

The activity we enjoyed most during "Intro to Surgery" was buying our very own surgical instruments to use in the coming year. Holding the shiny polished implements in our hands for the first time was exhilarating, even if their price tags took some of the wind out of our sails. By the time our surgical packs were completely outfitted we had spent well over $200, and this was in 1984. Still, a strong feeling of satisfaction and anticipation welled up as I gazed at my collection of new playthings. My hands itched to hold these finely crafted pieces of steel and use them to conquer disease in my patients. Nor was I alone. I saw some of my classmates stroking their instruments like long-lost lovers. It sounds weird (and probably was), but don't be too quick to judge. When you are overworked, you obtain gratification where you can—and it was healthier than alcohol.

CHAPTER THIRTY-FIVE

In the evenings I continued to huddle under my heated blanket as I studied my class notes. Sometimes I would take a break and share the couch with Jake as we watched the small battered television in the living room. It perched in one corner on a rickety stand that also had seen better days. Our reception was poor and only three stations were available in Tullville.

Changing channels meant having to walk over and manually move the rabbit ear antenna on the top of the set, to try to pick up each new station we were viewing. Our efforts met with variable success. Most of the time the picture remained grainy or had lines running through it. On school nights that didn't bother me, since there was little to watch other than sitcoms.

The weekends were another story. Jake and I both loved college football, and Saturday morning was our time to indulge. We were intent on having a quality viewing experience despite the primitive audiovisual equipment. Meticulous preparations would be made before the game began, including a trip to the supermarket to stock up on edibles. On the little coffee table we spread out our selected snacks which varied week to week. The only constants were beer and potato chips, two of the essential food groups for football viewing.

We'd kick back on the couch in worn jeans and T-shirts plus a sweater or two (after all, this was Jake's trailer, and it was still winter). Jake would set a six-pack of beer just outside the front door, and the brews would be icy cold when we grabbed one to drink. The funny thing was they didn't seem to warm up much even after sitting in the living room awhile.

After all the amenities were in place, we'd settle in for a nice long game, relaxed and smiling. Jake would grab the remote control and switch on the television. That's generally when the cursing would begin.

As chance would have it, the football games were carried on the channel with the worst reception. The color was so bad that the uniforms of the opposing teams were often hard to distinguish, and the players' faces looked decidedly jaundiced. Sometimes the picture was skewed diagonally so everyone appeared to be running up a steep hill while stretched impossibly tall. We'd watch the game this way for a while until our necks began to kink from holding our heads sideways. Eventually Jake would slam down his beer and exclaim, "Enough of this crap! Watch the picture while I adjust the antenna."

Then would begin the game within the game, as he attempted to move the two antenna arms into that magical alignment that would yield a viewable picture. I would drink my beer and offer a running commentary, something like, "Yeah that's got it—oh wait, go back to where you were! No, the other way, oops too much, oh right there! No the *other* right there! That's better, now step back...

hmmm, it gets worse when you let go of the antenna, it was okay while you were holding it!"

Jake would fume as he would nudge the antennae in tiny increments back and forth, occasionally losing his self-control and wrenching the two thin rods into extreme positions in the hope that something good would result. One day this process went on for a good fifteen minutes, and several times he had achieved a good picture, only to have it fade to an indistinguishable blur as he let go and stepped back to view the screen. In the end he threw up his hands in exasperation and said, "I give up. There is no way this will work. I could pass a bladder stone easier than I can get a picture on this piece of junk." He looked at me, utterly defeated, and said, "Have you got any ideas?"

I pondered the problem as I took another pull on my beer, and offered some simple alcohol-inspired wisdom. "Well, it works better when you hold onto the antenna...."

Jake snorted. "I can't see the screen when I hold the flippin' antenna! What good will that do me?"

"Well, you could stretch a bit and maybe see the picture."

"I'm not built like a gorilla! My arms aren't that long!" Jake retorted. "You need to slow down on your beer intake and come up with something better than that!"

"I wasn't thinking of your arms," I calmly replied as I reached for a handful of popcorn.

Jake stood frozen for a minute, pondering, and then said, "Oh, no, there's no way I'm going to do that! That's ridiculous! I'd rather go without seeing the game!"

I grinned slyly. "Are you sure about that, Jake? It's a really big match-up, remember. You've been talking about it all week."

He stood like a statue for a minute longer, a sour look on his face, then slowly sat on the floor and peeled off his shoes and socks. And for the remainder of the game we enjoyed a reasonably good picture on the TV screen. I sat on the couch sipping beer and munching snacks, and Jake lay on the floor near the television, his leg propped over the top of the TV stand as he gripped the antenna between his toes. I wish I'd had a camera with me, though I might have been found stuffed into a curbside garbage can if Jake had caught me snapping a photo.

At school my good humor, and that of my classmates, was tempered by work and more work. The most challenging class that semester was small animal medicine. This was a meaty subject which covered essentials we would need as practitioners of the healing arts. It began spring term of our sophomore year, and would continue well into our junior curriculum. "Medicine" was a word that encompassed many diverse areas of knowledge.

We began with an overview of infectious diseases, some of which was a rehash of freshman microbiology. In addition, we spent much time on clinical pathology, the science of evaluating specimens of blood, urine, pus, and any other appetizing bodily fluids that might be obtained. Blood and urine samples told us much about what was happening internally in a patient. There were chemistry tests to determine if organs were functioning normally or were being damaged. A complete blood count (CBC) looked at red blood cells, white blood cells, and the like. This could tell us, for instance, if a patient had leukemia (cancer of the white blood cells), anemia (too few red cells), or was battling an infection.

Other exudates were also of interest. If a dog was breathing poorly because of excessive fluid in the chest, we could obtain a sample with a needle and see what sort of material it was. Pus would suggest an infection, clear watery fluid might indicate heart failure, and fluid with bizarre abnormal cells floating in it could indicate cancer.

Making a diagnosis was like putting together pieces of a puzzle. The age and type of animal was the first piece of the puzzle. A fourteen-year-old female poodle named Fifi would have different disease risks compared to a six-month-old male cat. Added to that information we would get a history as observed by the pet's family—how long had Fifi been acting ill, what the signs they had observed, the other animals that Fifi regularly contacted, was their dog properly vaccinated, and so forth.

When the history and a thorough physical exam were not enough to answer the riddle of the illness, then we would perform a CBC and blood chemistries, urinalysis, or any other tests that seemed reasonable. Of course the radiologists would be screaming, "X-ray! X-ray!" and sometimes that made sense as well.

I found clinical pathology fascinating. These tests represented an elegant and noninvasive way of assessing what was happening inside our patients. The investigational aspect also challenged our minds: could we figure out what was wrong? It was a thought-provoking and important subject, and the more I studied, the more I liked it.

Immersed in the intense curriculum far from home, it was easy to lose myself in work. I would awaken early, attend classes all day, come home in time for dinner, and then squeeze in a little studying before crawling thankfully into bed. The next day the cycle would be repeated. Every minute of each day seemed used up, and I had to make a conscious effort not to neglect my personal life.

As the weeks passed I stayed in touch with my parents and with Cindy as best I could. Letters were slow and cumbersome, but I wrote down my thoughts and sent them to Cindy regularly. Mom and dad were likewise treated to a note every so often, mostly updates on how my classes were going with a couple of funny stories thrown in. I would always get a letter back from mom thanking me for writing, and encouraging me to keep applying myself in school. Sometimes the letter came with a box of home-baked cookies which I made short work of.

But the times I looked forward to most eagerly were those precious moments I was able to spend on the phone with Cindy each week. I loved listening to the music of her voice as she told me of her studies, her feelings toward me, her hopes for the future we would share once we both finished our education. She took me far away from my cramped cold trailer, and made me feel that everything was right with my world.

I like to think that I did the same for her. When she first answered the phone, I could hear the excitement in her voice. As we talked, her mood would change from animated to softer, more affectionate, more intimate. Then when the time grew near to end the call, I would catch a hint of sadness in her words, though she tried to hide it. Another person might have missed it altogether, but I knew her well enough to catch every nuance.

Those brief interludes were a tonic that helped me persevere through the long dark months in Tullville. Though I was often lonely, I was never really alone. I clung tightly to that knowledge as the work and the isolation bore down on me.

CHAPTER THIRTY-SIX

It was March and midterm exams had arrived. Once again I found that I struggled with radiology more than any other course. It was the one subject where no amount of memorization or note-reviewing could guarantee a good grade. You had to be able to interpret X-ray images, and no matter how many films you looked at, it seemed there were always more things you hadn't yet seen. I came out of the radiology exam with my head swimming and eyes crossed, black and white images still dancing on my retinas. Blinking, I saw a few of my classmates standing together nearby and walked over to join them.

Stan Hulbert was in the group and he grinned forlornly as he saw me. He didn't look very confident about his test results. Kristina Albright, another of our Oregon class, was talking to him as I came within earshot. She had long wavy brown hair that swirled about her shoulders as she shook her head. Her usually cheery features were downcast, and she glanced at me as she continued, "I just know I blew it on this exam. I was sitting in front of one of the X-ray stations, looking at the film with no idea of what I was seeing, and I thought to myself, 'I'm going to fail for sure.' Then Dr. Parry came up behind me and glanced at my exam sheet to see what answers I had written for the previous stations. Do you know what he said?" She looked around at us and we all stared back blankly.

"The pompous little so-and-so just shook his head and said, 'Good God, girl, don't guess!' Then he walked off!" She threw up her hands and looked around at us. "What if I don't pass this course?" she asked plaintively. "What will I do then?"

"You could find work cleaning horse stalls," Ed Martinelli offered. His advice was followed with an emphatic *"Ow!"* as Amy Baker punched him.

Kristina's eyes narrowed and she growled, "Be thankful we haven't learned how to perform castrations yet, Ed." This was met with chuckles from the other students, but the fire in her eyes was short-lived and soon she slumped back dejectedly in her seat.

The rest of us stepped in to offer our moral support. Looking contrite, Ed said, "Aw, Kristi, don't worry; you know you'll pass. You always do."

Amy added, "We're all in the same boat. I doubt that any of us feel good about this test, except maybe Mike." A murmur of amused agreement swept through the group; no one had yet seen Mike Callahan break a sweat in any exam.

Stan piped up, "The test is graded on a curve, and you can be certain that no one aced it. Your grade will be better than you think. Heck, if the rest of the class performs like I did, you might get an 'A'!"

Kristina giggled at that and thanked us for trying to make her feel better. I smiled at her and said, "It's a struggle for everyone, you know."

At that she snorted and replied, "Oh, that's easy for you to say. You always do well without even studying much. That's simply abnormal."

I grinned, for she was beginning to recover some of the spunky good humor that we expected from her. I retorted, "Well, if you think intelligence is abnormal, it says something about the people you hang out with, doesn't it? Does the term 'inbred and brain dead' possibly apply?"

"Oh! You…!" she sputtered. The others were laughing, and she could only maintain her stern look for a few moments. A grin finally broke through and she said, "Well, at least your humor's slightly more enjoyable than the radiology exam."

"Oh, now *that's* a glowing endorsement," I answered, rolling my eyes.

Gazing around at my classmates, I noted that they all looked as weary as I felt. Stan apparently had made the same observation and he spoke up, "Say, we're all a bit strung out. How about we go get a beer? It's Friday, so we have the weekend to study before the medicine exam."

His idea was endorsed enthusiastically by most of those present, now seven or eight in all. We discussed where to go and eventually ended up at the Den, which despite its name was not a study hall or library, but a pub that catered to the college student population. As I heard tell, the place had a long history and was a local fixture in Tullville. We found it easily enough, a small, weathered brick building facing the main street. Its front reminded me of a quaint nineteenth-century shop. The large rectangular window was a checkerboard lattice of smaller panes. A dark green awning arched out over the glass, providing some protection from the weather. Lacy curtains veiled our view of the interior, but warm yellow light leaked beckoningly onto the darkening street outside. We approached the front door, which sported a black wrought iron handle jutting from its worn wood surface.

Inside the décor was rather unique for an alcohol-serving establishment, since there were, in fact, rows of shelves lined with old books on every wall that I could see. Booths and small tables were scattered randomly around the room. A server wearing a neat brown vest and faded blue jeans walked by balancing several beers on a tray. Seeing us, he nodded and said, "Welcome, folks! Please, go ahead and find a table. I'll be with you shortly."

We found a booth against the back wall, grabbed menus, and ordered nachos and drinks. Once the pony-tailed waiter had taken the orders, I looked around the pub's interior. The place had a nice feel, and I thought that this was the way I'd want my bar to look if I were to own such a business. I had expected a rowdier atmosphere, knowing that the college crowd comprised much of the clientele.

But the people who frequented this pub seemed a quieter lot, perhaps graduate students and other mature-minded types. I saw chess boards on a couple of the polished wood tables along one wall, and patrons nursing drinks while they enjoyed a leisurely battle of wits. This pub had a distinctive flavor, and I was glad I had finally made it down here.

Settling into the cozy mood of the establishment, I took a sip of my beer and turned back to my friends, all too happy to join in a conversation which for once included absolutely no medical terminology. It was shaping up to be a good night.

Rest was a fleeting thing for the sophomore students, and after that much-needed break I spent the weekend studying for the small animal medicine test. On Monday morning I walked into class confident that I knew the material well. The professor handed out the tests and I grabbed mine, noting that there were enough pages to make the exam feel substantially heavy. I sighed and went to work.

Most of the questions were multiple choice. I read the first one which said, "A five-month-old unvaccinated dog is presented with high fever, crusty nasal and ocular discharge, hardened foot pads, and tremors. Which of these infections would be likely?" There were four possible answers: A) Canine parvovirus, B) Leptospirosis, C) Canine distemper, or D) Rabies. I marked "C" and proceeded to the next question.

It asked, "A microcytic hypochromic anemia would most likely be caused by which of the following?" The choices were: A) Acute blood loss due to trauma, B) Bone marrow damage with loss of erythrocyte production, C) Intravascular hemolysis, or D) Chronic blood loss with resulting iron deficiency. I nodded to myself. I knew the answer was "D".

Then it was on to the next question, and the next, circling the appropriate responses, occasionally filling in a written answer, page after page. My universe shrank and I lost track of time as I poured out all of my knowledge onto the papers in front of me. So focused was my concentration on the task at hand that I was only dimly aware of the world around me. Each new question rose up in challenge and was vanquished, only to be replaced by another, and another. Time passed, but I took no heed of the clock. Finally I completed a particularly difficult question and realized that there were no more to follow. I had finished the exam.

I closed the final page and took a long slow breath. Like a diver surfacing from the deep, the sights and sounds of the classroom burst into my awareness. I heard papers rustling, the scratching of pencils, someone coughing behind me. Looking about the room, I saw that a few of my classmates had finished their exams and gone, but most were still hard at work, heads bent over their desks with brows furrowed in concentration.

I grabbed my coat and book bag, dropping the test on the professor's desk on my way to the door. On this particular day I walked out knowing I had not missed more than a handful of questions. It was a great feeling, one that I wished I could replicate on my radiology exams. But no matter: small animal medicine was one of the most important courses I would study in vet school, one that would provide a core of skills I would use every day in private practice. And I had nearly aced the test. I felt like I was walking on air as I left the building to head home. On days like this, exams were almost fun.

Not long after midterm examinations were completed, my parents decided to pay me a visit in Tullville. I was excited to see them, as it had been months since I'd been home. They were arriving on Friday afternoon and had made reservations at the Star Light Motel, just a half mile from my trailer park. I walked right by it on my way home from school.

I had told them to call me at the trailer when they were settled in and we'd get together for dinner. At 7:30 P.M. that evening the phone rang and I ran to pick it up. I was relieved to hear my dad's voice in the earpiece; they had made the trip without any delays and he wanted directions to my trailer. He said that mom was curious to see where I lived, and then they would take me to dinner at a restaurant. I described my location and went outside to watch for my parents' car.

The trailers on my lane mostly looked alike and after dark it was difficult to discern the address numbers. In about ten minutes I spied my family's car creeping slowly up the drive. I went to the roadside and waved until my parents saw me in their headlights. Their car sped up and came abreast of me, and when dad rolled down his window, I showed him where to park.

When they got out of the car, we exchanged quick greetings in the chill night air, and then I led them up the narrow steps. "Watch the footing, mom, it's slippery," I said, taking them through the front door and into the relative warmth inside.

Then I gave them a brief tour. Given the diminutive size of the living space, I suppose even a wheelchair tour would have been quick. My mom laughed at the jail cell-like confines of my tiny bedroom, saying, "I don't suppose you'll be complaining much about the size of your room at home after this."

We returned to the living room and discussed where to eat. I told them I knew of a nice restaurant close to their motel. It was an elegant-looking building with stained glass windows all around its walls; I cut across its parking lot when walking to or from school. The graceful calligraphy on the midnight blue sign spelled out the name "Scallion."

Passing by the place so many times had made me eager to see inside. This was an opportunity to satisfy my curiosity, and frankly I knew of no other restaurant in Tullville that didn't fit the "Fast 'n' Fatty" or "Joe's Greasy Spoon" genres. I kid you not, this town actually offered an eating establishment named the Char & Chew Diner. Mike Callahan and I planned to outdo them by opening an eatery directly across the street called Hal's Slurp & Burp. It probably would have been an overnight success.

Weighing the alternatives, the Scallion sounded like a good bet. We arrived at the restaurant after a brief drive, and it turned out to be everything I could have wished for. The interior was elegant in a rough-hewn rural style and the food was well above average. The waiter brought freshly baked wheat bread with honey butter, and salads with a variety of crisp vegetables, bacon bits, and crumbled cheese sprinkled over the top. Dad and I both had filet mignon which was beautifully done.

Over dinner we conversed about vet school and life in the Palouse region. My parents in turn caught me up-to-date on current events back in Medford. My youngest brother Ted was doing well in college in nearby Ashland. Dad was thinking of retiring this year, and the Oregon Grape in the back yard was growing like, well, a weed. Mom told me she would rely on my grooming skills to tame it once again when I visited. I promised I would break out my axe and chainsaw at the first opportunity.

Most of my cherished childhood memories include my parents and fun things we did together, whether it was enjoying holidays, camping in the summer, or just sharing life at home. But the times I spent with mom and dad as an adult are perhaps the most meaningful. With maturity I could finally appreciate all that they had done for me, what they had sacrificed, and how their daily lives had taught by example. That night in the restaurant, when they had traveled far to be with their son, was one of those times I remember fondly when I think of them now.

CHAPTER THIRTY-SEVEN

The weather finally offered up some milder days in April, and I felt a touch of spring fever. I missed the outdoors and longed to hike and explore the countryside. Classmates who had cars sometimes drove into Idaho for day trips, as Tullville sat within a few miles of the state border. I had heard that as you headed east, the terrain became more hilly and forested, producing some very picturesque landscapes.

One Friday I overheard Arnold Harriman saying he was planning such an outing that weekend. Arnold was one of the elder students in our Oregon class, his "old man" status reinforced by his receding hairline and black-rimmed spectacles. Realistically, he was probably all of twenty-eight or -nine.

Hearing his getaway plans made me hungry to get out of town, and I approached him and asked if he wanted some company on his adventure. He grinned and invited me along, and Amy Baker managed to get herself included as well.

The three of us met at the vet school Saturday morning and piled into Arnold's car with excited anticipation. We drove out of Tullville, and in less than fifteen minutes we had reached the Idaho border. At first the landscape looked much the same as around the college, but as the miles passed, the hills grew higher and cultivated fields became interspersed with stands of pine trees and brush. The trees grew more robustly as the elevation increased, and the sporadic clumps of vegetation gradually merged into one continuous forest.

Arnold finally parked the car where the highway cut through a small hilly meadow. Here the shoulder widened into an area where we could pull off the main road and easily turn around. The sky was clear but for a few wispy clouds, and the day was bright and delightful to behold.

The car had barely stopped rolling before we grabbed our cameras and shot out of the doors. Once outside, I quickly discovered the pale sunlight carried almost no heat. Shivering, I pulled my coat close around me. At this elevation and early in the year, the breath of winter still lay on the land.

Scanning the hills around me I took in the crisp green of the pines, and the small patches of snow still persisting in the deeper shade beneath the trees. True spring was still many weeks away in this place. Beneath our feet the wet grass was mostly brown and crushed flat where the weight of snow had recently lain atop it. The wan rays of the sun struck steam off the cold dew on the meadow, creating a pale mist that hung over the scene with an ethereal beauty.

We walked here and there, breathing the virgin air, taking photos of the hills, the trees, and each other. Amy had brought a few granola bars and fruit drinks to snack on, and we gobbled them up quickly as the exercise and the cold whetted our appetites. While we munched quietly gazing at the scenery, Amy put her hands over her head and shouted, "Woooo-hooooo!" Her high pitched cry echoed off the surrounding slopes and she laughed, her face flushed and eyes dancing. "Isn't this great, guys?" she breathed. "What a wonderful day to be out!" Arnold and I enthusiastically agreed, grinning at each other. I was happy that Amy had come along; her unabashed love of life always made her fun to be around.

We hiked and explored for an hour or so until the chill began to penetrate our bones in earnest. Finally we returned to the car and headed back toward Tullville. On the way we stopped at a tiny tin-roofed café just inside the Idaho border to grab some hot cuisine. Afterward we rode back into town with the car's heater turned up high, each of us lost in quiet thought as the scenery rolled by. Basking in the drowsy warmth with a stomach full of a toasted ham-and-cheese sandwich, I mused that life at school didn't get much better than this.

A few weeks later I was sitting in class reflecting on the truth of that statement, and thinking that life could, on the other hand, easily get worse. The coursework had been piling on at an amazing rate as the spring term lengthened, and the professors had verified that yes, final exams would cover the entire year's worth of material. My small animal medicine notes alone had accumulated enough bulk to resemble a phonebook from a decent-sized city.

The weather had soured as well, returning to cold dreary days with few sun breaks. The entire month of May was pretty much this way, which effectively cured my case of spring fever.

On days when classes finished early and I was bored, I would head to the small animal hospital in Aimsley Hall to see cases. For a teaching hospital the caseload was surprisingly small. Surprising until one remembered that this was Dullville, I mean Tullville, and for all intents and purposes it was still winter in the middle of nowhere. This time of year few people wanted to make the trek unless their pet urgently needed help that no one else could provide. So I saw what patients I could, looking at the dogs and cats in their kennels and reading the chart notes on each animal.

As the year had progressed, I'd begun to make sense of the lab tests and much of the medical terminology written on the charts. What had previously been incomprehensible gibberish now became clear, like learning a second language. Henceforth I could nod knowingly as I reviewed a case, stroking my beard and frowning in concentration just like a veteran practitioner. Of course, I was simply reading someone else's chart comments and interpretations. I had yet to diagnose my own patient, which was an entirely different proposition. But that didn't deter me; right then I was full of my own accomplishments and I felt very knowledgeable and doctoral. All I really needed now was to develop the indecipherable handwriting of a true medical practitioner, perfect for filling out prescriptions.

Unfortunately, veterinary school was taking care of that issue as well. It seemed that as my education progressed, each new class brought with it larger amounts of information to learn. Correspondingly, the lecturers rattled off the material ever faster in order to cover the subjects. As I struggled to jot down notes more and more quickly, my handwriting deteriorated in direct proportion to the increased speed of my scrawl. By the time four years had passed and I graduated, I would indeed have a doctor's handwriting. And all without ever having to take "Bad Penmanship 101" as a required course.

As the semester moved toward its conclusion, I discovered that Mother Nature had a twisted sense of humor. She heaped blustery cold weather upon us from late April onward, locking us in a never-ending winter when the calendar said it should be well into spring. It was so bad that on the first day of June I awoke to find snow falling! Even the locals were shaking their heads, saying things like, "It's usually a bit nicer outside by now." On the positive side, poor weather meant fewer distractions when studying for final exams, right?

Actually, no—and that's when I decided that we were cursed. Finals were held the second week of June, and as I buckled down for the last days of serious note-cramming, the sun suddenly emerged in all its glory. Temperatures shot upward and we skipped over spring, jumping headlong into summer. Birds chirped ecstatically from budding trees; insects buzzed around newly opened flowers. Outside my window balmy breezes teased me as I sat in my tiny room trying desperately to focus on my notebooks.

The sudden heat also turned the tin can which Jake and I called home into a massive sauna. The lack of insulation had made life unpleasant enough in the winter, with an underpowered furnace as our only source of warmth. But now I realized that summers in this trailer must be nearly unbearable. Even this early in the year the heat beat down from the ceiling in stifling waves, and there was no cooling unit at all.

I studied for much of that week stripped down to a pair of old gym shorts, trying not to drip perspiration onto my notes as I squinted down at the pages. Every so often I shook an impotent fist at the trailer and cursed the fates for having the indecency to visit this upon me.

Nonetheless, I managed to put the distractions aside well enough to commit my notes to memory. I survived finals week, doing pretty well in the process, and I walked out of the last exam a free man until the coming fall.

Outside the exam auditorium many of the Oregon and Washington students were mingling one last time before they left the campus for the summer. Looking around, I saw a familiar trio standing not far from me: Amy Baker, Molly Boyer, and Mike Callahan, the classmates I had been grouped with freshman year. Those first days in vet school seemed far behind us now. We had learned so much since then, and still we had a lot of school ahead of us.

I smiled as I approached the others, and they greeted me heartily when they saw me. Amy shouted, "Do you realize that we're halfway done?!" I had to smile at that, as Amy had a talent for putting things into great perspective. I joined my old companions and we laughed and talked, sharing our individual horror stories about the examinations. Mike was energized as usual, confident that he had done well on all his tests. Molly wasn't so sure, but she felt that she had passed. She was mostly thinking about seeing her family again; her husband was due in town that afternoon to help her move back home. Amy was just thrilled to be done with school and her broad smile was contagious.

When the time came to say goodbye we all wished each other a great summer. "Until next year, my friends," Mike said, and he waved over his shoulder as he turned to head down the hall. The group split up then, each of us eager to start our summer break. I looked back as I slowly walked away. Seeing the happy faces of the students milling about in the corridor, I smiled to myself. There was much to feel good about. We had faced another challenging year of the curriculum and had survived. We were in fact halfway to being veterinarians. As I turned and headed for the door I had a strong feeling that the next two years would be even more interesting.

CHAPTER THIRTY-EIGHT

Getting home after finishing school was a problem I had mulled over for weeks. I could take a bus, but it would be a long slow trip. It would be faster and cheaper to hitch a ride with a classmate as we headed back to Oregon. After asking a handful of students, I finally found a ride with Kristina Albright, the classmate who had agonized over her radiology exam. I would return the favor by splitting the fuel bill with her.

Our last exam had been on Friday, and Kristina was leaving town that Saturday. I made certain that all my meager possessions were packed, my trunk and suitcase filled until they bulged at the seams. A couple of cardboard boxes held an overflow of items I had accumulated during the school year. I was worried about fitting everything into the car. I breathed a sigh of relief when Kristina pulled up in a sedan with a huge luggage rack on top. Much of her baggage was roped there, leaving plenty of room for my belongings in the rear seat and trunk of the vehicle. I returned to the trailer for a last look around. Delores was curled up on the couch and I gave her a fond stroke on the head. She stretched and began purring as she looked up at me.

Just then Jake came out of his room and saw me. "You heading out, Mark?" he asked.

"Yes, I'm all set to go," I replied. "Have a great summer, and thank you for putting up with me these past months. This place was a life saver compared to that freshman dorm!"

He laughed and said, "No problem at all! Your rent came in handy this year." He paused, looking wistful. "I do wish I was going with you, though."

"Are you staying here all summer then?" I asked.

Jake shook his head. "No, I plan on visiting Seattle in July to see my parents, so I'll be gone for nearly a month this summer. I'll keep the trailer as I'll need it for school the next two years. I have friends in town who can look after my animals while I'm away. I really need to get out of Tullville for a while."

"I can appreciate that," I laughed. We shook hands and bid each other farewell, and I descended the front steps of the trailer. Kristina was waiting in the car, the engine idling. I got in the passenger seat and we chugged down the driveway between the rows of trailer homes. I glanced in the rearview mirror and saw Jake standing in his doorway waving goodbye. I stuck my hand out the window and waved back.

We cruised out of Tullville and into the open countryside. Before long we rolled the car windows down, and the fresh spring air blew through our hair. Kristina proved to be a good conversationalist and she helped the hours fly by. We stopped twice for food and gas at towns along the way. Despite the length of the trip, she refused to let me spell her at the wheel, so I relaxed and even dozed a couple of times while she drove. Before I knew it we had arrived in Corvine, a meager eight hours after leaving Tullville. I was ecstatic, and thanked Kristina so many times that she finally told me she would slap me if I did it again.

Once we were in town, Kristina followed my directions to Cindy's apartment. We pulled up to the building and I practically flew up the long flight of steps to her door. After I rang the bell, I looked down at my classmate who was waiting at her car. Leaning over the railing I called to her, "I'll help unload my stuff in a moment; I just want to be sure someone is home before lugging the heavy pieces up these stairs."

As I turned around to face the door again I was hit by a warm avalanche crowned with flowing brown hair. Cindy's arms wrapped around my waist before I could even react and I was pinned against the railing at my back. Her lips found mine and I concluded that surrender was sometimes the wiser choice when confronting an overwhelming force. That decided, I gave in with enthusiasm.

After an undetermined length of time, Cindy happened to glance over my shoulder and abruptly she straightened, looking embarrassed. Straightening her clothes, she giggled and said, "Oh, who's your friend by the car?"

That reminded me that Kristina was still waiting for me, and I said, "Oops, I've got to unload my luggage so she can go. That's Kristi, one of my classmates. Come on down and meet her while I get my things."

Cindy followed me down and I introduced them while I was grabbing my trunk and suitcase. Kristina's eyes twinkled with mischief as she said, "It's really nice to meet you Cindy. I've heard so very much about you on the trip down!"

Cindy looked at me curiously and then said to Kristi, "Please, do tell!"

I had unloaded my things from the car and decided it was a good time to intervene. I quickly said, "Another time, ladies! Another time! Kristina has to be getting along now, don't you Kristi?"

Reluctantly she agreed, but she mimed holding a telephone, and mouthed the words "Call me!" to Cindy. I shook my head in resignation and they both giggled.

Cindy said, "It was nice meeting you, Kristina. Thank you for giving Mark a ride!" I thanked her as well and we wished each other a great summer. She drove off and Cindy helped me get my luggage up the stairs and into her apartment.

It was early evening by the time I unpacked. Cindy's roommate Stacy was out of town for the weekend. Whether that was good fortune or an arrangement of Cindy's design she wouldn't say. But we made use of the solitude, staying in for dinner and spending most of the evening getting reacquainted after our long time apart. I planned on taking the bus to Medford on Monday morning, so we had a day and a half to spend together.

We managed to pack a lot of fun into those thirty-six hours, including a hike in McLain Forest and a dinner on the town. In between all the activity we found time to talk about the future. Cindy excitedly told me of the job offer she had received. It was from a small pharmaceutical firm not far from Portland, and it offered good starting pay and benefits. She wanted to know what I thought and I told her that it sounded like a great opportunity. She agreed and said she would contact the company on Monday to accept the offer. We were both excited at her first step into the world beyond school, the beginning of her career.

With employment on the horizon we could discuss other plans. Cindy's graduation ceremony had already been held, though sadly I had been in Tullville and unable to attend. Soon she would look for an apartment in Beaverton where her job was located.

Everything seemed to be falling into place, and the time had arrived for the big question to be answered. When, where, and how would we be married? Both of us had thought about it at length, but living apart had made it hard to discuss our future in detail. I would not be out of school for another two years and we agreed that we didn't want to wait until then. So when?

We were lying on the sofa together on Sunday evening, Cindy's head on my chest as I stroked her hair. I said, "What do you want to do, hon? I can't see getting married during the school year while I'm in classes. We also need decent weather, if you want to have an outdoor wedding like we talked about. So that means we set a date for this summer or next summer, right?"

I felt Cindy nod. There was a long silence and then she said, "I don't want to wait for next summer. That doesn't leave us much time to plan if we want to do it this year."

A thrill coursed through me at the thought. Getting married this year…why, that would be within the next two months! Summer break was short between my sophomore and junior years, and I would be back in class by late August. As I mused I could feel Cindy shift positions and she turned to look up at me. Her eyes searched mine as she asked, "What do you think? Do you want to marry me this summer? Say, mid-July?"

"Do you have to ask?" I answered with a broad smile. "As far as I'm concerned, the sooner the better!"

She giggled with glee, and just like that it was set. After all the months of wondering and waiting, the occasion was upon us in a rush. Cindy ran off to call her mom with my lips still tingling from her touch. She talked rapidly and excitedly and her voice carried from the kitchen. I heard snippets of the conversation, "Less than five weeks away…not much time…invitations printed…guest list… outdoors…house in Bend…." I waited until she hung up the phone an hour later, then got the short version.

"Mom says it's a go, she'll take care of the arrangements," Cindy announced breathlessly. "We'll have an outdoor ceremony in Bend at the house if that's okay with you. We can do it on the front lawn; it'll be beautiful with the rock garden all around and a view of the Cascades behind us."

"I love it," I replied. "It seems like the perfect setting for a summer wedding."

She smiled and continued, "We'll get invitations done and mailed within the next week or so. Mom's working on a guest list; she'll invite our side of the family, the ones who live close enough to come. You'll need to give me a guest list from your family, plus any friends you want to be there. Oh, and decide who you want as a best man."

I nodded numbly, as it sank in that this was really going to happen in just a few short weeks! That thought led to another, and I said, "We need to decide on a date right away."

Cindy was ready for that one, too. "Mom and I talked about it, and I wanted to be sure we had time for a little honeymoon after the ceremony. How does the Fifteenth of July sound to you?"

It sounded great. She hugged me, and I could feel her body trembling with excitement. I smiled as I looked deep into her eyes and saw my hopes and dreams contained therein. Our time was upon us.

CHAPTER THIRTY-NINE

The wedding was a storybook affair, something I could not have envisioned until it happened. Much of the credit went to Cindy's mom and dad, who created a wonderful occasion with very short notice. We held the ceremony on the lush green lawn in front of Cindy's house just as planned. The day was sunny and bright, the air clear and full of the warm scents of the high desert. Cindy's mom had planted flowers throughout the natural rock garden beyond the grass. Their bright red, yellow, and purple blooms provided a colorful backdrop for our vows.

Snippets of that day stand out clearly to me even now. I can recall looking out from our hilltop vantage and seeing the vista below, with the Cascade Mountains rearing in their jagged grandeur in the hazy distance. My best man was my childhood friend, Daniel Weidler. He stood at my side and we chatted quietly while we waited for Cindy to walk up the path between the assembled guests. When she did appear, she was absolutely the most beautiful thing I had ever seen, stepping gracefully in a flowing white wedding gown. I can still see my mom sitting in the front row of little white chairs that had been set up on the lawn. My dad was there too, of course, but I recall mom so clearly because she was crying as she watched.

I also distinctly remember the little white-haired reverend who performed our ceremony. Cindy's mom had found him, and he had been performing local marriages for nearly fifty years. He was a dear old man and very kind, but he was near retirement and becoming a bit forgetful. Ironically, it was that particular trait that made him memorable.

When the moment of truth came, Cindy and I stood beneath a decorated arbor before our families and friends. The reverend smiled sweetly and proceeded to perform the ceremony as he had a thousand times before. In the process he neglected to read a large portion of the personalized passages we had written for the occasion. Hence we were through with the preamble in a jiffy. Before I knew it, I was slipping the ring onto her finger and saying "I do." But those two words were the most meaningful and most heartfelt of my life, and the look on her face when she saw the ring sent a thrill clear though me. By the time I pulled up the lacy veil and kissed my bride, the rest of the world didn't matter at all.

Such was my bliss that I didn't even notice the gap in the proceedings until we were walking hand-in-hand down the aisle. Just then I overheard one of the guests saying, "Wow, that was fast!" My new wife and I looked at each other in dawning realization and then we both started to giggle. What else could we do?

From there it was on to the reception, or as anyone who has attended a wedding would say, "Time for the fun part!" Tables and chairs had been set up in the back yard and everyone headed that direction. Celebration and merriment abounded, fueled by the occasion and by abundant food and drink. A wedding brings together friends and relatives who may not have seen each other for years, so the day was full of reminiscing and the renewing of old ties. Although Cindy and I were the center of attention, the reception had the feel of a big family reunion. Cameras flashed incessantly, as everyone seemed to be taking pictures of everyone else. After the first half hour my retinas had permanent spots burned into them.

I had the chance to meet many of Cindy's relatives that day, since her family was well represented at the wedding. Her uncle Gene stood out from the crowd, mainly because he was a real-life backwoodsman and looked the part. Attending a formal event like the wedding, he appeared completely out of his element. Whereas most of the male guests wore suits, he attended the wedding dressed in a casual sport coat and blue jeans. To his credit the jeans were clean and his leather boots sported a fresh coat of polish. His rather shaggy brown hair was neatly combed and his weathered face clean-shaven, but he seemed a bit uncomfortable even in the sports jacket.

I struck up a conversation with Gene about an hour into the reception. He had an endless supply of intriguing stories about living in the wilderness. Of course his day-to-day existence was not the struggle to survive that had confronted early settlers. Even remote properties usually had modern amenities such as electricity and running water. But outdoor life could still have its occasional drama.

Gene's cabin stood at the end of a lonely gravel road outside of the small town of Tumalo. The previous summer he had gone berry-picking one August day in the Cascades, and that evening his wife Abigail had baked a huckleberry pie. For those of you unfamiliar with huckleberries, they are round purple fruits resembling small blueberries, but more tart and flavorful, making them ideal for pies and cobblers. They grow wild throughout the Pacific Northwest, mostly in mountainous terrain. Wild animals relish them as well, which brings me to the story at hand.

After Abigail had baked her pie, she left it sitting on the kitchen counter near the sink. Just over the sink was a small window which provided a scenic view of the woods outside. On that warm summer evening the window was open. As a result the smell of the pie wafted tantalizingly out into the night air. Gene and his wife were morning people and retired to bed early in the evening as was their habit. On this particular night they didn't stay asleep long.

Around 10 P.M. they were abruptly awoken by a loud rending sound. Gene bolted from his bed and rushed to the darkened kitchen from whence the noise was originating. When he turned on the light switch he found himself face to face with a large black bear tearing furiously at the window in an attempt to enter. Its powerful thick claws had shredded the window screen and were tearing out large chunks of wood from the frame. Gene approached yelling loudly and waving his arms to intimidate the animal, but the bear was having none of it. It opened its mouth wide in a fearsome snarl, and Gene could see its long white teeth dripping saliva as the bear smelled the fruit pie.

I was mesmerized while he told me this story, and when he paused I prompted, "Well, what did you do then? Did you have a gun?"

Gene flashed a lopsided grin. "I have a rifle but it was in the gun rack in my truck, not much use to me right then. I grabbed a broom from the utility closet and jabbed the handle at the bear's head, but it bit the end clean off and wouldn't back down. I think I just made it angry."

I shook my head, admiring his spunkiness. "So then what?" I asked.

"Well, the bear's claws were dismantling the wall of my house. I had to do something before the animal caused even more damage, and before it got inside. So I did some quick thinking. You'll never guess what finally made it leave."

I was clueless, so I shrugged and shook my head.

"Pepper! I grabbed a jar of ground pepper from the wife's spice rack and dashed the entire contents in the bear's face. It opened its mouth to snap at me and the pepper went right in. I think some of it got in the beast's eyes too." He laughed then, saying, "You'd think it had gotten sprayed by a skunk. It just shook its head and yelped, and it disappeared from the window just like that!" He snapped his fingers for emphasis and then chuckled again. "I could hear it crashing through the brush at breakneck speed as it ran off."

"Wow! Was that the most dangerous wildlife encounter you've faced?" I asked him.

"Oh, no." He shook his head. "I was never really in serious danger unless the bear had managed to get all the way into my house. And I wasn't going to let that happen. You know, black bears are usually shy and avoid people. I was surprised this one was so bold. It may have been a camp tramp, a bear that was used to begging from humans. When people feed those animals at campgrounds, they lose their natural fear of us, and they get more assertive, even dangerous." I nodded in agreement.

"Of course the berry pie was an awfully big enticement too," Gene said, rocking back on his heels. "In hindsight it was foolish of us to leave it near an open window like that." He pursed his lips in thought, adding, "You should have seen the side of the house. My outside walls are finished with heavy cedar planks, and the boards were torn clear off in some spots. The wood had deep gouges nearly an inch wide carved in it. My window frame was mostly ripped apart; I had to completely rebuild it. All in all it needed nearly $1,000 worth of repairs."

It sounded like an incredibly intense experience to have lived through. All of which piqued my curiosity and I had to ask, "So what *was* the most dangerous encounter you've had, if it wasn't the bear?"

"Ah." Gene nodded. "That's an interesting story. It wasn't like the episode with the bear at all. There was no face-to-face showdown, no growling beast coming at me with claws bared. But it's probably the closest I've come to meeting the grim reaper nonetheless."

He paused for effect, taking a swallow from the beer in his hand. When he saw that he had my undivided attention, he smiled and continued, "I was fishing in the mountains a few years back, catching trout in a small stream my buddies and I frequented. You could only reach it via a winding little gravel road, not much more than a cow trail. There were two other guys with me that day. It was June, so the days were long, and fishing was especially good as the afternoon lengthened. We were pulling some nice fat trout out of there. None of us wanted to quit, but as dusk approached my buddies decided to go into the nearest town to grab some chow before the diner closed. They were going to order take-out and hustle back so we could eat while we fished.

"I stayed behind, working the stream where it bent close to the road so I could hear their truck when they returned. But as it turned out the drive was longer than we remembered and the diner took forever to prepare the orders. The end result was that my companions didn't return until well after dark.

"As the light faded and I could no longer see to fish, I climbed back up to the roadside and stood under a gnarled old pine to wait for them. The night was clear, but there was no moon, so it was soon pitch black; I could barely see my hand in front of my face. I lit a cig and waited, bouncing in place and rubbing my arms to stay warm as the temperature dropped.

"The air was dead still, and other than a couple of crickets chirping there was not a sound to be heard. It was so quiet that when a pine cone came rattling out of the tree above me it made me jump. Just about then I heard the faint whine of the truck's engine coming up the road, and I could see a glow from around the bend where the headlights were approaching. The glow got stronger and in a minute the truck came round the corner. When it did the headlight beams suddenly lit up the entire road to the spot where I was standing. It was blinding after being in near total darkness for so long.

"With the illumination came a sudden thrashing in the tree above me. I quickly looked up but could see nothing. My friends pulled alongside me a few moments later, and both of them were excitedly pointing and saying, 'Did you see the mountain lions? They were right there above you in that tree! Two of them! Did you see them?'"

Gene gazed at me soberly and said, "The truth was, I never heard or saw anything before the truck came around the bend. Aside from that pine cone falling there was not a hint of anything amiss. I don't know why there were two of them together; cougars are solitary beasts. It could have been a mother with one of her older offspring. But I know why they were there. If they were that close and moving with that much stealth, then they were hungry. They were hunting."

He shook his head, and studied his boot tops as he said quietly, "I have no idea how long I was being stalked. But if the guys had arrived a minute or two later, I might not have been around to tell this story. It still gives me the shivers whenever I think about it."

The tale sent a chill up my spine as well, even on that brightly-lit afternoon. I couldn't imagine what it would have been like to have stood in his shoes. Gene moved on to other stories then, and even his more mundane experiences were fascinating to an average suburbanite like me. Eventually Cindy joined us, smiling as she snuggled against me and listened to her uncle's tales.

Awhile later when he took his leave, Gene turned to her and said, "Thank you for inviting me today; it's been really nice to see you again, Cindy." With that he gave her a fatherly hug, then turned to me and shook my hand. As he did so he looked me straight in the eye, saying, "It's a pleasure to finally meet you as well. I've heard nothing but positive things. Take good care of my niece, young man," he added sternly. "If I hear otherwise, well, Cindy can tell you how good I am with an axe."

I must have looked a bit wide-eyed, because after a moment he winked and chuckled. Cindy scolded him for his lack of manners, and Gene tried unsuccessfully to appear contrite. Then he bid us farewell and headed for the driveway where his truck was parked. We looked at each other grinning, and I told Cindy that I thought her uncle was quite a character. She laughingly agreed, and we turned back to mingle with the crowd.

When the evening had grown late and all the guests had departed save immediate family, Cindy and I finally found some time to be alone. We slumped back on the couch in the living room, she in her dress and I in my tuxedo, and smiled wearily at each other. The gifts we had opened earlier lay strewn about the floor of the room. Cindy wriggled up next to me on the couch and I slid my arm around her to pull her close. She laid her head on my shoulder and said, "It's been quite a day."

I sighed and nodded. "You can say that again! I'm glad we're not celebrities; it's tiring being the center of attention." I kissed her forehead and said, "The night's not over yet. Are you coming to bed, Mrs. Bridges?"

She sat up then, smiling at me, and replied, "Mister, I thought you'd never ask!" Our parents had retired earlier, so we turned off the lights on the ground floor and fumbled our way to the stairs. My mom and dad were in the guest room that I had stayed in previously. That left one room available, and I followed Cindy upstairs quietly to avoid waking anyone. She walked through her doorway and turned, beckoning me with one finger. Grinning, I followed her lead and stepped into her bedroom. She closed the door firmly behind me and wrapped her arms around my neck. As I kissed my lovely wife, I had time to briefly hope that I wouldn't appear too tired come morning. Then I stopped worrying about the future and started enjoying the present.

CHAPTER FORTY

Two days later we left on our honeymoon. My mom and dad had stayed the weekend at Cindy's house to visit with us, so we said goodbyes and thank you's to both sets of parents. Then my wife and I drove off together on our first trip as a married couple. We spent a week touring the Oregon coast, enjoying the postcard beauty of un-blemished sandy beaches, barnacle-encrusted cliffs, old lighthouses, quaint coastal towns. When the mood struck us, we would pitch a tent and stay overnight in one of the small campgrounds that dotted the coastline. Other evenings we found lodging in nice hotels, enjoy-ing a hot bath after a day spent hiking the beaches, followed by a fresh seafood dinner at a local restaurant. The days were nonstop fun, and the nights—oh, the nights!

One especially warm evening we built a small driftwood camp-fire on the beach, watching the orange and red sunset slowly sink and fade down into the ocean. The sound of the surf was hypnotic, and as night fell we soon nodded off to a peaceful sleep. It was so comfortable there that we ended up staying until morning, wrapped in a warm blanket and each other's arms.

The following day as we traveled the central Oregon coast south of Florence we encountered the extensive sand dunes that border the ocean there. Several local charter services offered dune buggy rides, and on a whim Cindy and I decided to try it out. Our driver was a cheery blond man in his twenties decked out in blue sunglasses, a yellow T-shirt, and patched jeans.

The cherry red buggy had an open chassis with heavy roll bars overhead. It was fitted with oversized tires that allowed it to grip the sand and not sink. As we climbed in the back, I took note of the ve-hicle's light build, basically just a framework of metal tubing with no doors or other unnecessary mass. Despite the big tires it sat low to the ground, making it very stable and difficult to flip over. It didn't take long to find out why those attributes were so important.

We headed out from the parking lot onto a dirt road that led to the beach. At first we bounced along at a sedate pace through a dwarf pine forest, the trees barely reaching fifteen feet high. As we approached our destination, the hard-packed soil turned to soft sand. The wind-sculpted trees faded away to reveal a pale tan landscape of undulating dune hills as far as we could see.

When the buggy hit the first dune, the driver gunned the engine and we were pushed back in our seats, the rush of air making our eyes water. We grabbed the roll bars and hung on for dear life. Over the next half hour our chauffeur put our vehicle through maneuvers I hadn't thought were physically possible. In any normal terrain we would have crashed or rolled on multiple occasions.

In one instance we approached a dune that had been sculpted by wind and erosion into the shape of a massive breaking wave. The buggy shot toward this intimidating formation at breakneck speed. The leading edge of the dune was so steep it was nearly vertical, and it looked like the driver was heading straight for it. I could not believe he would drive up and across that impossibly sheer face. We would roll over and down the hill if he tried. I knew that he had to turn away at the last second. Then I saw that we were following previous tire tracks in the sand and realized that they did not veer off.

I gripped the roll bars tightly and heard Cindy shrieking as the right side of the vehicle lifted up, up, the sand beneath us tilting crazily until we were shooting sideways across the face of the immense dune like a spider scuttling across a wall. I glanced to my left over Cindy's shoulder, and I was looking nearly straight down at the ground far below. It seemed impossible that the buggy could grip the sand that well.

In a few moments we were off the cliff-like face of the dune and roaring across more level ground in search of another thrill. I worked to dislodge my heart from my throat and hung on, grinning at Cindy. She was a bit pale, but she gulped and returned a pretty good facsimile of a smile. It almost looked like she was having fun. I imagine that I appeared in similar condition to her eyes.

We streaked along at high speed, the wind rushing through our hair and blasting our faces, until the driver abruptly slammed on the brakes. In another moment we were perched on the edge of a sandy cliff even larger than the dune we had just sideswiped. I don't know how high we were, but it looked like a long way down. The sand face below us was nearly a straight vertical drop; I was amazed that such loose material could hold a steep slope so well. We sat there at the top a moment, admiring the vista of the surrounding dunes and the ocean in the distance. I assumed that this was why our driver had brought us here, for the view that our high position afforded.

Then he looked back at us with a huge grin and said, "Are you ready?"

Cindy barely had time to squeak, "Ready for what?" and then the buggy shot forward and right over the cliff face. In a split second we were facing straight down, rocketing toward the ground below at a breathtaking speed. It almost seemed like a free fall, but when Cindy screamed, the driver laughed and abruptly we stopped. Dead still, right there in the middle of the cliff, hanging seemingly in mid-air. I looked over the side of the buggy, and sure enough, there was sand beneath our wheels; the tires were buried in it up to the hubs. The slope was extreme, but apparently there was a big difference between "almost vertical" and "truly vertical."

"See how the tires grip?" the driver grinned at us. "I can stop anytime I want, even on a really heavy slope. I have to give it the gas to even make it move downhill." Cindy and I both nodded, bemused and more than a little relieved. No sooner had we done so, than we were once again propelled downward, the rear tires kicking up fountains of sand. It looked as if we would crash directly into the flat ground at the bottom, but at the last minute he turned the wheel and the buggy skewed sideways. We leveled out running parallel to the hill. Cindy threw her arms up, yelling, *"Yaaaaa!"* Her energy was contagious and I broke out laughing. From then on we relaxed, both of us whooping as we continued our thrill ride through the dunes.

We returned to our motel room later that afternoon. Then we discovered the other side to the day's entertainment as we began the lengthy process of trying to divest ourselves of sand. I hadn't known that so much loose material could stick to a person. Our arms and necks were coated where perspiration had glued the tiny bits to us. My pockets were full, my shoes were full, even my socks were full. We had sand in places where sand was never ever intended to be.

When we showered the water ran brown and the bottom of the bathtub was covered with dirty sludge. I shampooed my hair three times and still had dark "dandruff" falling in the sink when I ran a comb over my head. Our clothes we shook out as well as we could, and put into a plastic bag pending a chance to launder them. When we ate dinner it tasted gritty; when I blinked I could feel a few grains fall into my eyes; when I lay down to sleep I had sand pour out of my ear onto the pillow. I sometimes wonder if I still carry remnants of that day's activities even now. The buggy driver's job had seemed like a fun summer gig during the ride. Afterward I wasn't so sure; it would take someone with true "grit" to stay with it.

Those were just a few highlights of our trip, but suffice it to say, the entire week was magical. Our honeymoon wasn't anything fancy; we had neither the time nor the money for an extravagant trip to faraway places. But it was spontaneous and carefree, full of love and discovery and hope for the future. It was a special time above and beyond our normal lives, a brief enchanted escape together.

Such moments are precious in part because they burn bright and then are quickly gone. It seemed like only a few heartbeats' time before our honeymoon was over and the responsibilities of living on our own loomed close at hand. We traveled to Cindy's apartment in Beaverton for a few days to regroup before school and work hit us. She would start her job at the beginning of August and had found a place to live near her work. I lamented the fact that I hadn't been there to help her move. She reminded me that she was a new graduate who owned little more than the shirt on her back. Moving was absurdly easy when there was nothing to carry. This was one time when it paid to be poor.

Regarding possessions, we had one other item to address before I left. Now that one of us was employed it was about time I had a car. Cindy and I searched the newspaper ads and located a sedan with low miles at a decent price. It was a light blue station wagon, definitely not sexy, but it was clean and it checked out fine when we took it to an automotive shop for a pre-purchase inspection. Everything went smoothly, and in two days we had secured a reliable vehicle that I could use when I headed back to school.

My time to leave came too quickly. Summer had rushed past with so many things happening to us, and this year my classes resumed at the inhumanely early date of August 20th. Cindy and I shared every possible moment together, but time rolled inexorably onward, and before we knew it the day had arrived when we had to say goodbye.

This time there was no waiting at the bus station. I packed my things into our new used car, and my wife bid me farewell in the comfort of our apartment. For awhile we stood toe to toe, arms around each other's waists, and she made me promise to call her when I got to Tullville. I said I would and she asked for one more kiss. An hour or so later I actually made it out the door.

As I slowly descended the steps down to street level, I reflected on how much harder it was to leave now that we had gotten a taste of life together. To know such joy briefly and have it ripped away was worse than not having been together at all. I had been single my entire life until now, but after being with Cindy, the bachelor existence seemed a miserable path.

I got in my car and I drove, somberly pondering what awaited me in Tullville. This year's curriculum would be new and exciting. On the other hand I knew these upcoming months were going to be long and difficult ones. Part of me feared that my prolonged separation from Cindy could somehow damage our still-growing relationship. I didn't look forward to living in isolation again, and that's where my car was carrying me now, each click of the odometer taking me further from my wife and closer to the Palouse country. Trips always seem slower when you are headed in a direction you don't want to go. I sighed and settled in for a really long drive.

YEAR THREE

CHAPTER FORTY-ONE

I pulled into Tullville around five P.M. and rented a motel room for the night. It was the fifteenth of August and I had five days until classes started. My main tasks before then were buying my textbooks and finding housing. I paid for one night's stay. The desk clerk gave me a key and I went to drop off my luggage in the room. When I entered the small quarters, the windows were closed and the hot musty air was stifling.

After turning on the air conditioner, I called Cindy to let her know I had arrived safely. We kept the conversation short due to the expense. Hearing her voice made me want to grab my suitcase and drive straight home. We did our best to reach out to each other across the tenuous lines spanning the distance between us. Then we had to say goodbye. After hanging up, I stared at the telephone receiver for several moments. The room was dead silent except for the hum of the air conditioner, and I was alone again. It was going to take some getting used to. After a minute I made myself get up off the bed and left to find dinner in town.

The following morning I picked up a copy of the local newspaper and visited Goltz Hall to check the bulletin board for housing ads. The latter source provided a couple of decent prospects. I called the numbers and reached one person who agreed to see me that afternoon.

A few hours later I headed out to find the house with the room for rent. It was located conveniently downtown, only a block off the main street. It was also just a quarter mile from the campus. At this distance I could easily walk to school and not worry about finding parking for my car every day.

The neighborhood was an older one, and the venerable shade trees along the avenue sported thick trunks and wide spreading branches. The house I was looking for sat at the first corner on my right. It was a white, two-story wood frame residence, with a steep roof and large front porch in the traditional farmhouse style. Stately old lilac bushes framed the main window, their glossy green leaves providing an attractive backdrop to the bright clumps of marigolds planted along the front of the house. I stepped up onto the porch and rang the doorbell.

After a few moments I heard the thump and creak of feet inside the house. The noises stopped and the lock rattled for a moment. Finally the door cracked open. A stout woman in her forties eyed me through the gap. Short-cropped brown hair hung limply about her broad face. For a moment we stared at each other in silence, and then she uttered one word, "Yes?"

Thus prompted, I cleared my throat and began, "Uh, my name is Mark. I'm here about the room for rent. I called you earlier and…."

Abruptly she swung the door wide and said, "Yes, yes, I remember. C'mon in and have a look-see, then." As I entered I got a full view of my potential landlady. She was a plain woman made more so by an unflattering ensemble of baggy jeans, suspenders, and a faded green shirt. Her lumbering gait would have fit well on a construction worker. She beckoned me into the house and I followed, closing the front door behind me. Just inside the entrance was a large foyer with a glass-paned door which let into a cozy living room. Through this door we went, and then Millicent (as she said I should call her) gave me a running commentary as we went room to room.

"This is the room I'm renting out right now," she told me as she showed me a corner bedroom just off the main bath. "I plan on renting out two more rooms upstairs as well, but this one is the best, so I figured you'd want it, as you are the first one to answer my ad."

"Why is it the best room?" I asked as I walked in and looked around. It was nicely appointed, with a comfortable-looking twin bed, a chest of drawers, and a small desk with a reading lamp. Lacy yellow curtains fluttered in the breeze from the open window.

Millicent scratched her neck and answered, "Well, it's near the bathroom; there are no facilities upstairs. Also, the upper floor is colder in the winter and hotter in the summer; this room's more comfortable in my opinion." I thought that her reasoning made sense.

She proceeded to show me the rest of the house. "Here's the kitchen and dining area, and you've already seen the living room. I have a small television in there, and you can watch what you want when I'm not using it, but please keep the volume low when I'm asleep. My bedroom is right off the main area." She pointed to an open door at the opposite end of the living room.

I nodded my understanding. "I'm going to be very busy studying, so I don't anticipate I'll be doing a lot of television watching," I assured her. She seemed pleased at the prospect of landing a quiet renter, and a trace of a smile momentarily played across her lips. We then got down to the nuts and bolts of the arrangement and she named a monthly rate for the rent. I thought it sounded reasonable and told her I'd like the room. And just like that it was done.

After parking my car in the wide driveway, I unloaded my things and was settled in by afternoon. Millicent directed me to a neighborhood grocery store just around the corner, and I walked over to stock up on food and other essentials. That evening I cooked my own dinner in the tiny kitchen and ate a relaxed meal in the adjacent dining nook. It felt really good to be situated.

I slept in Friday morning and the house was blissfully quiet. The simple absence of bird squawks at dawn was enough to justify the rent in my mind. After a leisurely breakfast I walked to the veterinary buildings to scout the locations of my upcoming classes. Most of the lecture portions were in the auditoriums in Goltz Hall, similar to the previous year. But many of the lab sessions, including junior surgery, would be held in the sister building, Aimsley.

I wandered through both buildings and located the rooms without much difficulty. On the way I said hello to a professor or two and also saw Molly Boyer in one of the hallways. She too was trying to find her way around before classes began. We shared the high points of our summer breaks, and of course I had the better story with the marriage and honeymoon. She congratulated me as her husband Terry approached toting one of their children, a wide-eyed little girl named Tammy. We exchanged pleasantries awhile longer and then they headed off to enjoy the day together. Molly said, "See you in class on Monday! Bright and early!" Her mischievous tone suggested that she remembered how I detested mornings.

I groaned and said, "Don't remind me!" She just laughed and waved as they walked away down the hall.

I didn't stay long in the buildings after I had accomplished my goals. The bright sunshine awaited, and soon I would be spending most of my time indoors. With that in mind I drove out to the cemetery and walked around the familiar grounds. Sitting in the shade of the ornamental trees, I watched the ground squirrels as I had a year earlier, enjoying the peaceful setting. Birds busily warbled and chirped their songs, hidden in the thick foliage above me. Warm air wafted in from the sun-baked hills nearby. It was going to be difficult sitting in a classroom during weather like this, so I enjoyed these last moments of rest before the toil. I was pretty sure that such opportunities would be hard to come by in the weeks ahead.

CHAPTER FORTY-TWO

Things really started getting interesting that fall semester. We had medicine lectures covering both small and large animals. The class we had all been waiting for, small animal surgery, was finally a reality. We were even treated to a short course with the eyebrow-raising title of "Large Animal Restraint." Yes indeed, learning how to not get maimed by animals who weighed ten times as much as you was an important facet of a veterinarian's skills. It was particularly useful for those who wished to practice without the aid of prosthetic limbs.

The medicine classes continued to provide the core of our curriculum, what we would need to know to diagnose and treat patients. They also were the courses whose notes accumulated at a prodigious rate. After only a few weeks of lectures, Mike Callahan came into small animal medicine class one morning and dropped his note binder onto his desk. The resulting boom turned heads and stopped all conversation in the room momentarily. Looking sheepish, Mike shrugged and commented, "There's some heavy material in this course."

Large animal medicine was the toughest subject for me. This was partly due to my inexperience with farm animals. All of my pre-veterinary observation had been done at a small animal hospital. Big herbivores were so different from what I was used to treating that they might as well have come from another planet.

For example, early on we learned about the horse and its complex fermenting hindgut. It was a great digestive system when it functioned properly, since it allowed these large animals to survive on feed such as grasses and hay, a diet that would starve a dog or human. The downside to such a large, complicated digestive tract was that it could easily be upset. Most gut disturbances in horses were lumped under the catch-all term of "colic." In reality the causes were numerous: eating indigestible objects, drinking excessive cold water, heavy consumption of rich foods such as oats or fruit, old age, intestinal worms, bad luck, all these and more were implicated as potential causes of colic.

Regardless of the cause, the signs were similar: pacing, pawing at the belly, sweating, and pain vocalizations such as groaning. If the colic was severe, the suffering animal would progress to violent contortions, often injuring itself trying to escape the pain. Shock and death could quickly follow on the heels of these symptoms.

The problem with having a big complex gut was not only that many things could go wrong with it. When an organ that large becomes ill, it also drags the rest of the body down rapidly. Look at a horse and appreciate how huge its abdomen is compared to the head and limbs. That's because it takes a cavernous belly to hold all those bowels. Indigestion in these animals was not a nuisance disease as with a human. Colic was often rapid and fatal, and was always considered a potential emergency.

Occasionally a horse actually managed to block its gut. Dr. Wilson, one of the instructors for the large animal course, brought a few hairballs into lecture while we were discussing colic. They were perfect spheres and varied from the size of a small orange to that of a large grapefruit. The objects varied in color depending on the coat of the horse, but they were all smooth, firm, and dry to touch. I thought they were oddly attractive, like works of art woven from thousands of short hairs.

Dr. Wilson explained that each of these had built up slowly in a horse's gut as it groomed itself, eventually causing an obstruction. They had been removed surgically, in one case during a necropsy after the unfortunate animal had suffered a rapid and painful death. It made me appreciate having a simple digestive system, even if I would starve when put out to pasture.

As essential as the medicine courses were, small animal surgery was the class that captured our imagination. Here was a chance to actually do something exciting, not just read about it. We hadn't handled a scalpel since freshman year, and back then our patients had been deceased and preserved. Now we had breathing dogs and cats whose lives depended on us performing well.

Early each week we sat in lecture, learning the details of various procedures. Thursdays found us in the surgery suites struggling to hone our skills. The simpler tasks such as spays, neuters, skin lump removals, and laceration repairs were performed entirely by the students. As I mentioned previously, we had teams of four, each with different jobs in a given surgery. The professors observed and offered advice, but did not actively participate unless absolutely necessary. Most of these patients were from animal shelters, and received discounted treatments prior to being adopted as pets.

Challenging surgeries were performed by the professors with the students assisting. These ranged from orthopedic procedures such as fractures and knee repairs to soft tissue surgery such as large tumor removals and caesarian sections. These surgeries were often referred to the teaching hospital due to their high degree of difficulty, and weren't necessarily a good representation of what we would be asked to do in general practice. I was relieved to know that, since some of the procedures I assisted on were hair-raising to observe, much less perform.

One of the first student surgeries that my team tackled was a tumor removal in an older Basset Hound. Her name was Maggie and she was a shelter dog. She was friendly and outgoing with a perpetual motion tail, typical of her breed. She also was fairly heavy set, a common problem with Bassets. Maggie's build, teeth, and graying muzzle all told us she was not a young girl any more. Her genetics combined with advancing age had possibly predisposed her to developing the large lipoma that protruded from her right flank.

We had covered neoplasia (abnormal growths or tumors) to some extent in our medicine courses. In my mind I could hear the professor droning, "Lipomas are very common in older dogs. They usually grow from the fat layer under the skin. These 'fatty tumors' are nearly always benign and most remain small. They are localized and not typically invasive. However, occasionally lipomas can become quite substantial over time." Looking at Maggie, I could vouch for that last statement, since her tumor was larger than my clenched fist.

We examined the cheery dog before surgery to assess her overall health. My teammates and I poked and prodded and listened. The lump on her side was easily palpated, very soft and pliable, and seemingly not uncomfortable to our patient. The mass appeared shallow and we could pull it away from the body wall easily, suggesting it was not deeply attached or invasive.

After scrubbing the area over the lump, we used a syringe to do a needle aspirate, sucking some material from the growth. We obtained several small clear drops resembling water. Microscopic inspection of the substance showed it to be fat droplets. The diagnosis of a lipoma was thereby confirmed.

Our surgical group consisted of two Oregon students and two from Washington. Fellow Oregonian Dan Alderman was chief surgeon for the day's procedure. The two Washington students I didn't know well. Danielle Peterson was a wiry, energetic lady who reminded me of a female Mike Callahan. Her classmate was Jason Thomas, a large, quiet man with long brown hair and a full bushy beard. At first glance he was intimidating, like someone you would find on a lonely piece of land in the mountains, brewing moonshine in his coveralls and smoking contraband. But he turned out to be a really personable fellow with a dry sense of humor.

After our examinations, Maggie was deemed stable enough for surgery, so we went ahead with the procedure. Her tail never missed a beat when a sedative was injected under the loose skin of her back. Life was easy when the patient cooperated.

Next we injected the actual anesthetic, a barbiturate, into a vein on the dog's forelimb. Or I should say we attempted to do so. Apparently Maggie had some objections to this particular endeavor. She was a very nice dog, but she was big and muscular with short crooked limbs. Every time Jason tried to insert the needle into her vein, she would jerk her leg just enough to thwart him. You would think that four young strong students could hold one dog's leg still, but apparently that was foolish optimism. Danielle had both her hands wrapped around Maggie's elbow to brace the leg, and Dan was lying across our patient's chest to pin her in place. I brought up the rear, literally, holding Maggie's rump so she couldn't back up.

The problem wasn't that Maggie struggled incessantly. Most of the time she just lay there wagging her tail furiously, and trying to lick whoever was closest to her face. But when she did feel a twinge from the needle, she moved so abruptly that we couldn't prevent her leg from shifting just a little. A slight movement is all it takes to keep a tentative student from threading a vein.

Our patient wasn't the only one unhappy with the proceedings. Between her body heat and our exertions, we were all getting sweaty and smelling more and more like dog. Eventually an anesthesiologist came around to help us with Maggie. Dr. Reiser was a tall, lanky guy with a disorderly mop of brown hair and a perpetually rumpled doctor's smock. The students joked that he always looked like he slept in his clothes. That may in fact have been the truth on nights when he was called in to assist with emergency surgeries. Despite his less-than-elegant appearance, he was highly respected among peers and students alike for his knowledge of anesthesiology and his commitment to his patients. He was a joy to work with, since he always seemed unruffled and had a smile for everyone.

Now Dr. Reiser approached our group and stood a moment observing our struggles with Maggie. Hands in his pockets, the doctor grinned at Jason and offered, "There's a big difference between sticking it 'in the vein' and sticking it 'in vain.'" He laughed fiendishly as we all groaned and rolled our eyes. After that he got more serious and settled down to the business at hand, talking Jason through the venipuncture.

"Okay now, you're right-handed, so hold the leg firmly with your left, close to where you want to thread the vein. That will help keep the leg still. Lay your left thumb alongside the vein, to prevent the vessel from rolling away from your needle as you insert it. There you go, now slide the needle in. Slowly! Slowly, or you will go right through and out the other side of the vein. Angle the needle a bit more shallowly, that's it. It looks like you're in. Pull back the plunger and see if you get blood. Ah, there it is! Now inject the drug steadily, watching how your patient responds. We only dose to effect; she is older and may not need the entire calculated amount. Good, good. There you go!"

So began the day's anesthetic procedure. The surgery that followed was equally shaky, but we muddled our way through and the end result was, in the supervising surgeon's words, "quite respectable." It was true that someone could have cloned a new body for Maggie in the time it took us to remove the mass. The incision also bore a close resemblance to the tortuous path of the Columbia River as seen on a map. Nonetheless, we felt quite proud of the fact that we had come, we had seen, and we had conquered. Best of all, our patient still had a pulse when we were finished. Not a bad day's work, all things considered.

CHAPTER FORTY-THREE

As we settled in to our new curriculum, I found that one of our biggest challenges was dealing with the unique personalities we encountered in school. Nowhere was this more evident than in our surgery class. Medical specialists tended to have big egos, with surgeons possibly being the worst. Two of our professors were such individuals; it probably didn't help that their statures were as short as their heads were large. They were impatient with students, demanding perfection and criticizing anything or anyone who didn't meet their standards. The junior class viewed them with a weird mixture of awe and distaste.

By far the worst offender was Dr. Payne. His demeaning manner was accompanied by a notoriously short temper. Students assisting him during surgery held their collective breath whenever he encountered difficulty. Being that he was called upon to perform some of the most challenging procedures, it goes without saying that difficulties often abounded. One could gauge how well things were going—or not—by how red his face became. When tensions ran high and his forehead veins were bulging, it was best not to speak at all, even if you were bursting with questions.

I was the main assistant for Dr. Payne during a particularly difficult orthopedic case. He was repairing a multiple fracture of a dog's femur, and the fragments weren't stabilizing easily. Intramedullary pins and cerclage wire were the methods of repair that day, but the bones kept shifting and destabilizing as he tried to tighten the wires around them. I could tell he was getting more frustrated as the clock ticked away the minutes and the fracture refused to cooperate.

Part of assisting a surgeon meant having instruments ready for him to grab when they were needed. Each doctor had different preferences, which made it all the more confusing. Experience helped, and with practice I learned to anticipate what might be needed during each portion of a procedure. But on this day I'm not sure there was any instrument in the pack that would have made Dr. Payne happy.

Midway through the repair he abruptly held out his hand, palm up. This meant he wanted an instrument, but he didn't say which. I hesitated and he shook his hand impatiently, never looking up from the surgery site. Guessing, I slapped a pair of scissors into his hand firmly, handles forward, as we had been taught to do. He brought them toward the open wound, then seeing what he held he snorted in disgust and threw the scissors onto the floor.

I cringed and he glared at me, growling, "What the hell are you thinking? Everyone knows that if a surgeon puts out his hand without specifying an instrument, then he wants a hemostat. Not a retractor, not a scalpel, and NOT a damned pair of scissors! Understood?"

I nodded mutely, handing him a hemostat. He grabbed it roughly from me, muttering, "Who taught you surgical assisting anyway? They should be castrated." It occurred to me that this was not the best time to mention that a large portion of that curriculum had been covered by Dr. Payne himself. Nor was it wise to point out that the "default hemostat" rule had never been brought up. So I simply bit my tongue and tried to appear attentive.

My classmates in attendance shot me looks of sympathy over their surgical masks. Mike Callahan winked and made a cupping motion with one hand, as if he were holding something. I frowned in puzzlement until he used the other hand to make a scissor motion over the top, nodding toward the surgeon as he did so. I suddenly realized he was miming a castration and I had to choke off a laugh.

Dr. Payne glanced up and I was ever so thankful that my mask hid my broad grin.

In all fairness, the teaching staff weren't the only individuals who had personality issues. Vincent Studebaker was one of my classmates from Oregon who came from a wealthy family. His way through school was greased by a total lack of worries about tuition. Student loans and summer jobs were foreign to him, and when he stayed in Tullville, his parents rented him an entire house to live in. This somehow made him better than most of his classmates, and he looked down his nose at those who were less fortunate. In class he maintained an air of detached superiority. You didn't call him "Vince" or "Vin," as that would be too informal. Ignoring the fact that no one needed to pull straight A's any more, he prided himself on having the highest grade point average in the class.

In keeping with his sparkling personality Vincent seemed convinced that he was the best junior surgeon. His group was stationed across the aisle from mine, and whenever we called a surgeon to our table for advice, he glanced over at us and shook his head disparagingly. I knew what he was thinking; far be it from him to ever need assistance.

People who know me can tell you that I am an easy-going person and can put up with a lot, but Vincent's smugness was annoying in the extreme. That is why the incident with the rebreathing bag was so hilarious.

On each anesthetic machine hung a large black rubber bag. It was connected with the oxygen tubes that provided gas anesthesia to the patient. During an inhale, the bag deflated. When the patient breathed out, the bag filled up.

One day in surgery Vincent was the anesthetist for his team. Besides monitoring the patient, the anesthetist was supposed to squeeze the rebreathing bag every now and then to give the animal a deep breath. While under anesthesia a dog would breathe shallowly, and we were taught that "sighing" the patient with a deep inhale every so often would make the lungs function better.

The anesthetic machine wasn't a closed system. New oxygen was constantly being pumped to the patient, so it goes to reason that the exhaled gas from the animal had to be vented off. There was a pop-off valve through which old gas was evacuated and taken out of the building, venting harmlessly into the outside air. This valve had to be closed when you squeezed the bag to inflate the lungs, otherwise the gas you pushed out the bag went mostly though the pop-off valve and was lost.

The important thing was this: after you gave the patient a big inhale, you had to reopen the pop-off valve. If you didn't, then no gas could escape the system. As oxygen kept getting pumped into the lines, the pressure would build higher and higher. This would continually expand the patient's lungs, making it impossible to exhale at all. Eventually the lungs could even rupture.

On this particular day Vincent wasn't paying close attention to his duties as anesthetist. He was busy watching his group's surgery, and offering a running commentary on how it should be done. Meanwhile he had "sighed" the dog and then forgotten to reopen the pop-off valve. The rebreathing bag became full, then overfull, then fuller yet. By the time I glanced over and saw their machine, the normally flaccid bag looked like a giant beach ball. My jaw dropped as I stared at the grotesque apparition. I hadn't realized the heavy rubber could stretch that far. At any moment I expected the distended shape to come flying off its moorings and shoot around the room like a sputtering balloon.

Just then Vincent caught me looking in his direction. Doubtless he assumed I wanted to overhear some pointers from the top student in the class. He gave me a knowing smirk and turned back toward his patient. That did it; I found I could not resist the temptation any longer. My evil genius compelled me to say, "Hey Vinnie, that's a whopper of a bag you have on that machine. I didn't know they made a jumbo size."

He glanced casually back at the rebreathing bag and the transformation in his face was remarkable. His look of disdain was wiped away by one of sheer panic. Bedlam immediately ensued as his team frantically scrambled to get the pop-off valve open. Finally Vincent's fumbling fingers turned the knob, and the dog said "*Huhhhhhh*" as it exhaled forcefully. I don't know how long it had been made to hold its breath with its chest expanded, but thankfully no serious harm seemed to have been done.

My group burst out laughing, along with students at several other surgery tables who were close enough to have seen the episode. Vincent's face was beet red. It got even redder when he was reprimanded by the supervising professor for not attending to his duties. As my old friend Daniel loved to say, karma's a bitch. From that day on Vincent lost a little of his swagger in the surgery suite.

Life at home was also becoming more entertaining. Millicent had followed through on her plan to have three boarders. I now shared the house with two female college students. Miko was an exchange student from Japan, petite and polite. She was also very shy, in part because she wasn't confident in her English skills. Later when she got comfortable with us, she became quite vivacious and was easy to understand. Sometimes she would apologize, "My English not very good." Whenever she did I would reply, "It's far better than my Japanese."

The other girl was a tall American named Molly. Her sandy blonde hair was trimmed short and framed a narrow but attractive face. She was a graduate student studying physiologic psychology, the chemistry behind the brain's workings. Due to our related areas of study, we could speak each other's language pretty well. Hence we shared many interesting discussions over the time we lived at the house. Our landlady was not the best conversationalist, so I enjoyed having Molly there to talk to.

In addition to our other subjects that term, there was that little matter of large animal restraint that we juniors had to tackle. This class was more hands-on than lecture-oriented, and we spent a lot of time in the hospital barns practicing handling of the big herbivores. Besides chemical sedation, there was an amazing array of tricks and methods used to bring an oversized patient under control. These helped level the playing field so we could come to the aid of these animals without becoming hospitalized ourselves.

We learned about twitches, hobbles, squeeze chutes, hoods, casting, and other arcane sounding methods of restraining a horse or cow. Some of them made perfect sense, such as a tight chute the animal could be led into that restricted movement and limited the ability to kick. But other methods left me scratching my head, wondering, "Why the heck does *that* work?"

As previously discussed, one example of such was the twitch, that simple piece of rope that was looped around a horse's floppy upper lip. The loop was then tightened down on the trapped lip by twisting the rope. With moderate pressure the horse would become almost tranquilized, relaxing and allowing routine treatments and examinations without fussing or kicking. It was strange, but it worked!

Another odd technique involved using fancy rope work to pull a standing cow over onto its side. This was called "casting." There were a couple of different ways to place the ropes, but essentially you ended up with a few linked loops around the cow's body, which would tighten and squeeze when you pulled hard on the rope's end. Normally cows are strong enough to easily withstand a person pulling them sideways. They simply brace themselves and look down on your puny efforts while chewing their cud. But with pressure applied properly, the ropes trigger the animal to give in and roll onto its side. It might take a couple of strong individuals pulling, but it was quite achievable. Watching a hulking bovine just fall over made me shake my head at the inventiveness of it. I had to wonder who had first come up with casting and how they had figured it out. I imagine that there was quite a bit of sweating, grunting, and cursing mixed in with the ingenuity.

CHAPTER FORTY-FOUR

That fall the passage of time became blurred by the torrent of class work thrown our way. Small and large animal medicine kept us scrambling to keep up, the volume of information made even more worrisome by the recognition that this was stuff we really had to know. There was no memorizing the notes just well enough to pass the test, then forgetting it a week later. From now on every item we learned could prove important, especially when we were on our own struggling to diagnose and treat patients.

Helping to ease the burden was the simple fact that not all of the material was really new. Much of what we were seeing now was built upon the foundations of our first two years of school. For instance, when small animal medicine turned its focus to ophthalmology, we had our first introduction to diagnosing and treating ocular disorders. However, we had covered eye anatomy in our freshman year, so when Dr. Brisbane talked about the lens and cornea and sclera, we all knew what he referred to. When he covered viral infections of the eye, we were familiar with the diseases from virology class. When it came time to discuss ophthalmic medications, we had already learned the drugs and their basic effects in pharmacology lecture.

The further we went in our education, the more we began to encounter familiar material; it was simply being approached from a different angle. Each additional time we saw it, our retention improved. Everything was beginning to coalesce into a unified picture, and it all was starting to make sense. Despite the frenetic pace of learning, vet school was becoming really enjoyable.

Adding to the fun were a few truly nice professors. Dr. Brakel, the surgeon who had helped me with my very first spay, was a silly man who loved to spread the joy. He was always joking with the students during his surgeries. Stan Hulbert remarked that assisting Brakel after sitting in on Dr. Payne's surgeries was like going to a Mardi Gras after having attended a wake.

One of Dr. Brakel's pastimes was collecting surgical mantras. He often used them as ammunition when debating with the medicine department about how to manage a case. I should explain that within the profession there is a good-natured running battle between "medicine" people and "surgery" people. If a case is hard to diagnose, an internist wants to run more tests. A surgeon may elect to go look inside to see what the problem is. A medicine person often prefers to be noninvasive and minimize stress to the patient; a surgeon wants to get an answer quickly and certainly, as well as having the opportunity to fix a problem while he's in there.

Each approach has its strength, of course, and each can succeed in helping the patient. Indeed, many cases need both medical and surgical treatments working in concert to produce a cure. But the discussions between internists and surgeons can be animated and grow quite heated at times. Dr. Brakel loved to throw out one-liners every now and then to illustrate his point during such debates. By our junior year we had all heard his favorite, "Grab a knife and save a life," but the good doctor had an endless repertoire.

He often shared these with the students to lighten things up. We'd be scrubbing and preparing a patient for a procedure, and Dr. Brakel would breeze into the surgery suite. He'd look around to see which students he had with him that day. Then he'd smack his hands together and offer a hearty greeting such as, "Good afternoon, guys and gals! Are you ready for some fun?"

We'd nod our heads and answer with an enthusiastic "Yes!"

He would open his instrument pack and grab a scalpel. Before making the first incision, he'd pause and look around, eyebrows raised. The room would be silent with anticipation as the students watched attentively. When he judged the moment to be just right, he'd raise his hands like a preacher and give us a surgical saying for the day.

There were so many I can't begin to remember them all. One day it would be, "A chance to cut is a chance to cure," and the next it was, "The way to heal is with cold steel." Other gems included "When in doubt, cut it out," "All bleeding stops eventually," and that old favorite, "Never let skin get between you and a diagnosis." He'd have us in stitches (pardon the pun) before we had even begun, and this set the tone for the rest of the surgery. Even when things went less than smoothly and tension mounted, there was a sense of camaraderie that we never experienced with some of the other surgeons.

Dr. Payne, by contrast, was an excellent clinician but didn't seem to care about teaching. He gave the required lectures in class, but in the surgery suite he couldn't be bothered. I respected his need to concentrate when struggling to perform a difficult procedure. But when the hard part was over and he could easily answer questions, I felt that it was part of his job description to help us learn. He never openly discouraged questions, but his demeanor made students reluctant to ask. He often implied that the questioner should already know the answer, so that his pupils were made to feel ignorant in front of their classmates.

As for me, I was paying good money to be in vet school and to learn, so I planned to get the best education that I could. If Dr. Payne didn't offer to teach, then I would make him do so regardless. I knew I was a good student; if he wanted to imply otherwise, it simply revealed a flaw in his personality, not a flaw in my intellect.

One day I was assisting Dr. Payne, and he had finished the strenuous portion of the surgery. He asked me to close the patient and I began suturing the incision. Halfway through I found that I was having trouble with the stiff nylon monofilament. Instead of nice square knots, I was often producing granny knots which were not as secure. As far as I could tell I was doing everything properly, but I was certain that the end result was not what I wanted. Grannies can untie themselves and aren't considered adequate for surgical closures.

Dr. Payne hadn't noticed anything amiss. He was chatting with other students in the room about surgical methods and wasn't even paying attention to my work. I had to bring his attention to my problem. When I did, he snorted and said, "Well, you're not throwing the knots correctly! Do it again so I can see what you are doing wrong."

I quickly threw another knot and he said impatiently "No, no, slow it down so I can see." I obliged, and he watched closely. "There!" he pronounced, pointing at my instruments. "You're not pulling the sutures the right direction when you tighten the knots. You have to pull in the same orientation as the knot is being tied, the same plane. You're pulling out to the sides, which flips the knot over. Do it the way you were taught in class!"

When I tied the next knot, I paid attention to which way I pulled the suture ends, and sure enough a nice neat square knot resulted. That little detail had never been mentioned in class, but it made all the difference. Dr. Payne knew his stuff, and if I didn't mind getting berated a bit, I could pull the needed information from him. The other students in attendance had fallen silent after the doctor's brusque correction of my technique. I just grinned to myself as I worked. I had made the crotchety professor teach me whether he liked it or not.

That evening I got a call from Cindy. We talked more often now that she was employed and we had money coming in. I heard the phone ring from my bedroom and jumped up to answer it. When I came into the kitchen, Millicent handed me the receiver, saying, "It's your lady calling."

My heart skipped as it always did when Cindy called. I grabbed the phone from Millicent and waited until she walked back into the living room. Then I put the receiver to my ear and said, "Hello?"

Cindy's sweet voice answered, "Hi baby! Oh I've missed you! How are things with my favorite man?"

I laughed and replied, "Aw, I miss you too, every day and even more at night! It's hard having a new spouse and then not having her."

She sighed and said, "Yeah, tell me about it. This separation is killing me. At least I have my job to keep me occupied. How are you holding up?"

I answered, "Well, things are going pretty well. I figured out how to deal with Dr. Payne, you know, the surgeon with the Napoleonic complex I told you about."

Cindy giggled and said, "Oh do tell! What happened?"

I related the story of my request for help in surgery, and threw in the episode with Vincent and his rebreathing bag as well. When she finally stopped laughing, she said, "I just love hearing your voice. You always make me smile, no matter what kind of day I've had. Having you makes life worth living."

Cindy's frank expression of affection touched my heart even from so far away. I struggled to find the words to return the sentiment. "Thank you for sharing that," I answered. "I love when you say what you feel, Cindy. It goes both ways, you know. Living up here is hard because I'm so far away from you. But knowing that I have you at my side makes the work and the isolation easier. Even when you're not at my side. If that makes any sense at all," I finished lamely.

Her musical laugh filled my ear and she assured me that it made perfect sense. We talked a bit more about life and daily events and how much we missed each other. Eventually I asked her how work was going, and she became quite animated. Cindy was just settling in after the initial training period, but it was obvious she was quite happy. She told me that she loved the company and her coworkers, and she was getting to do research which was her dream. Cindy hated being bored, and this job was intellectually stimulating enough to keep her interested. I was happy for her and I knew she would do well in her new career.

Finally we had to say goodbye, since it was getting late and we had been on the phone for nearly an hour. Reluctantly I said, "Get some sleep, baby. You've got work in the morning. I'm glad things are going great for you. Just don't forget about me while I'm stuck here in Dullville."

She said, "Oh, don't worry about that. What you should be worried about is what I'll do to you when we get together. We've been apart far too long. Get plenty of rest before you come visit. You'll need it!"

"Ohhhh!" was all I could manage.

She laughed and said, "Good night, darling. Sleep well and dream of me. I miss you."

"I miss you too, more than I know how to say," I told her. "Sweet dreams."

A moment later she was gone. After she hung up I replaced the receiver on the wall and slowly walked toward my room, my head down. Halfway there I paused, then took a deep breath and straightened my back. By the time I returned to my bedroom I was smiling to myself. And why shouldn't I? In truth I was incredibly lonely away from my young wife, but I also felt that I was the luckiest man alive. Not a bad place to be, when everything was considered.

I had other reasons to be happy that fall. Life in my new home was quite an improvement over my previous year in the trailer park. There was no frozen fog from my breath in the bedroom and no birds waking me before the sun came up. In the evenings when I wasn't studying, I spent time getting to know my housemates. If our schedules allowed, we sometimes had dinner together or stayed up in the evenings chatting in the living room. Initially I had been leery of having to share living space with two other students. To my delight I found that Miko and Molly made the house feel warm and alive. Molly and I thought a lot alike, and Miko had fascinating stories to tell of her life in Japan. They were both great companions and made my time there much more enjoyable.

On the other side of the coin, our landlady was a bit eccentric. Maybe downright strange was a better term for it. Some days she acted like an average person, quite talkative and even funny. Other times she was morose and withdrawn and had behavioral quirks. I thought I might be imagining things, but Molly mentioned it as well while we were eating dinner one evening. Millicent had gone to bed early as was her tendency. Miko was upstairs studying so Molly and I were alone in the dining nook.

"Say Mark, have you noticed anything unusual about Millicent?" Molly asked me between bites of a muffin. "She's been acting more peculiar lately. I mean, she's a bit of an odd bird anyway, but these past few days I just don't know."

I nodded and swallowed, then said, "Yes, she's been restless, unable to sit still for more than a minute. She also seems distracted. Half the time when I speak to her I get no response."

"Exactly!" Molly replied. "I was trying to talk to her today, and it was like I wasn't there. Then when I did get her attention, she practically bit my head off."

I frowned. That didn't sound like Millicent. She could be a bit reserved and gruff, but was never volatile. "What do you think is going on?" I asked. "You're the psych major."

"Physiologic psychology," Molly reminded me. "I don't study behavioral psych very much. But I do think something is wrong with her. She's not acting right. And she's changed in the past week, which is peculiar as well. People's personalities and behaviors don't just shift for no reason. She hasn't mentioned anything to you about a family problem or anything that would have made her depressed?"

I shook my head. "No, nothing at all. Of course there could be something and she's just not telling us."

Molly pondered that for a moment as she sipped her drink. Eventually she shrugged and said, "Well, there's no way to know without asking her, and I don't want to do that right now. But I'm worried about Millie. Let's both keep an eye on her, okay?"

I promised her that I would and we finished our meal. Then we headed to our rooms to study, and for the moment the puzzle of Millicent was shelved as the demands of school took over.

CHAPTER FORTY-FIVE

Fall lengthened toward winter and the days grew chill, the deciduous trees lining the avenues dropping their autumn finery to stand starkly naked. The first sprinkling of snow fell in early November. My walks to school, though shorter than in the previous year, were becoming less enjoyable as the cold deepened. Helping to hasten my pace was the seductive promise of heated comfort at the end of the road.

Midterms had come and gone, and I had achieved good marks as was typical of my stay in Tullville. In my comfortable housing I found that studying was easier than ever, especially when I didn't have to huddle under a blanket to keep from freezing. The weeks passed slowly that November, with no major exams and nothing exciting happening in class or at home.

Millicent continued to be predictably unpredictable, some days being outgoing and other days quiet and withdrawn. But overall she was easy to deal with, giving Molly and me no real cause for concern. The one new twist to my housing situation came not from the landlady, but from her elderly father.

Dick was a sweet old man who had lived most his life as a farmer in the Palouse area. His once solid frame was now thin and frail, and he walked with the uncertain shuffle of the infirm. Most mornings he donned coveralls with suspenders just as I imagined he would have worn in younger days. His bald pate sported wisps of snow white hair matching the stubble on his weathered face. Deep-set hazel eyes and arched brows gave his features an aspect of focused intelligence. When I met him I had to wonder what life experiences those eyes had beheld, what wisdom he might have been able to impart with all the history he had seen. But wondering was all I could do, since it was all gone now.

You see, Dick had advanced Alzheimer's disease and was barely able to recognize his own daughter. Usually he lived at a local nursing home due to his need for constant supervision. I've had family members who developed this condition, and it is heartbreaking to experience. Not so much for those afflicted, as they don't remember what they have lost. But for those who love them, watching a spouse or mother or sibling fade away until all that is left is a vacant shell is devastating to deal with.

The affected individuals are also a difficult burden to care for. As the illness progresses, they often become a danger to themselves and others. Left alone for even a few minutes, an Alzheimer's patient may wander out of the home and into a busy street, or worse yet attempt to drive a car. He or she may decide to cook dinner but forget to unwrap the food, setting a cardboard box directly on a stovetop and starting a house fire. Attempting to shave with a razor becomes a hazardous endeavor. The list of potential daily disasters is endless. Caring for such a person is a twenty-four-hour-a-day job with no breaks. Even the most devoted relatives often are forced to seek professional supervision for their loved one sooner or later.

Millicent obviously shared a close connection with her father. Consequently she missed him and would bring him to the house for days at a time, occasionally for as long as a week. I quickly found out that there were problems with that arrangement.

Most of the time Dick sat in an easy chair in the living room, not moving and rarely responding to what went on around him.

Molly told me over dinner that she could get him to answer questions sometimes, and that he could recall things from long ago. But recent memories were difficult to dredge up, and his periods of lucidity were brief.

The first hint I had that Dick's presence might be problematic occurred one evening when had I stayed up late pouring over class notes. I came out of my room to get a snack just in time to catch Dick heading out the side door of the house. Millicent was nowhere to be seen; I assumed she had fallen asleep in her bedroom. I knew her father wasn't supposed to go anywhere on his own, so I put down my notebook and hurried over to intercept him. He paused as soon as he felt my hand on his shoulder. I asked him, "Dick, are you going somewhere?"

He shook his head vaguely and mumbled something which I didn't catch. Then he turned back to gaze out the open door, apparently oblivious to the harsh bite of the freezing night air swirling in around us. I noticed that he was dressed only in flannel pajamas and soft slippers.

I continued, "Where would you be going at this hour? It's cold and dark outside and you don't even have a sweater on. Come on back and sit down where it's warm; we can watch television together."

Dick nodded and allowed himself to be led back into the living room, where he soon occupied his familiar spot in the recliner. I made sure the door was locked and remained in the room with him while I studied. Fortunately Millicent later got up and came out to relieve me of guard duty. She helped Dick to his feet and took him into her room where she had a guest bed set up for him. I could hear her lock the bedroom door behind them. I headed off to my room to sleep, but it took awhile for slumber to overtake me. My ears perked up at every creak of the old house around me, imagining I heard the shuffle of slipper-clad feet wandering in the night.

As November neared its end, I counted the hours until Thanksgiving holiday. This year more than ever I yearned to get away and share precious days with Cindy. She and I had discussed vacation plans and had decided to spend Thanksgiving at my parents' house. Her mom and dad were traveling back east to visit Cindy's brother, so they wouldn't be around for the holiday.

The drive home for vacation was easy and relaxed, the roads were clear, and the fact that I wasn't on a crowded bus made all the difference. With no need to stop in multiple towns along the way, the trip to Beaverton went quickly. Around six P.M. I pulled into the apartment complex that Cindy and I called home. After grabbing my luggage from the trunk, I turned and walked up the stairs to the second floor apartment, wherein awaited the person who could make me whole again.

CHAPTER FORTY-SIX

The days following were a much needed break, wherein the only task to be accomplished was relaxation. I treasured every minute I got to spend with Cindy. Our time alone in our apartment was wonderful beyond description. Equally enjoyable was sharing the big holiday dinner with my parents in Medford that Thursday. I loved my family and my wife, and getting to have them all together was the nicest gift I could have asked for.

Cindy and I were thankful that we were now able to stay together in the same room under my parents' roof. Being apart for months had created a "feast or famine" pattern to our relationship. Our times together were intense and carried a sense of urgency, knowing as we did that they would end again so quickly.

Late Thanksgiving night we lay in bed talking, our stomachs still full from the banquet we had enjoyed hours earlier. Cindy laughed she recounted the day's events. "Your parents are both so nice," she said. "Your dad was telling me war stories before dinner; he's got an endless supply of them."

"Yes, I think I've heard just about all of them over the years, mostly around campfires in the mountains," I replied. "He was a fighter pilot in World War II and the Korean War, so he had a lot of adventures. He's very skilled at story telling, setting the scene and making you feel like you were actually there."

Cindy agreed. "He was quite entertaining to listen to," she said. "But it's your mom who really loves to chat. I had a hard time getting a word in edgewise. I got to hear all sorts of stories about you as a child. It seems you were a prankster and trouble maker even then!"

"I deny all charges," I replied emphatically, waving my hand in denial. "I was a complete angel...by the way, which pranks did she tell you about?"

Cindy giggled. "Oh, there were the bumper stickers, of course. And what's this about terrorizing your little brother with the toilet troll?"

I laughed and shook my head. "Oh, that was my older brother Stan's brainchild, not mine. I just helped sell the idea to Ted. As I recall, he was afraid to sit on the toilet for quite some time after that."

Cindy rolled her eyes and shook her head at me. I grinned and tried to look innocent. She hesitated a moment, as if debating whether to ask anything more. Finally she said, "How about when you scared Ted in his bedroom at night? That was all your idea, wasn't it?"

I chuckled then nodded sheepishly. "Yes, I guess I have to take credit for that one," I admitted. "Stan approved of my work though!"

"Yeah, I'll bet he did," Cindy retorted. "It sounds like you were two of a kind. Your mom said you rigged things in Ted's room that moved. How did you do that?"

"Ah, the engineering was surpassed only by the ingenuity," I began, but as I waxed eloquent, Cindy made a gagging motion with her finger down her throat. I feigned offense and drew myself up, saying, "Will the peanut gallery please refrain from disparaging gestures while I tell my tale."

Cindy pasted an attentive look on her face, and suitably appeased I continued, "Now, then, let me entertain you with glories from my youth. When we were kids my little brother and I each had our own bedroom. Ted would often visit a friend's house during the day, and on occasion I would take advantage of his absence and rig pranks in his room. The bedroom floor was so strewn with toys that you could hardly see the carpet. A simple trick I liked to pull was attaching a string to one of the toys and running it across the floor under all the clutter. There was a rear entrance to Ted's room that we never used; I'd slide the loose end of the string under the door's edge where it would barely protrude on the other side. At night when Ted went to sleep, I'd creep up to his door and select a string (there were usually several to choose from). I'd pull it slowly and you could hear the sound of Ted's toys going 'clank, clank' across his floor."

Cindy tried to put on a disapproving expression, but the effect failed due to her laughing at the same time. "What did Ted do?" she asked, fascinated despite herself.

I grinned back at her. "Well, he had a light on the headboard of his bed, in case he needed to get up at night or was scared. He could reach up and hit the switch and it would click on. As soon as I heard that sound I'd stop pulling the string. Ted would look around his room and there'd be nothing to see. After a minute or so the light would click off and a few seconds later I'd begin to pull the string again. *Clank, clank,* would go the toys; it was actually pretty loud. *Click* would go his light, and I'd pause again while he looked around…and so on. Even when I stopped for the evening, his light would click on repeatedly for quite some time. I think that some nights he didn't sleep very well."

"You were evil!" Cindy laughed. "I'm glad you weren't my brother!"

"Yes, I've had other people tell me the same thing. I can't imagine why," I answered, putting on my best angelic expression.

"I'm glad you've found a more constructive use of your intellect," Cindy declared. "Don't you try any of those pranks on me, mister! I'm a big girl and there would be payback!"

"Oh yeah? Like what?" I challenged her teasingly.

"Like this!" she replied, and then she jumped on me, pinning me down as she tickled me ferociously. I squirmed frantically but it was no use; she had the advantages of surprise and motivation. She only stopped when she had me totally subjugated.

As I caught my breath I said, "What was that for? I haven't even done anything to you yet."

"Yet? YET?!" she replied menacingly.

"I meant, I would never do anything like that to you!" I clarified instantly. "So no payback was needed!"

"Well, that was for your little brother then, and long overdue," she declared. She looked stern for a few seconds before the smile broke through again and she started to laugh. "Oh, but you were a wicked child!" she scolded, smiling at me.

"I'm still wicked, milady," I said as I reached for her.

"Oh, do tell me more. You've piqued my curiosity," she replied, and then I don't remember much conversation after that.

On Saturday Cindy and I left Medford and drove back to Beaverton. We spent one more night together in our apartment before I had to head back to Tullville. Neither of us wanted to say goodbye again. We consoled ourselves with the knowledge that in a few short weeks we would have a long Christmas break together. I kissed away my wife's tears and promised to be back very soon. Then I was off again to the land of dust and snow.

CHAPTER FORTY-SEVEN

Our December class work seemed to rush ahead double-time toward an early conclusion. This year our schedule was different, due to the Oregon students' need to cram in all the small animal courses prior to returning to Corvine. We had started the semester in August, which meant that the dreaded final exams would be coming in late December, not January. When our tests concluded, we could go on our holiday break free of the burden of studying.

Better yet, after Christmas vacation we entered the phase of our education called "small animal blocks," a series of short courses mixed with actual clinical experience in the teaching hospital. By all accounts the blocks were both fun and educational. Things were looking up for the junior class, but first we had to finish out the fall semester.

The medicine and surgery courses had proven to be both relevant and interesting, but they also presented copious masses of information to learn. Our first two years in vet school had helped prepare us for this, so we mostly took it in stride. Small animal medicine ranged far and wide, jumping around from subject to subject. Cardiology and ophthalmology took center stage late in the term, and I enjoyed both subjects. Perhaps it was because each focused on just one organ, which made it easier somehow in my mind. Also I found the intricacies of the eye and the heart intriguing. Each was a critically important organ and each was a wonder of elegant design.

Dr. Brisbane taught ophthalmology, and he reminded us of somewhat of the surgeons: short in stature and in patience, large in self-importance and ego. Maybe that stemmed from being a mini-surgeon, since he did perform some eye procedures in addition to practicing medicine. Despite his personality I found that I liked his class. He was organized and had extensive printed notes that covered everything in logical detail. I didn't have to write much at all in his lectures. For many years after graduation, I referred to Dr. Brisbane's materials whenever I needed a question answered about the diagnosis or treatment of an ocular disorder.

Cardiology captured my interest as well. We learned about how the heart functioned normally, its intricate anatomy, and all the various ways problems could develop in animals. Aside from humans, few species seemed prone to cholesterol-induced disease or heart attacks. Most heart disease in our pet animals was due to other problems, and usually caused a slow deterioration. Symptoms were often absent until the disease was advanced. It was only when the heart was truly failing to perform that the animal (and the family) began to realize that something was amiss.

By the time I see a cardiac patient with lethargy, wheezing, or a bloated appearance from retained fluid in the body, I know that I'm dealing with the final phase of a long-term illness. The survival time of those late-stage patients is often measured in weeks to months rather than years. All the more reason to have regular checkups for a pet, since heart conditions can sometimes be detected early just by listening with a stethoscope.

I found the EKG (electrocardiogram) to be one of the most fascinating aspects of cardiology. The little squiggly lines looked remarkably similar to what I had seen on television in human medical shows. These waves represented the electrical impulses shooting through the heart. By measuring the size, shape, and speed of those impulses we could diagnose cardiac enlargement, rhythm disturbances, fast or slow heart rates, abnormalities in electrical conduction due to disease, and so on. It was a powerful tool which was both inexpensive and non-stressful. Nearly all animals could have an EKG done while wide awake.

As with ophthalmology, I liked cardiology partially because of the presentation. The professor, Dr. Simpson, was a young, long-haired man from Southern California who looked like he had arrived on a surfboard. In fact he was a board-certified veterinary cardiologist, and although he retained a casual beach bum persona, he was razor sharp when he donned his doctor's smock. His lecture notes, like those of Dr. Brisbane, were typed out for us and well organized. That was the only similarity I could find between the two professors, since Dr. Simpson was as congenial as Brisbane was aloof.

Despite the appeal of the medicine courses, small animal surgery still held our interest better than any other subject we studied in vet school. It was really hard to be bored when handling a scalpel. Dr. Brakel continued to make his surgeries fun, although late in the semester he was running out of surgical mantras. Nonetheless, his sense of humor was boundless. I recall one day when we were working on a difficult bowel resection in the operatory. An old male Airedale had a malignant tumor of the small intestine, and Dr. Brakel was attempting to remove it when he called for a Balfour retractor.

The retractor was a steel instrument with small arms that could spread an incision wide open, making it easier to see inside the patient. In surgery class we had learned about retractors, but this particular type hadn't been mentioned. The doctor also didn't use the word "retractor." Instead he just said, "Give me a Balfour, please."

One of the vet students assisting him, a girl from Washington named Shirley Hand, looked totally bewildered and said, "What's a Balfour?"

Then, right in the middle of the difficult procedure, Dr. Brakel looked up at her with his eyes crossed and in a goofy voice said, "It's for pooping." It took me a moment to get the joke and then I burst out laughing, joined by the other three students who were assisting. Shirley looked like she was frozen in surprise. I don't think her brain ever successfully made the transition from life-and-death seriousness to joviality. Such was life in the operatory when Dr. Brakel was presiding.

After school I headed home each day to eat dinner, and then my evenings were mostly occupied with studying. Occasionally I spent time with Miko and Molly when I needed a break from my notes. But with final exams approaching, I found myself sequestered in my room for long hours each night, the door closed, my universe narrowed to the lines of print on the page I was struggling to memorize.

There were some distractions arising on the home front, however. Millicent was more erratic than ever and was becoming progressively more irritable. I thought maybe she was feeling the strains of caring for her dad and having three boarders in her house. Molly and I also noticed that our landlady wasn't monitoring her father as well when he visited. We all worried that Dick would get himself into trouble if left alone. It was a strained atmosphere, and I found myself avoiding Millicent while also trying to keep an eye on her father. I made an effort to coordinate my meals with Miko and Molly; I enjoyed their company and they were a healthy buffer against the malaise that seemed to have settled over our little home.

Then in mid-December one of the problems resolved itself. Sometimes it takes a situation becoming really bad in order for it to improve. Dick had been getting progressively more disoriented as time went on, to the extent that I could notice the difference even in the relatively short time I had known him. Most of the time his eyes were unfocused and he rarely responded when spoken to. His movements were more tentative, and he seemed to lack volition to do anything without guidance.

On the occasions where Dick did walk around, he needed constant supervision. One evening he tottered into the kitchen for a drink of water and tripped on the small floor mat in front of the sink. He fell hard and was fortunate not to break bones, receiving only a nasty gash on his forehead. It seemed obvious to me that he was not well suited for a household living situation, but I knew that Millicent would have to come to that conclusion herself before anything would change.

I happened to be there for the proverbial straw that broke the camel's back. On a cold December evening Molly, Miko, and I were making a shared dinner in the kitchen. Millicent and Dick sat watching television in the living room. As we chopped vegetables the girls and I were quietly discussing the situation in the house. All of us felt that Dick needed professional care beyond what his daughter could provide. We also agreed that something was amiss with Millicent. Whatever it was, she seemed affected enough by it that she wasn't a reliable caretaker for the old man.

We talked quietly so as not to be heard over the television. "What you think we need do?" Miko asked in her faltering English. "We no tell Millicent how to care for father. And besides, she is landlady. I don't want upset her and then have no house to stay."

"We should make more of an effort to socialize," Molly insisted. "She is aloof and shy, but she likes it when I sit and chat with her. Except for when she is in one of her real quiet moods."

"I agree," I said. "Our being friendly will make her more comfortable with us. Then she might be more forthcoming about what's on her mind. Having people to talk to can really help when dealing with stress. She doesn't work and has no close friends that I know of; we're about the only people she interacts with."

Molly nodded. "I'll bet she's lonely," she offered. "Dick's not much company to her now, and she mostly lives through the television. It's not much of an existence."

"Okay then, so we can try to make overtures," I said. "It's worth a go, though I think we need to be selective about when we do it. If she's in one of her sullen periods, I don't think I'd want to approach her."

Molly chuckled and agreed. "I still think something's not right with her," she added. "I just can't put my finger on what it is yet."

Just then Miko shushed us, whispering, "She coming now!" Looking up from my food preparation I smiled as Millicent walked into the kitchen. We all said hello and she acknowledged us gruffly as she opened the refrigerator to rummage inside.

Molly glanced at me and shrugged, then said to Millicent, "We're making dinner and we're about to sit down to eat. There's plenty if you want to join us."

Millicent looked around at us and her expression softened. "Why, that's nice of you to offer, sweetie," she replied. "I think I'll just get a snack, though; I'll eat more later when dad is in bed. Until then I have to watch him."

As she spoke, she peeked around the corner of the kitchen door into the living room, and her expression immediately clouded. "Where did he go?" she asked. "He was in the recliner a moment ago." She quickly ducked through the doorway and we crowded close behind. I scanned the living room and Dick was nowhere to be seen. The sofa and two chairs were empty. I knew he hadn't snuck past us to the bathroom or the upstairs, since he would have had to go through the kitchen. There were three other doors he could have exited through. These led to Millicent's bedroom, her sewing room, and into the foyer by the front door.

Millicent called out, "Dad? Where did you get off to?" We all listened for a reply or any noise that would tell us where he was. Just then I heard an odd sound, as of water running, but not coming from the bathroom or kitchen. It emanated from Millicent's bedroom. It took a moment of pondering, and then I looked at Molly. She returned my gaze, and by her appalled expression I could tell she also realized what was happening. It appeared Millicent knew as well judging by how fast she ran into her bedroom. She vanished inside and I could hear her exasperated words, "Dad, stop it! Oh, you had to go and try things on your own, didn't you? Well you really missed the pot this time! What a mess, and all over your shoes too! C'mon, don't step in it, sit on the bed and let me get some rags. You'll have to change. The carpet is completely soaked! What am I going to do with you?!"

The rest of us just stood silently in the living room, unsure of what to say. We all felt sorry for both Millicent and Dick. Whatever their relationship had been in the past, they now had problems that made it hard for them to enjoy each other's company. Dick wasn't mentally competent at even the most basic level, and his daughter wasn't emotionally able to deal with him on a continual basis.

As I said, sometimes things have to get worse in order to get better. The incident in the bedroom proved to be the catalyst for Millicent's decision to move her father permanently into a nursing home. She brought him to visit the house after that, but only occasionally and never for more than a couple of hours. Mostly she went to see him at his residence, which was easier for both of them. Part of me was saddened to see this transition, since I knew they had been close before his illness. It would never be the same for them again and I felt her loss. Millicent was an odd sort, besides being plain in appearance and socially inept, so she had few friends on this planet. With her father's progressive dementia, she was losing one of the few people who had really cared for her. It's a sad fact that life isn't always fair or happy, and people often don't deserve what fate hands them.

On the more positive side the household was less stressed, and a bit more sanitary, once Dick had moved out. I was able to study without constantly worrying about the feeble old man coming to harm. Even Millicent seemed less on edge with the daily responsibility of her dad's care lifted from her shoulders.

The resolution of this difficult situation came just in time for me to buckle down and focus on final exams. The amount and importance of the information the junior class had been given this term was considerable. My classmates and I were all feeling the strain of meeting the demands placed on us. The mood in class was somber, with little of the good-natured banter that usually characterized the students' interaction. Everyone was getting serious as the semester drew to a close.

It seemed that each individual had a unique approach when it came to studying. Stan Hulbert and Special Ed often got together after classes to quiz each other on their notes. Vincent Studebaker always studied alone; I suspect that in his mind no one else could teach him anything. Amy Baker and Molly Boyer retained their study partnership that had started way back in freshman anatomy class. Mike Callahan bounced around helping people when they asked for it, and pursued his own studies in his spare time. He was sharp enough to excel without really exerting himself.

As for me, I had always found that the most efficient way to learn was by myself. When it came time to study the material, I had a system that worked. My notes were logically organized in outline form, making them easier to memorize. In addition, I knew what I needed to learn, what the key points were that really counted. From there it wasn't a matter of tricks or gimmicks. Memorization was just hard work, pure and simple. It required concentration and discipline, reviewing the notes over and over again until the words became ingrained in my brain. There was no easy way around it, and I plowed headlong into the task night after night.

A student can experience a large range of emotions during finals week. In the days leading up to the exams I lived and breathed nothing but veterinary medicine. My days were spent in class, and my nights were lived on my bed pouring over notebooks. I was intensely focused, and I pushed myself until the pages blurred and my thoughts ran ragged from exhaustion. When I slept I dreamt about EKG's and arrhythmias, cataracts and retinal atrophy, horse twitches and hobbles. I had the classic stress nightmares wherein I somehow had forgotten to study for a test and sat in class totally unprepared.

At times I felt like I was mastering the material and could handle whatever the exams threw at me. Other times, especially late at night, I despaired of ever learning it all. When I left my friends and classmates at school and went home to study, it came down to just me against the notes. There was no one who could make it easier or help carry the load. As I stared at page after page late into the night, my wife and family were far away and probably sleeping comfortably in their beds. There is no lonelier feeling than struggling in solitude to excel.

Then came the exams themselves and the rush of anticipation, filled to the bursting with hard-won knowledge humming along the synapses of my brain. The adrenaline flowing as I reviewed key points in the hallway one final time before stepping into the classroom, seeing the line of classmates waiting their turns at the door of the usually vacant men's room, bladders twitching from the combined effects of stress and caffeine.

Best of all was that sense of triumph partway through an exam when I realized that I knew the material, really *knew* it, and that success was mine for the taking. I loved the rush of supreme confidence that came when even the trickiest of questions seemed simple, and the answers rolled off my pen onto the paper as if I had known them all my life. Knowing how much work I had put in to get to that point made it all the more satisfying.

Lastly, there was the utter peace of mind I felt when the final page of the last exam had been completed, and nothing remained but the promise of a well-deserved vacation. Especially when I could take that break knowing I had done well. It made the hard work, the stress, and the separation I endured while pursuing my dreams all seem worthwhile.

CHAPTER FORTY-EIGHT

Christmas break was everything the holidays should be. By that I mean it was lazy, lengthy, and entirely devoid of work. It also was a time for me to again spend quality moments with Cindy and with both our families. Fortunately, Cindy's employer let her take a vacation between Christmas and New Year's, so she was able to travel.

In Bend we enjoyed again the brisk, dry days of the high desert winter. Christmas morning we opened gifts with Cindy's family, sitting around the big tree in the living room, sharing the warmth and giving of the season.

We drove to Medford the day after Christmas and had a fabulous time there as well. My mom and dad were delighted to see us, and we had another round of gift-opening the evening we arrived. I also was treated to my mother's cooking which tasted even better than I remembered. Absence, it seemed, did make the heart grow fonder, or at least it had that effect on the stomach.

We spent several days with my parents, resting and visiting as I soaked up the ambience of my childhood home. One afternoon dad and I puttered in the garage together working on little home projects. He wagged his finger and told me, "Now that you are married, son, you can officially 'putter.'"

Cindy and I headed back to Beaverton before New Year's Day since we wanted to have some time alone before I traveled to school again. Once there we made the most of our opportunity, dining out and sleeping in, browsing through quaint little antique shops in the town of Aurora one afternoon, and enjoying quiet time together in the evenings.

One other noteworthy event happened that holiday. Cindy had been wanting a pet, and we had talked about what sort of animal to get. The apartment wasn't spacious, and neither of us had time for a high-maintenance animal. My older brother Stan had had an albino ferret when I was a teenager. I had played with it on many occasions, and had found its silly antics very appealing. Cindy was intrigued by my descriptions, and thought that she would like one as well. We searched the want ads in the local papers and soon found an owner with a young female ferret for sale.

We drove out to a residential area on the west side of Beaverton and located the address we had been given. The house was a modest, ranch-style place set well back from the road behind a large front yard. A stately old oak tree stood in the middle of the lawn, one of its thick branches supporting a car tire swing dangling from a length of heavy rope. We stepped around two bicycles piled on the ground near the front door and rang the bell.

A frenzied barking immediately erupted from within the house, and I heard a woman's voice yell, "Sadie! Knock it off!" The barking subsided except for an occasional yip, and in a moment the door opened. A petite brunette woman in her mid-thirties looked out at us and said, "Yes, what can I do for you?"

I answered, "Hi, we're here to take a look at your ferret that's for sale."

The woman smiled and said, "Oh, yes, you're the one I talked to on the phone. C'mon in!" She backed up to allow us to squeeze past her, and then closed the front door behind us. Once inside, we were confronted with a large Dalmatian whose tail wagged incessantly as she pushed her way forward to greet us. "Never mind Sadie; she'll do you no harm other than licking you to death," the woman said. "She's not got a bit of common sense, and I'm sure she'd invite a burglar right in as well. But she sounds impressive when she barks at the door, so I figure maybe that's good for something."

The woman led us back into the house, chatting all the while. "Excuse the mess, I've got three kids and they never clean up after themselves. They're at their friends' house for the afternoon; it gives me a break from the noise," she laughed.

We followed her into a small bedroom and saw a wire cage sitting in one corner. "Here's the little one you're interested in," the woman said, gesturing at the cage. "She's only about five months old and she's a sweetie. She was given to us by friends who were moving away, but we have too many pets already. Ferrets tend to be nocturnal, so she sleeps a lot during the day. We call her Bandit, but I'm sure you can come up with your own name for her."

Peering down at the enclosure, I couldn't see the animal in question. The woman opened the cage and reached in under some old towels that covered the bottom. When her hand emerged, it held a slender fuzzy bundle that squirmed and opened small, round, black eyes at us. The animal's fur was lovely, with long, charcoal-colored guard hairs sprinkled over a white undercoat. Its feet and tail were solid black, and the tiny eyes were framed by a dark mask similar to that of a raccoon.

As we stared at the beautiful creature, a narrow pink tongue licked the pointed nose, and then it yawned wide, showing off tiny canines like those of a kitten. It stretched its front paws out in a human-like gesture, and then proceeded to wiggle in its owner's grip. "I think she wants down," the woman told us. She set the little animal on the floor and it immediately began capering around, bouncing up and down on its four short legs like it was on springs. The ferret made little excited grunting noises as it explored the room, pushing its elfin face into a pair of shoes on the floor and tipping a garbage can over to investigate its contents. Cindy and I laughed with delight at the odd manner in which the animal moved. Its long body walked humped up in the middle like an inchworm caterpillar, with the front and back legs seeming to move independently of each other. The effect reminded me of two men inside of an animal costume, neither one knowing what the other was doing, so their legs were unsynchronized and at times they pushed close together or lagged farther apart as they tried to walk as one.

"Can I pick her up?" asked Cindy, her eyes dancing with amusement.

"Oh yes, just grab her, she won't bite or anything," the woman said with an offhand wave.

Cindy bent down and grabbed the little furry creature around the middle. The pointed face swiveled to look at her hand but otherwise did nothing. She brought the ferret over for me to see as well, and we took turns holding her. She was warm and soft, slender but lithely muscular in our hands. A faint musky smell reached my nose, and I remembered my brother's ferret having a similar scent. Neutering greatly reduced a ferret's odor, as well as preventing some health problems, and I knew that I would need to take care of that when she was old enough.

With that thought I realized that I was already imagining the little animal as my pet. I looked at Cindy inquiringly and said, "Well, what do you think?"

She nodded and smiled at me. "I like her a lot." Turning to the woman, Cindy asked, "How does she interact with other animals?"

Our hostess grinned broadly. "She seems to like everyone okay. I'd be careful with dogs, since they could easily harm her. Sadie is curious, but she's so big I'm worried about her stepping on Bandit. I don't leave them unattended together. The adult cats mostly stay out of the ferret's way, since she likes to jump on them to play. That offends their sense of dignity. The kitten on the other hand...well let me show you!"

The woman took Bandit and led us down the hall to the living room. There we found a tabby kitten maybe three or four months old curled up on an easy chair. The woman picked up the kitten and put it on the floor, where it stood and stretched just as the ferret had done. Then she put Bandit down and when the ferret's legs hit the floor she made a beeline for the cat. The two animals came together and immediately transformed into a single ball of fur, rolling around wrestling and playing as if it were the most natural thing in the world. We watched fascinated for quite a while before the woman separated the two and handed the ferret back to us. "Well, what do you think?" she asked us. "We're asking thirty dollars for her."

Cindy and I looked at each other and we both nodded. "We think she's great!" I said to the woman. "Yes, we'll take her." And so it was that Cindy and I found our first pet.

The woman included the ferret's cage, water bottle, and food dish in the purchase price, so we came home fully equipped. We stopped at a pet store and got a bag of good quality kitten food, which is what the owner had been feeding her. Back then there were few ferret diets available in stores, but kitten kibble was a decent alternative, since it approximated the nutritional needs of these tiny carnivores.

The remainder of my vacation with Cindy was highlighted by watching Dixie (our new name for her) frolic and play in our apartment. She was friendly, spunky, and charmingly clumsy. If we waved our hands and got her excited, she would hop and spin around wildly, often running headlong into a wall or piece of furniture. When we passed by, she would jump out at our feet in a play attack. We quickly learned not to walk barefoot unless we were prepared for an occasional nip on our toes.

Finally the time arrived for me to return to Tullville. This would be my last stint in the eastern Washington town. When I came home to Oregon again, it would be for good. Cindy was quiet as I packed my suitcase, and as I prepared to depart, I held her close for a moment and lifted her chin with my finger. She looked up at me, her expression glum. "Hey now," I chided her. "Let's have none of that. I'll be back before you know it, and no more of these trips to Tullville ever again."

"No, you'll be off to Corvine for another year instead," she pouted.

"That's only ninety minutes away instead of six hours," I reminded her. "I'll be able to come home on the weekends, classes permitting. Two days all to ourselves, every week." She brightened up at that, and I kissed her goodbye.

When we pulled apart she smiled bravely and said, "Good luck in school. Call me when you arrive in Tullville, please! I worry about you driving those winding country roads in winter."

"I'll be careful," I assured her, and I gave her one last hug before I headed down the steps to my car. I toted Dixie's cage in one hand; she needed to be spayed, and I had a small animal surgery block coming up. The professors had told us that if our pets needed surgeries we could perform them ourselves, provided the procedures were within our capabilities. It seemed a perfect opportunity. Dixie would get her spay free of charge and I would get some much-needed practice with the scalpel.

The trip to Tullville that day was blissfully uneventful. Traffic was less than usual, and the skies spit nothing worse than rain showers. I hit my destination at the refreshingly early hour of five P.M. When I phoned Cindy, I noted with wry amusement the surprise in her voice when she realized what time it was. We talked for awhile, and then I got busy unpacking my clothes and checking the coming day's schedule. I would be starting the small animal medicine block, which would include examining new patients as they were checked in, feeding and treating hospitalized cases, and working side by side with the staff clinicians. After a few weeks of this, I would begin my small animal surgery block, again assisting with real hospital patients. When that was finished, my Tullville curriculum would be completed and I would leave this town, never to return. There was finally light at the end of the vet school tunnel, and I couldn't wait to come out the other side.

CHAPTER FORTY-NINE

The Doberman pinscher looked half-dead when they rushed it into the ER. The big male dog was only five years old, and was a beautiful example of his breed, deep-chested with narrow hips, his sleek frame covered with rippling muscles. But his eyes were glazed and staring unseeingly at the wall, his breath coming in agonized wheezes as his head lolled weakly side to side. One glance at his abdomen told the story: it was grossly distended and the skin was stretched tight as a drum. He was suffering from an acute gastric dilatation, commonly called a bloat.

When the dog was brought into the teaching hospital, the admitting veterinarian had taken one look at him and had sent the critically ill animal straight up to the emergency room. We placed the patient on the treatment table, and the supervising doctor directed the student assistants to get a TPR (temperature, pulse, and respiratory rate) stat. While this was being done, I helped shave and scrub a forelimb to place an IV catheter. The ER veterinarian that day was Dr. Deborah Torrey, a slender young veterinarian from Texas who spoke with a southern drawl. This was her first job after completing an internal medicine residency. She was energetic and quick thinking, and the students looked up to her as an example of what they might someday become.

The ER used staff technicians and junior students to assist the doctors. Dr. Torrey directed the proceedings while she did a quick assessment of the dog. "His gums are pale and tacky," she muttered. A frown creased her forehead as she quickly poked and prodded, moving from head to tail in her examination. When she flicked her finger against the turgid flank, I heard a distinct echo from within the animal's abdomen. "Wow, he's tight," the doctor remarked, shaking her head. Raising her voice she called out, "What's the TPR?"

"He's cold, the temp is ninety-six," the student with the thermometer answered.

"Pulse is one-sixty and weak," another student piped up. "Respirations are around ninety-five and shallow."

The doctor nodded. "Put a mask on him and give him oxygen; he's not down enough to intubate him. And get a liter of Lactated Ringer's warmed and ready," she instructed. "Add five milliequivalents of sodium bicarbonate per kilogram of body weight to the Ringer's. Also give him two milligrams per kilogram of dexamethasone sodium phosphate. How much does this boy weigh?"

"Forty kilograms [about ninety pounds]," came the answer.

"Fine. We'll run a shock drip rate to start. Give me a twenty-gauge IV catheter. Then find an eighteen-gauge needle and a large stomach tube quickly." She turned back to me and surveyed my shave and scrub of the dog's forelimb. "Good," she said. "Let's see if we can find a blood vessel; this guy's in shock and likely has no blood pressure. Hold off the vein for me."

Grasping the dog's leg at the elbow, I used my thumb to clamp down on the cephalic vein which ran from the elbow to the wrist. With the blood flow occluded, the vein reluctantly stood up under the shaved and alcohol-wetted skin. The doctor grabbed the IV catheter from a student, and as I watched, she deftly threaded it into the vein on her first try. Dark red blood came welling up the needle. She quickly taped the catheter in place and attached the IV line from the bag of Ringer's. She started the IV pump and we watched the liquid begin to run from the bag into the patient. Shock fluid rates are aggressive and this was no slow drip. The solution was being pumped in rapidly, to stabilize the dog's blood pressure and correct the electrolyte imbalances he was likely struggling with. The bag had been preheated in a microwave, but we also ran the IV line through a bowl of hot water to keep it warm on its way to the patient.

"Okay, we've got a line in," the doctor declared. "Use one of his other veins and try to get blood to check chemistries and electrolytes. While you're doing that, let's get the stomach decompressed if we can. Prep a spot here," she said, pointing to an area of skin directly over the bloated flank. The students rapidly shaved a patch about a hand's breadth in diameter, and then scrubbed it with iodine soap and alcohol. As soon as the last scrub was completed, the doctor took the eighteen-gauge injection needle and stabbed it into the turgid stomach. A hiss and foul smell erupted as the accumulated gas vented through the needle.

"Phew!" gasped a female student who was bending over to observe the procedure. "That would gag a maggot!"

A second student chimed in, "Smells like Dr. Payne's cologne."

Dr. Torrey smirked despite herself. "I'll tell him you said that," she threatened with a twinkle in her eye. We watched as the pressure was relieved and the stomach became visibly less distended. The doctor gently pressed on the dog's abdomen to help evacuate the gas. When stomach fluid began to drain from the needle, the doctor attached a large syringe to suck out as much as possible. Despite her efforts, the flow soon became clogged with bits of food and hair in the stomach contents.

"That's all we're going to get with the syringe," Dr. Torrey said as she pulled the needle out. "Give me the stomach tube."

A student handed her what looked like a length of rubber garden hose. She applied lube to one end and said, "Someone find me a mouth gag. Our patient is only semi-conscious, but he still has some jaw tone, and I want to go home with all my digits attached."

A steel mouth gag was found and used to jack open the Doberman's jaws. He barely reacted as the doctor slid the tube down his throat and attempted to empty the stomach. "Damn," she exclaimed after she tried several times to advance the tube. "It's not going past the cardiac sphincter. The stomach must be torsed."

My heart sank at those words. A gastric torsion was worse than a simple bloat. When a dog's stomach became overly full and heavy, such as after consuming a large amount of food and water, then it could occasionally twist on its axis, flipping over inside of the abdomen. When that occurred, the entrance and exit to the stomach were twisted shut, much like twisting the end of a plastic bag to keep it from leaking. A torsed stomach could not empty. As gas was produced from fermentation of the ingested food, the bloating would get worse, with no chance of relieving the pressure. The dog couldn't vomit, nor could he eliminate the fluid and gas via the bowel. Worse yet, a stomach tube couldn't be passed to drain the contents.

A short time later we viewed the radiographs that had quickly been taken of the dog's abdomen. Sure enough, the stomach not only was distended, it also lacked the typical shape I had grown accustomed to seeing on X-rays. The reason: the organ was twisted completely out of its normal position.

"We don't have a lot of choice here," Dr. Torrey concluded. "We're going to have to cut him to relieve the torsion and empty the stomach. How's his color? Recheck his temp while you're at it."

"He's pinker now," came the reply.

"Temp is at 98.5," another student chimed in a moment later.

"Good, we're making some progress," the doctor nodded. "Someone run down to surgery and see who's on. Let them know we've got a torsion that needs a laparotomy pronto." She took out her stethoscope and listened to the dog's heart for a minute, then frowned. "His rhythm is irregular. I think he's throwing PVC's. Get an EKG on him right now; I want to see what his heart is doing."

A technician ran to one of the cupboards, and quickly returned with a machine. They ran electrical leads to the dog's four limbs and turned on the readout. I looked at the now familiar waves of the heartbeats depicted on the graph paper as it rolled off the spool. My eye caught the problem right away: interspersed with the normal electrical complexes, I saw large bizarre waves that looked totally out of place. "See here," Dr. Torrey pointed at one of the interlopers. "This wave came before the next normal beat would have happened; it's a premature ventricular complex or PVC. This dog is sick enough that his heart is being affected; the muscle is contracting spasmodically before the pacemaker is telling it to beat. If this happens too frequently, the heart chambers could become totally uncoordinated. Then the heart might abruptly stop."

"What do we do?" asked Bruce Braden, one of my Oregon classmates in the group.

"You tell me," Dr. Torrey replied, turning to look at him. "You've all had cardiology, yes? What's the treatment for ventricular arrhythmias?"

Bruce hesitated, looking uncertain. After a moment Mike Callahan spoke up, "You can treat it acutely with intravenous lidocaine, followed by quinidine or procainamide for longer-term maintenance if needed."

"Very good!" the doctor replied. "Someone's been paying attention in class. Get me some lidocaine and we'll infuse a small dose into his IV drip. Monitor the EKG and we'll see how he responds."

The calculated dose was injected into the IV line, where it mixed with the fluids being pumped into the dog. Over the next few minutes we watched intently as the drug took effect. Initially the PVC's were occurring with every third or fourth heartbeat; there were even some clusters of several abnormal beats in a row. But as the lidocaine distributed into the bloodstream, it began to inhibit the random contractions. Slowly, gradually, the PVC's tapered off until we only saw one every thirty beats or so.

Dr. Torrey sighed and nodded. "That's much better," she proclaimed. "Now at least he's got a chance of getting through surgery. Let's get him up there; leave his IV line attached and bring the pump as we move him."

A stretcher was brought alongside the table and we gently slid the ailing dog onto it. He whined and tried to lift his head as we handled him; he was definitely more aware than when he had come in. I took one end of the stretcher and Mike Callahan took the other. Another student rolled the IV pump on its stand alongside us to keep the fluids running. We moved the patient quickly down the hallway to the surgery department. A technician waved us into a surgery prep area where they rapidly shaved the dog's entire belly.

Once our patient passed into the surgery ward, he was under the care of the surgeons and of the students in the small animal surgery block who were assisting. I was taking the medicine block at the time, so I couldn't participate in the procedure. However, the surgeon allowed Mike and I to stand in the operatory and observe while they tried to save the dog.

In surgery everything was a blur of coordinated movement. The surgeon scrubbed and gowned while the technicians prepped the patient on the table. An instrument pack was opened and waiting as the doctor pulled on his gloves. He grabbed a scalpel as soon as the dog was draped and made a bold incision that would have laid open my arm from wrist to elbow. Once through the skin the surgeon quickly found the white center line of the muscle layer and cut through it to enter the dog's abdomen. As he did the bloated stomach tried to pop up through the incision.

"Retractors, please," the doctor said, holding out his hand. A student handed him the instrument, and he pulled the skin open wide to allow us to see into the body cavity. Most of the abdomen was filled with the still-distended stomach which looked to be several times normal size. The organ was blotchy and dark red in places, entirely unlike the healthy light pink I was accustomed to seeing. It also seemed to be sitting backwards, at least from the angle I was viewing it, and I had a hard time orienting myself as to what went where.

"He's definitely torsed," the surgeon commented. "The stomach wall looks fairly viable; we may have caught this one in time. Now we've got to straighten this guy out." So saying, he grabbed the enlarged organ and gently lifted it. The stomach did a slow flip and suddenly everything made sense again. The restored anatomy looked like the drawings in the books and I could easily get my bearings.

"Pass the gastric tube now, slowly," the doctor instructed. "We'll see if we can empty this stomach."

The student who was assisting him looked up in surprise and asked, "Aren't you going to open the stomach to drain it?"

"Not unless I have to," the surgeon answered. "Why make an incision on a less than healthy stomach which might not heal readily? And at the same time let out a ton of nasty material to contaminate our surgery site? If we can flush and drain the stomach non-invasively, then that's what we'll do." I nodded at the simple logic.

It made perfect sense now that he said it, but I have to admit I had been expecting the stomach to be opened as well.

A technician slid the stomach tube down the dog's throat and slowly advanced it. With the torsion relieved, the tube passed easily through the esophagus and into the stomach. We could see the end of it moving within the organ like a finger probing the inside of a cloth bag. The doctor said, "Okay, it's far enough in. Hook up the pump and pull out what you can."

The tech attached a hand pump to the stomach tube, assisted by a student who held a bucket under the pump. As the tech worked the handle, the pump began to spew foul brownish liquid and solid chunks into the bucket. The acrid odors of fermented food and gastric juices immediately permeated the room. The surgeon massaged the dog's stomach, working its contents toward the tube which then sucked the material away. The bloated organ held an impressive amount, and the bucket was filled and emptied again before the surgeon said, "Okay that's got most of it out. Flush warm water through the tube now and we'll lavage the stomach."

The technician reversed the pump flow and sucked clean water from a bucket into the stomach. The surgeon massaged the organ, sloshing the liquid around to loosen any retained food particles. When he was done, the technician aspirated the contents back out again. "There, it should be pretty clean now," the doctor pronounced with satisfaction. "How's our patient doing?"

The anesthetist said, "His vitals are good. Strong steady heart beat, good oxygenation. His color is nice and pink now."

"Great," the surgeon said. "I'd better do a gastropexy on this guy or he may torse again. He sounds stable enough to keep down a little longer. Hand me some suture."

It's well known that dogs who have had a torsion are highly prone to reoccurrence. A gastropexy is a procedure where the stomach is surgically fastened to the body wall. This holds it in its normal position so that it cannot flip over in the future. I watched as the surgeon used heavy gauge suture to attach the stomach to the inner abdominal wall, anchoring it firmly. When he was done, he briefly inspected the rest of the organs in the abdomen and pronounced, "It's time to get out of here!"

He grabbed suture for the closure, then he paused and cocked his head. He looked around at us and winked, saying, "I'm no Dr. Brakel, but my mantra for the day is, 'You've got to have guts to be a GI surgeon.'" We all groaned in unison.

Once our patient was out of surgery, he became a ward of the medicine department again. Mike Callahan and I were among those assigned to treat the dog post operatively. He continued on an IV drip for two days, and also received pain medications and antibiotics twice a day. We learned from his chart that his name was Adolph.

Adolph showed amazing recuperative powers and was standing the morning after his surgery. Looking at him, you would never know that he had been inches from death twelve hours earlier. Fortunately for us he was also a very nice dog, stoic and well-mannered. His incision looked great and he didn't seem to be licking it excessively. The surgeon checked in on him that morning and pronounced him to be "in excellent shape, considering his ordeal." The internist who was managing Adolph told us to give him small amounts of water throughout the day. If the dog was able to drink without problems, then a watery food gruel would be offered starting that afternoon.

Later that day Adolph's family came to visit. They looked like a typical suburban American family, a thirty-something mom and dad with two excited little boys in tow. I showed them back to the kennel, and when the dog saw them he leapt to his feet, legs prancing and rear end wagging furiously. The family poked fingers through the kennel bars and Adolph licked them, whining. The father said, "He looks good! How is he doing?"

I answered, "So far he's recovering nicely. We've not got him on food yet, but he came through the surgery with flying colors. You can tell that he feels pretty good today. Would you like to pet him?"

One of the boys clapped his hands and said, "Yeah! Can we?"

I knelt down to face him and said, "Well, we'll have to keep him from getting too excited. We don't want his IV line getting pulled out! I'll open the kennel door and hold him so that he stays put. Then you can all say 'hi' and pet him, okay?" The boy nodded, his eyes wide as he looked at my smock and stethoscope. He probably thought I was a doctor and he appeared quite impressed.

I grinned and opened the kennel door, catching the dog by the collar so he couldn't leap out. The family took turns greeting their pet, and the little boy who had spoken wrapped his arms around the animal's muscular neck and said, "We love you, Adolph!"

The mother said, "I can't believe how much better he looks now. He was so sick I was afraid we were going to lose him. The kids just adore Adolph. Thank you all so much for saving his life." She wiped away a couple of tears from her eyes, and I smiled back at her. It felt great to help save a patient, and it was obvious that two little boys were going to be very happy having their companion around for years to come. I had worked hard and sacrificed much to reach the point where I could begin to make a difference. Adolph was one of the first patients I had a direct hand in treating. Seeing his outcome reaffirmed the conviction I had felt when first embarking on my career.

CHAPTER FIFTY

The weather in January was typical of Tullville in winter: bitterly cold and blustery. Several snowstorms hit within a two-week span of time, cloaking the town in frozen precipitation. On these midwinter days the chill was pervasive. As I walked my breath crystallized on my face, forming a crusty layer of ice on my beard by the time I reached my destination.

One frigid afternoon I arrived home, rubbing my hands and stomping my feet as I closed the door. The house was empty and quiet. I removed my coat and got a snack from the fridge. Awhile later, with my hunger curbed, I opened a notebook and sat in the living room studying.

After an indeterminate time the front door opened and Millicent walked in, snow swirling around her. She came through the door from the foyer and just stood there, saying nothing. I glanced up curiously and noticed that she was staring blankly straight ahead. An alarm bell rang in the back of my head, and I asked her, "What's wrong, Millicent?"

She said nothing for a minute, her face devoid of expression. Finally she looked at me and in a voice equally lifeless said, "He's dead."

I sat up abruptly, my studies forgotten. "Who is?" I asked.

Again the hesitation, then, "My dad," she said softly.

Stunned, I put the notebook down and blurted, "How can that be? What happened? He looked just fine yesterday!"

She shook her head and looked down at the floor. "Oh, he's alive, I guess you'd say. But he didn't even know who I was today. He's gone. I can see it in his eyes. He looks like my dad, but there's no one inside anymore."

Once again her normally gruff voice was a hollow monotone, like all the life had been drained from her. She looked devastated standing there with her arms at her sides, her hands clutching her leather gloves as if they didn't know what else to do. I felt that I should say something, but my tongue stumbled on the words. Finally I said, "Millicent, there's nothing you could have done to prevent his illness, no way to anticipate such a thing happening. I'm sure he's getting the best of care and he's not suffering at all. Remember that he cares for you, even if he can't express it any more."

She nodded and stood there for a moment longer, then shuffled slowly into her bedroom. I sat on the sofa dazed, wondering if she was going to be all right. In truth her father's decline was beyond her control, but I knew how much she cared for him. I was concerned over how she would handle this latest blow. Doubtless she would feel more alone than ever now. I wasn't sure what I could do, but I vowed to help her in any way that I could.

The next day before school I talked to Molly and Miko at breakfast, and they agreed that we should keep an eye on Millicent and try to be supportive to her during this emotionally difficult time. For once we were able to talk freely in the dining nook, since our usually early-to-rise landlady was still asleep in her room when I left for school.

Once at the vet building, I had to refocus on the tasks at hand. That week my medicine block included a stint with Dr. Brisbane treating ophthalmology cases. His interactions with me varied, but tended to fall into two basic patterns. The first was ignoring the fact that I existed, which probably constituted ninety percent of our doctor-student collaboration. Interspersed with this quality time were occasional sermons from the mountain wherein he expounded on the depth of his ophthalmologic experience and knowledge. There was only one right way to do things, and Dr. Brisbane would show me the error of my ways if I contemplated any deviation from his teachings.

My days were spent trailing behind the aloof little man and trying to absorb some ocular wisdom. Sometimes I would take in a new case, greeting the client in the exam room and checking the pet's weight and temperature. I'd also talk to the family and get a case history. This included asking what signs the patient was exhibiting, and reviewing any prior records or treatments done by the referring veterinarian. Then when the groundwork was laid, Dr. Brisbane would enter the room in all his glory and save the day. Our clients loved it.

The junior students were less enthralled. However, we did manage to have some fun at his expense. In addition to his arrogant perfectionism, Dr. Brisbane had certain attributes that made him an easy target for jokes. He was tiny in stature, and his delicate facial features were offset by (ironically, to my mind) disproportionately large, bulging eyes. The effect reminded me of a hatchling bird, the ones that don't have proper feathers yet and sit with their mouths wide open while the mother drops in a worm.

The bug-eyed look was enhanced beyond belief when Dr. Brisbane donned his ocular loupes. These were magnifying glasses that attached to headgear, and could be flipped down in front of his eyes when he examined a patient. He wore them almost constantly during clinical rounds, and whenever he looked at you through them his eyes were like two moons. When he blinked, it was enough to make you cringe reflexively.

Unlike the other clinicians who often chose colorful doctors' smocks, Dr. Brisbane always wore a long white lab coat. Combined with his nervous energy and twitchy mannerisms, his appearance closely approximated that of a mad scientist as featured in old horror movies. Amy Baker coined the name "Dr. Greeble," and for some odd reason it fit perfectly. She would bob her head and wring her hands together, blinking fast as she said in a thin reedy voice, "There is only one way to treat a severe glaucoma case, and I'm going to share with you that knowledge, yes I will. Please take notes!" She had the professor's mannerisms down pat, and the students around her would break into laughter at her antics. I had to watch myself though, as I nearly addressed the good doctor by the name of Greeble on a couple of occasions.

Despite his eccentric ways, Dr. Brisbane knew his ophthalmology, and I learned a lot during my days spent at his side. The following week I was walking down a hospital corridor when I passed a clinician and two students examining an Akita. The large dog looked up at me as I walked by. As it did so the ceiling lights glinted off its eyes.

Many species have reflective surfaces on the back of their retinas which helps their night vision. This is what we see when a car's headlights make a forest animal's eyes light up. Seen at close range this reflection is usually blurred into a smooth glow by the eye's lens; you can't see any details of the back of the eye without an ophthalmoscope. But when the Akita glanced at me its right eye reflected back a bright glitter and I could have sworn I saw its retinal blood vessels for a brief instant. The only way that could happen would be if the lens was no longer obstructing my view.

I stopped in my tracks and exclaimed, "That dog has a luxated lens!"

The doctor who was working with the patient looked surprised and said, "How could you know that?"

"I saw the retina clearly as I walked by," I replied grinning. "That's not possible unless the lens has moved out of the way."

"Very good!" the doctor complimented. "My students took a while with the ophthalmoscope before they came to that conclusion."

I walked off feeling quite confident about my clinical skills. My self-esteem was still flying high later in the week when I was brought abruptly and jarringly back to earth. One of the cases I was helping with was an old Australian Shepherd with chronic bloody diarrhea. Antibiotics had provided only temporary relief, and the clinicians were worried about a serious lesion in the bowel. The case was being handled by a young doctor who was doing her residency at the university, preparatory to becoming certified in internal medicine. Dr. Tamara Harris was quick and energetic, and her enthusiasm for medicine was unbounded, but as a recent graduate her communication skills weren't her forte, as I was to find out.

Dr. Harris approached me one afternoon and said, "Mark, I want you to assist me with doing an endoscopy on the bowel case. We'll need to perform an enema beforehand to clean out the gut so we can see what's going on in there. I'll meet you here around ten A.M. tomorrow to do the procedure, okay?" That seemed straightforward enough, so I agreed and jotted a reminder to myself in my pocket notebook.

The next day at the appointed time I waited in the staff lounge adjacent to the hospital wards. Dr. Harris arrived shortly after ten o'clock. Looking a bit harried she said, "Okay, we've not got a lot of time, so let's get going. You got the enema done earlier, I assume?"

I stopped and stared at her, and managed to say, "Umm, no, I thought we were going to do that now."

She gave me an exasperated look and exclaimed, "You can't do an enema right before an endoscopy! It will inflame the gut lining and affect the biopsy results. I told you to get it done ahead of time! That's just marvelous. Now we can't do the procedure at all this morning; we'll have to reschedule it. Can't I rely on you for anything?"

Her voice rose angrily as she spoke so that everyone in the lounge, faculty and students alike, were staring at us. I could feel my cheeks burning up as I stood and listened to her tirade. She had quite a few choice words for my perceived shoddy performance. I stood silently until she was done talking, nodding occasionally, and wishing that we were somewhere much less populated.

When my tongue-lashing was over, I slunk off to the hospital ward to check on my other patients. Instead of strutting proudly down the corridors I now tried to appear as inconspicuous as possible. But the word spread of my supposed mistake, and I was the recipient of more than one disapproving scowl from other clinicians in the days following.

I did learn one thing from that episode, and it has proven true through my entire career to date. Any time you feel that you have achieved a mastery of the medical arts, something will come along to dispel that notion and bring your ego crashing down. Maybe that's why they call it medical "practice." You never get it perfect no matter how long you work at it, and you eventually retire knowing that there was still more to learn.

CHAPTER FIFTY-ONE

My housemates and I were growing more concerned about Millicent as the days went by. She spent most of her time sleeping or brooding silently in the easy chair in the living room. Though often brusque, she had always been active and full of life. Her current behavior was a major shift from the norm. "She isn't doing anything but sitting all day long," Molly whispered to Miko and me over dinner one evening. "I had no classes today so I've been home the entire time. I can't recall seeing Millicent eat anything since I got up this morning. She's taking her father's decline hard, and I don't think she's looking after her own health. It's got me really worried."

Miko added, "She not speak now, just sit. Sometimes with no television on, just sitting. Very strange."

I agreed that Millicent was in need of some help, but what exactly we should do was uncertain. Both Molly and Miko had exams coming up over the next two days, so we decided to keep a close eye on our landlady for now, and see if she could work through her emotional turmoil. For our part we would be friendly and try to involve her in activities such as preparing meals together.

The following morning I was up and off to school early. Over the next couple of days the demands of veterinary education occupied most of my waking hours. Molly and Miko also led the busy lives of graduate students. Since Millicent hadn't done anything to catch our attention, I must admit that she went mostly overlooked until three days later.

On the evening of the third day I arrived home late from school, brushing off the snow from my coat and ice from my hair as I entered the house. Millicent sat in her rocking chair in the living room and I said hello to her. She nodded but gave no verbal reply. I smiled at her and then proceeded into the kitchen, since I was famished. The hospital had had several high-maintenance patients, including an old tomcat with severe heart and kidney disease. It had taken longer than usual to do all the patient assessments, treatments and chart write ups.

I fixed myself a quick dinner and ate alone at the dining table. When I was done, I cleaned my dishes in the kitchen sink. It was then that I noticed dishware from a meal Millicent had prepared days earlier. The plate and glass still sat in the sink unwashed. This was totally unlike her, since she always insisted on a neat and tidy house. Moreover, I could see that no new dishes had been added since. It seemed unlikely that Millicent would have cleaned up after recent meals while leaving older dishes soiled. I had to conclude that she had not prepared any food for herself for several days.

I contemplated that sobering fact for a moment, then I walked into the living room to talk to her. She sat rocking and staring straight ahead at the opposite wall. I moved around to stand in front of her and asked, "Are you feeling all right, Millicent? Do you want something to eat?"

I got no response, just the same steady gaze while she continued rocking in her chair. I tried again, "Millicent, can I get you anything?"

After a moment she shifted her eyes to look up at me, and she said, "You can get me my money back."

That threw me off stride for a moment, but after a surprised pause I asked, "What money, Millicent? Are you missing some money?"

She nodded slowly, still rocking, and said, "Molly made some cash disappear out of my purse. I had twenty dollars in there and it's gone."

"I can't imagine Molly stole from your purse," I told her. "It's probably just misplaced, or maybe you spent it and forgot about it. Molly's not a thief."

"I didn't say she stole it," Millicent answered. "She made it disappear. I watched her. She made the bills float up into mid-air and disappear right in front of me."

Suddenly I felt reality become disjointed and a small chill ran up my spine. With those few words, so matter-of-factly stated, it became clear to me that Millicent was not well, not well at all. I struggled for something to say, finally managing, "Well, I'm sure the money will reappear soon. For now try to get some rest, okay? I'll check in on you later."

I backed out of the living room and headed upstairs to talk to Molly and Miko. There was no light shining from under their doors and I remembered that this was Friday. They had planned to go to a party together and would not be back until late. Until then I was completely on my own. I descended the stairs and headed back to my bedroom.

Not knowing what else to do, I studied alone in my room until the hour was late. It was difficult to concentrate, as Millicent's eerie comments kept intruding, the scene in the living room replaying over and over in my head. Finally I called it quits when I realized I was too tired to remember what I had just read. Closing my notebooks, I got up and headed into the bathroom to prepare for bed. After brushing my teeth I hesitated, torn between the tantalizing escape of sleep and the need to check on Millicent once more. My conscience won out and I walked slowly down the hall, through the kitchen, and into the main room.

The lights in the living room were off and I breathed easier, thinking that Millicent had gone to bed. I took a few steps into the darkened room to check for light under her bedroom door. Just then a faint sound behind me made me whirl, my heart pounding. The dim outline of a figure sat in the rocking chair, backlit faintly from the hall light. I could see that she was looking directly at me but the details of her face were hidden, her eyes two black hollows. She said nothing, just sitting there staring at me in the dark.

I licked my lips and tried to slow my breathing. Clearing my throat, I ventured, "Hi Millicent, I see you're still up. I was just heading to bed myself and thought I'd come say goodnight."

She stirred but didn't reply. I tried again, "Can I get you anything before I turn in?"

Another pause, and then she spoke. "I know what you're up to."

"What do you mean?" I asked, feeling apprehensive as I waited for her answer.

"You and that girl, Molly. I know what you two are doing."

"What are we doing?"

"Making my things disappear." The words were spoken softly, but they made the hairs rise at the nape of my neck. I didn't know how to respond, so I just stood there speechless. Millicent began rocking in the chair, the *creak, creak* of the springs grating on my ears in the dead silence of the room. I felt an icy flicker of fear brush my thoughts. It was odd, as I was still standing in the mundane confines of the familiar living room, but confronting that strangeness in the darkness was enough to raise my primal alarms.

I drew a deep breath and broke the tableau by saying, "Well, I'm going to bed now. I hope you get some sleep. It's important to look after your health. We all enjoy having you around, you know."

Millicent made a noncommittal noise and I waited for her to speak but nothing was forthcoming.

"Well...good night then," I said awkwardly and stepped out of the room back into the kitchen. The brightly-lit hallway leading to my bedroom beckoned like a sanctuary. I had to force my feet to walk at a calm steady pace until I got into my room. Once there I closed the door and prepared for bed, climbing in under the blankets and switching off the light. I huddled there waiting for sleep to come and wondering what to do about Millicent. It was nearly midnight and the girls still weren't back from their party.

As I lay there I heard a creak of floor boards and the scuff of feet just outside my door. I cocked my ear to listen and for a moment there was complete silence. Then the noises resumed, moving past my door and up the stairs toward the second floor. After a few minutes I heard someone descend the stairs and pass slowly by my room again. Was it my imagination, or did the footsteps once again pause at my door before moving away toward the kitchen?

My imagination was running amok as I considered possible scenarios. Millicent was a strong woman, but I was a young healthy man, and I wouldn't be an easy target if she decided to try something. Something? What exactly was I thinking? Surely she wasn't dangerous, probably just suffering from depression and food deprivation. What could she do really? Of course, if she found me asleep...and then the image of her long-bladed kitchen knives sprang into my mind.

I can tell you happily that sanity and logic won out eventually, and slumber caught up with me soon after. In fact I slept peacefully until morning, with no worries about my own safety. One simply has to face one's concerns and take steps to overcome them. Rational thought is what separates us from wild animals in the jungle. Well...that, and our ability to make and use tools. Speaking of which, it's amazing what assurance a strong wooden chair can offer, provided that it's wedged securely under the doorknob.

The following morning was thankfully a Saturday, and I knocked on Molly's door early. She came to the door clad in candy cane-striped pajamas, looking very drowsy and more than a little surprised to see me. The sleepy look quickly vanished when I told her of the previous night's events. We went next door and roused Miko, filling her in as well. Then the three of us sat on Molly's bed and planned a course of action.

"Millicent is obviously suffering from delusional episodes," Molly stated. "She seems very depressed from dealing with her father's deterioration and having to make the decision to institutionalize him. She's not taking care of herself because right now she doesn't care what happens to her."

"Why she talking strange?" Miko asked. "If just depressed, she shouldn't see odd things like she say."

Molly nodded. "You're right, Miko. I think she may be getting ill from food and water deprivation, possibly becoming hypoglycemic or worse. That can certainly mess with your brain. Maybe she's got other health issues we know nothing about. But what is certain is that we can't stand around and wait to see if she gets better. We have to do something, and now!"

"What do you suggest?" I asked her.

"Well, the first thing is to get her to eat and drink something. We can make a nice breakfast and tell her that we want her to join us. If all of us invite her together, she might have a harder time saying no. There is strength in numbers."

"It sounds like it's worth a try, but what if she won't come to breakfast?" I countered.

"Let's cross that bridge when we come to it," Molly replied. We all agreed and set out to make an appetizing breakfast spread. After the girls threw on day clothes we met in the kitchen and got to work frying eggs, bacon, and hash browns. Enticing aromas soon filled the kitchen and, we hoped, wafted into the living room as well. Millicent had awoken while we worked and had come out of her bedroom to sit in the rocking chair. We let her remain there undisturbed while we finished our preparations.

I sliced some apples and oranges and we set the table. Molly poured four glasses of orange juice, and Miko brought the hot food over on two platters. When it was done we stepped back and surveyed the results. My stomach grumbled appreciatively and I said, "Yum, that looks great to me! Let's eat!"

"Let's go get Millicent," Molly said, glancing toward the living room. I sighed and nodded. The three of us walked together into the main room and stood smiling in front of Millicent. Molly spoke first. "Hey, Millie, it's the weekend and we thought it would be nice to have breakfast together. We made a lot of food; come share some with us! It's really good and you won't have to cook. What do you say?"

Millicent looked up momentarily, then shook her head and looked away. I pitched in then, saying, "Oh, come on and try some food. The girls worked hard on it just so you could have breakfast with us. You'll hurt their feelings if you don't even have a bite."

That last statement seemed to get through to Millicent. Whether or not it was because she identified with being hurt I'll never know. But she looked me in the eyes and nodded, then heaved herself up out of the chair. Unfortunately that simple effort taxed her remaining strength to its limits. She swayed on her feet for a moment, suddenly glassy-eyed, and then began to slump sideways. I was standing right there so I reached out and caught her as she fell.

Even people of modest stature are surprisingly heavy when they become dead weight. I grunted as I strained to lower Millicent's limp body carefully to the ground. She was pale and completely unconscious. Molly and I checked for a pulse and found it. She looked up at me and said, "Call 911 right now! Get an ambulance over here!"

She didn't need to ask again. I ran into the kitchen and dialed. After a short interval that seemed like an eternity, I heard a siren outside announcing the paramedics' arrival. They quickly assessed Millicent's condition, pronounced her stable, and wheeled her out in a gurney to the ambulance. As I followed them outside I saw curtains drawn back in several neighboring houses with curious faces peeking out at the flashing lights. One or two were braving the cold and stood on their porches observing the show.

I watched by the door as the crew bundled Millicent into the back of the waiting ambulance. Molly got a phone number from one of the paramedics so we could check on Millie's condition later in the day. Then the ambulance sped away down the snow-covered road and rounded the corner out of sight.

We headed slowly back inside to eat our breakfast. The house seemed oddly vacant even with three of us around the table. Our anticipated feast was a subdued affair and the food didn't taste as good as I had thought it would. We each picked at our plates and said little, contemplating the morning's events. Molly occasionally glanced to my right, and I knew she was looking at the empty seat in front of the fourth place setting. I shivered, but the cold I felt that morning had little to do with the weather outside.

CHAPTER FIFTY-TWO

We called the hospital late that afternoon and got a report on Millicent's condition. The attending physician said she was stable and conscious, though a bit disoriented. She had been examined and the initial diagnosis was dehydration and mild malnutrition. Preliminary blood tests had revealed moderate hypoglycemia as we had suspected. In light of the history we had provided, the doctor suspected that she suffered from clinical depression as well. The doctor thanked me for our prompt response in obtaining medical assistance for Millicent. "She was quite ill and would have gotten steadily worse; you may have saved her life."

After I hung up from the call I gave the news to Molly and Miko. My housemates were relieved to hear that our landlady appeared to be all right, at least physically. With that load off our minds, the three of us were able to relax and turn our attention back to our studies.

At that point I was just finishing the medicine block. My next and final block rotation in Tullville was small animal surgery. I would work side by side with the staff surgeons, assisting in the operatory as well as handling some of the postoperative patient care. It would also be my chance to spay my ferret.

On the very first day of my surgery block, I scrubbed in to assist with a spinal surgery on a paralyzed Dachshund. This breed of dog has a strong tendency for back problems. It's not due to having elongated bodies, as is often thought. In reality their backs are normal length; it's their legs that are disproportionately short. The same dwarf trait that stunts the legs also causes the intervertebral discs in the spine to degenerate, leading to a higher incidence of disc ruptures.

The discs are like jelly-filled capsules that sit between the spinal bones, acting as soft cushions and shock absorbers. When they degenerate and become hardened they can easily rupture, leaking disc material which pushes up into the spinal cord itself. Mild pressure causes only pain, but severe pressure can crush the cord just as with a spinal fracture. The result can be partial or total paralysis of the body behind the damaged disc.

The surgeons were worried because Hans, the patient in question, had presented with acute paralysis of the rear legs. The five-year-old dog was active and in good shape, but when he had tried to jump up onto his owner's couch he had cried out and fallen to the floor. Jumping puts a lot of pressure on the spine, so it is common to have a degenerated disc rupture at the instant the dog leaps upward.

The concern with Hans was the severity of his injury. He not only lacked voluntary movement of his lower half, but testing revealed he could not feel his rear legs at all. From neurology class I knew that this was a bad sign. The nerves that transmitted pain sensation were located deep in the center of the spinal cord. A total loss of feeling meant that the cord was severely injured to its core. Hans could be a paraplegic for life and might not be able to urinate or defecate normally. The outlook was grim.

Hans was admitted to the teaching hospital within hours of his injury. Radiographs confirmed that he had ruptured a disc between the first and second lumbar vertebrae. "See here," the radiologist told the surgeon, pointing to the region of the injury. "The two vertebrae are nearly touching; the space between them is narrowed due to the disc having ruptured and collapsed. The neighboring disc between L-2 and L-3 is also degenerated; you can see mineralization of the disc material which makes it visible on the X-ray. It will be prone to rupturing in the future also; I'd recommend you fenestrate this disc while you're in there." His advice made sense to me; fenestration meant extracting the disc contents to prevent future leakage of material. Fortunately dogs can do without their discs, so if one appears problematic you can remove it.

The surgeon handling Hans's case was Dr. Brown, the other half of the diminutive duo in the surgery department along with Dr. Payne. They were both vertically challenged and had similar personalities as well. Dr. Brown was often gruff, impatient, and egotistical in his interactions with students, though his instruments were less prone to flying across the room than Dr. Payne's.

With all that said, I can tell you that I was happy to see him in charge of Hans. Despite his interpersonal shortcomings, Dr. Brown's surgical aptitude was second to none. His fingers possessed a skill and dexterity that was almost magical, and I found him inspiring to watch. He could make the most challenging procedures look incredibly simple, as if anyone could step up and do it. I knew enough to realize this was just an illusion; a measure of true mastery is being able to make the difficult look easy.

Dr. Brown listened to the radiologist's interpretation, nodding from time to time. Then he said, "We'll need a myelogram to characterize the extent of cord compression and to know which side to do the laminectomy on."

The radiologist agreed. "Yes, I'd say we should proceed with that now, and then head directly into surgery. He's got a severe herniation and needs the pressure taken off that cord, or he'll continue to suffer more damage."

Dr. Brown quickly met with Hans's family in the waiting area and made the recommendation to do immediate surgery. They gave us permission to proceed.

The doctors had drawn a blood sample when the little dog first was admitted, and the organ functions all looked good, so we anesthetized him and shaved his back. Once Hans was prepped and his IV line was in, the radiologist performed a myelogram, carefully injecting a contrast dye directly into the spinal column. As the liquid flowed up and down the spine, it made the normally invisible cord show up clearly on X-rays, allowing us to see just how it had been pinched.

After the myelogram was performed, Hans was wheeled into radiology for quick spinal films. When we viewed the developed images, we could see that the cord had narrowed severely, and that it was more compressed on the right side than the left.

"Okay, it looks like the disc blew out more to the right, so we'll decompress the cord on that side," Dr. Brown decided. The radiologist agreed, and off to the surgery suite Hans went. I joined Dr. Brown at the scrub sink just outside the operatory, and lathered my hands and arms with disinfectant soap. Another student from the Oregon class joined us, due to the doctor wanting two sterile assistants for this procedure. We scrubbed in silence and then donned surgical gowns and gloves.

The doctor began the surgery by making a long spinal skin incision that opened the dog like a split melon. Reflecting the muscles back he revealed the vertebrae, with my fellow student providing suction to keep the area free of blood. I handed instruments to the surgeon as he called for them. The spinal bones stood out cleanly white against the deep red of the muscles. The doctor identified the first lumbar vertebra and said, "All right, we need to do a hemilaminectomy on the right side of this bone. Give me the air-powered drill and a round burr."

I handed him the sterilized drill which had an air hose leading from it. A technician grabbed the other end of the hose, and plugged it into an air supply outlet in the wall. Now the surgeon had a sterile, air-powered tool which could drive a grinding burr at high speeds, like an overgrown dental drill.

The high-pitched whine of the drill filled the surgery suite as the doctor carefully ground away the bone covering the spinal cord. The

delicate cord ran through a round tunnel in the center of each vertebra, and it fit tightly into that space with no room to spare. Therein
lay much of the problem. When disc material pushed up into the canal, there was nowhere for the cord to move, so pressure mounted in
the confined space and the nerve tissue was pinched and narrowed.
This quickly led to cord damage and loss of neurologic function.

The hemilaminectomy the doctor was performing was simply a
removal of some of the overlying bone to give the soft tissues room
to "spread out," thereby relieving the pressure. Because the spinal
cord was directly under the bony layer, you had to proceed very
carefully with the drill or you could punch right through the cord
and paralyze the patient.

The pungent smell of vaporized bone hit my nostrils as the surgeon ground away layer after layer of the vertebra. Beneath the
shriek of the air-driven motor I could hear the lower-pitched vibration of metal biting into living tissue. Finally Dr. Brown said,
"There we are!" and I saw a moist white substance glistening
through the gap he had created in the bone. It was almost gelatinous
in appearance, and I knew that I was looking at the naked spinal
cord of the dog.

The doctor carefully enlarged the window in the bone until he
deemed it satisfactory. Then he grabbed a small instrument shaped
like a miniature scoop. Probing gently around the cord he removed
bits and pieces of the disc material lying in the narrow canal. The
spinal cord in these regions was darkened and blotchy, in contrast
with the smooth white of the undamaged tissue.

Eventually all the wayward bits of disc pulp were extracted and
the canal looked clean. The doctor then directed his attention to the
joint space between the vertebrae. He located the ruptured disc and
removed it to prevent further leaks into the canal. He also removed
the neighboring disc that the radiologist had pointed out as being at
risk for injury. When he was done, there was no remaining pressure
on the spinal cord and a reduced chance of disc problems in the future.

After that it was a simple matter of closing the tissues that had
been laid open during the procedure. Simple for Dr. Brown, at least.
His hands were a blur as he flew through the closure, suturing layer
after layer with incredible speed. In surprisingly short order we were
out of surgery and observing Hans in recovery. He was stable and
breathing steadily, his body shivering strongly to warm itself as the
anesthetic wore off. The question that remained was how much had
been accomplished by the procedure. The spinal cord was severely
traumatized and there was no guarantee it would heal. We had done

everything possible to maximize the little dog's chances of recovery; the rest was now up to Hans.

In the days following I checked on our little patient regularly, since I was one of the students assigned to his case. He was quite a sight to behold. With his brown shaved back sporting a long line of stitches he resembled an elongated American football.

Every day when I opened his kennel door he would push his slender pointed nose into my hand as if to remind me that my responsibilities included petting him. I suspect his tail would have been wagging furiously as well if only he could make it move. Sadly, there was no sign of motor function in his back end. He seemed comfortable and willing to walk, but his rear legs dragged limply as he pulled himself along.

Predictably, Hans had no control of his bowel or bladder, so he often was coated with his feces when I came around to assess him. Then I'd have to lift him out of his kennel and rinse his rear end off, being careful to avoid wetting the fresh incision along his back. I also had to squeeze his full bladder at least twice daily to empty it for him. He didn't mind, as he could feel nothing from his ribcage to the tip of his tail.

All the while we watched and waited for any sign of returning function in his spine. On the tenth day postoperatively a neurologist came and rendered an opinion. After a thorough examination of Hans, he shook his head. "It doesn't look good," he concluded. "He's got absolutely no deep pain response back there, and this long after surgery his chances of improving are slim to none." Dr. Brown nodded resignedly; he hadn't expected to hear anything different.

The dog's family was apprised of the situation and they elected to keep Hans at the hospital for awhile longer. They were devoted to their companion, and wanted to explore the possibility of him living at home as a paraplegic. There was a chance he might be a manageable patient if he wore doggy diapers. We also discussed fitting Hans with a small wheel harness that strapped to his rear end. This could allow him to regain some mobility and move around the home, even go for walks. The man of the house was a machinist, and he was confident he could fabricate a suitable cart for Hans. After discussing design parameters, he told us he would produce a prototype within the next week or so. Until then all we could do was watch and wait, hoping that Hans would find a way to come home.

My thoughts were occupied with another homecoming as well. That evening Molly and I talked on the phone with Dr. Brenda Meyers, who was supervising Millicent's care. She assured us that our landlady was physically stable and recovering well. "She's basically healthy, but had neglected herself to a point where she was severely weakened," the doctor told me when I got on the phone.

"What about her emotional state?" I asked the doctor. "I'm worried about the fact that she let herself get sick in the first place."

The doctor's tone turned serious. "Yes, I agree. Millicent was evaluated by our staff psychiatrist, and she is suffering from clinical depression."

I said, "Millicent seemed very close to her father. I suspect that his decline probably played a role in her collapse."

The doctor agreed. "Recent events have been hard on her, and she has no support group to lean on; no immediate family, few friends, and no spouse or children of her own. This makes it harder to handle adversity."

I tried to imagine dealing with tragic events entirely alone, having no one who really cared about me. I shuddered; it was not a pleasant image to contemplate. "So what happens now?" I asked the doctor.

"Well, I've recommended to Millicent that she undergo some counseling. Fortunately, she seemed receptive to the idea when I broached it with her. I think this episode scared her a bit and she knows it would be good to talk to someone."

"Do you know when she'll be coming home?" I asked.

"She's doing very well. Come tomorrow she should be discharged," she replied. "If you have any concerns later on, you can call me or the counselor that I've assigned to her."

That night I slept well, comforted by the knowledge that my immediate universe, and those within it, seemed to be back on the path to health and stability. It felt good knowing that my efforts had made a difference in Millicent's life. Sometimes things do work out for the best, if one is willing to step in and give fate a nudge here and there.

CHAPTER FIFTY-THREE

The next day I downed a quick breakfast and headed out the front door. The young morning was bright and clear and I burrowed deep within my heavy coat as I walked toward campus. Although the snow had melted away over the past two weeks, the relentless winds of the Palouse still carried a bitter edge. Discomfort always skewed my perception, and I could swear that the distance was twice as long as it had been during milder weather.

When I arrived at the teaching hospital, I passed through the main entrance and felt a rush of pleasure as the heated interior surrounded me in a cocoon of warmth. I threw back the hood of my coat and rubbed my hands and my face to regain feeling in my extremities. As my tingling skin returned to life, I made my way to the surgery ward and quickly checked on Hans. After that I found Dr. Brakel and tagged along as he headed into an exam room. It was there that I met the second memorable patient I dealt with during my surgery rotation.

Charlie was a big, friendly Old English Sheep Dog with a perpetually lolling tongue and an endless supply of drool. He appeared well cared for, and his five family members were crammed into the small room to be with him. One week after Charlie's eighth birthday, his owner had noticed a small swelling on his face. The mass had rapidly enlarged, and by the time he was referred to us he presented with a nasty-looking growth that had severely deformed his lower jaw.

The referring vet had biopsied the lump and it had turned out to be an osteosarcoma. This was an aggressive cancer that arose directly from the bone and could spread rapidly. Being deeply imbedded in the jaw made its removal via surgery nearly impossible. The dog's regular vet had been happy to refer him to us, so the tumor and its treatment now became our problem.

When I saw Charlie firsthand, I was appalled at the extent of the growth on his face. The dog was a big male of his breed, weighing around forty kilograms (ninety pounds). Even so the tumor looked disproportionately large, extending from the right side of his lower jaw around to the front of his chin. Externally it manifested as a cluster of bulging nodules that altered the contours of his face into a hideous caricature of his former appearance. It also had grown deep into his mouth, and many of his teeth had disappeared inside the spreading mass of tissue. When he chewed food, he often bled profusely due to his upper teeth lacerating the tumor below. It was only a matter of time before the expanding growth made it impossible to eat at all.

The internists in the medicine department said that there was not much they could do with a mass of this size and type. An osteosarcoma would not respond well to chemotherapy, nor would radiation treatments be likely to stop a tumor this large. Their recommendation was to surgically debulk the mass or remove it entirely if possible. Only then might they follow up with medical therapy to treat any remaining traces of the cancer.

Thus Charlie made his way to the surgery department, with Dr. Brakel being the lucky recipient of the case. For once he was at a loss for words and no surgical mantras rolled off his tongue. He simply shook his head as he opened the dog's mouth and saw the extent of the growth. "The mass extends across the mandibular symphysis and involves both sides now. A hemimandibulectomy won't suffice," he decided. "Damn. I was hoping we could just remove one mandible and be done with it. This is going to be difficult, really difficult."

Radiographs of Charlie's face confirmed the doctor's observations. There was visible bone destruction on both lower jaws; removing the right side alone wouldn't cure him. That led to a debate over what to do next.

There didn't seem to be an easy solution. Removing one mandible was feasible; the remaining jaw would lend some stability and provide a fairly normal shape to the face. But with both mandibles gone the lower face would be nothing but a flaccid mass of soft tissue without form. There also would be no lower teeth to oppose the uppers, so chewing would be impossible.

After extensive discussion among the surgeons, a compromise procedure was decided upon. They would remove the front half of both mandibles, leaving the rear portions (and some molars) in place. This was an unconventional procedure, and they were only attempting it because, in Dr. Brakel's words, "We've got nothing to lose. He'll die if we don't try something, and at least this gives him a chance."

Charlie's surgery was scheduled in an early afternoon time slot. I quickly gulped down a brown bag lunch that I had brought from home, and then I scrubbed in on the procedure alongside Dr. Brakel. Of course it was not just the two of us; as usual, there were a lot of helping hands involved. By the time two other students, a technician, and an anesthesiologist crowded into the surgery suite, the usually spacious room was filled to capacity. We arranged ourselves in our designated positions and settled in for a long afternoon.

Mike Callahan and I stood across the table from Dr. Brakel as his assistants. Mike provided instruments as needed, slapping them into the surgeon's hand with practiced confidence. At this stage we were becoming experienced enough to feel pretty comfortable in the operatory.

The early phase of the surgery involved dissecting the dog's lower lips and skin away from the jaw. As the surgeon slowly peeled the flesh back, I used electrocautery to control bleeding from the numerous small arteries that were severed. Whenever blood welled up into the surgery field, Dr. Brakel would dab it away with a gauze square, and I would quickly touch the metal tip of the cautery wand to the spot that bled. With the push of a button a surge of high voltage current cauterized the vessel closed. The tiny zap of the electric spark was followed by a small puff of smoke and the faint whiff of cooked flesh.

Control of hemorrhage made everything easier to see and Dr. Brakel steadily progressed with his dissection. Soon the dog's outer facial tissues had been loosened from the underlying mandibles. With the skin flayed back, the osteosarcoma was revealed as a hulking pale mass with a lumpy irregular surface. It clung to the dog's lower jaws like an invasive parasite. I could see that fingers of the tumor extended deep into the face.

The doctor explored the area until he found the margins of the large growth. Carefully he began to separate it from the normal tissues around it. The task was made more difficult by the need to preserve as many structures in the mouth as possible, especially the tongue. In several areas the doctor had to cut close to the edge of the tumor to avoid damaging vital oral anatomy. This was not ideal, as it increased the risk of cancer cells remaining behind after the surgery. But he had no choice; removing too many structures would leave Charlie without a functional mouth. There was little margin for error.

Finally the front portions of both lower jaws stood out starkly bare from the softer tissues, the ugly mass clinging to the bones with nowhere to hide. It was time to remove the forward halves of the mandibles and the tumor along with them.

Once again the air-powered drill came into play, this time with a tiny saw blade attachment. The surgeon severed each mandible between the premolar teeth, trying to avoid damaging tooth roots in the process. The lower jaws came free and were tossed with a heavy sounding thump into the medical waste container on the floor. The deed was done. Now we had to salvage as much as we could of Charlie's face and hope that the end result was functionally and aesthetically acceptable.

The closure was a challenging bit of surgery in itself. Dr. Brakel adroitly sutured the soft tissues in the mouth to cover up the raw ends of the cut bones. Likewise the skin and lips were pulled forward and reattached to the underlying tissues, in an approximation of their original orientation.

When it was all done, we took a collective deep breath and surveyed our handiwork. The tumor was gone. What we had left was a severely shortened lower face with loose skin hanging limply where the dog's chin had been. The appearance reminded me of a saggy-faced Bloodhound with a severely undershot lower jaw.

Charlie recovered smoothly from surgery and was slated for feedings of liquefied gruel, pain medications and antibiotics until his mouth healed. I added him to my daily log of treatment responsibilities, and hoped that he would reward us with a positive outcome. Just as with Hans, we had done all that we could. Only time would tell whether we had salvaged a good quality of life for our patient.

I didn't have to wait as long for home life to take a good turn. That evening I found myself standing on the front porch with Molly and Miko, welcoming Millicent home from the hospital. I had no idea what to expect, and waited with some trepidation for my first glimpse of her since she had been wheeled away in a stretcher.

I needn't have worried. When Millicent stepped out of the cab she was alert and lively, her face flushed a healthy pink as she hailed us. For all appearances she seemed as sturdy as when I had first met her, bustling up the sidewalk through the cold morning air and taking the steps up to the porch with confident strength. She shooed away our attempts to lend her a hand, but her usual gruffness was tempered by the warm smile of gratitude she gave all of us. It was obvious that she was happy to be home, and that was a sentiment we all shared.

Later that evening we sat down to dinner as a group. This time the fourth seat at the table held its rightful occupant. Ignoring the lateness of the hour we had prepared a sumptuous spread of bacon, eggs, hash brown potatoes, and sliced fruit. That meal was one of the best I can remember from my time in Tullville. Like the food we shared, Millicent's homecoming was seasoned with the flavor of caring. We laughed and ate and talked, learning more about each other than we had in the long months preceding that day. The most rewarding thing of all was seeing our landlady smiling, really smiling, for the first time that we could remember. It had been awhile coming, but at last we had our breakfast feast with Millicent.

CHAPTER FIFTY-FOUR

The day eventually came when I got to spay my little ferret. Dixie had been a fun and affectionate companion for the past month since I had brought her to Tullville. We had grown comfortable with each other, and she loved to play with me when I let her out of her enclosure. When I set her down, she would hop and wiggle around the room in her silly uncoordinated manner, investigating every nook and cranny along the way. After she grew tired, she sometimes would climb up in my lap and sleep while I sat on the bed studying. The sight of her elongated body curled into a tight ball always made me smile. I would look down and watch the slight movements of her chest as she breathed, her legs occasionally twitching in response to secret ferret dreams.

When the big day arrived, I drove to the teaching hospital rather than walking. Dixie's cage sat on the back seat and she peeked out curiously at the scenery flashing by. When I parked at the school, I grabbed her from the cage and stashed her under my coat to keep her warm on the short walk to the building.

Once indoors I let Dixie come out and carried her in my arms. Predictably, she got a lot of attention from students and professors alike as we made our way through the hallways to the surgery ward. I found a kennel with small enough bars to prevent her from wriggling through. After I stashed her within, I marked the cage card with her name, and provided her with a blanket and litter box. On the patient instructions I noted that food and water should be withheld prior to surgery.

Later that morning I performed my first ferret spay, assisted by one of the staff surgeons. Actually, I did all the work and the doctor provided only verbal advice. By now I was comfortable doing routine spays, but the species differences in size and anatomy warranted having an advisor on hand. When it came to finding surgical assistants, I'd had plenty of offers from classmates who were eager to see a procedure involving an exotic species.

Dixie's uterus turned out to be a Y-shaped organ just like that of a tiny cat. The only significant difference in her anatomy was that her ovaries were encased in heavy sheaths of fat, making them difficult to see. The surgeon watched closely, talking me through the process. "Be sure you can visualize both ovaries before you clamp and cut the vessels; you don't want to leave a piece of ovarian tissue behind. There's the left one—see that pink spot in the fat of the pedicle? It's not as distinct as in the cat due to the adipose surrounding it, but you can see the color difference. Clamp and ligate at a safe distance beyond and you'll be sure to get it all."

I did as she said, and before long I had the entire uterus and both ovaries removed, and hardly a speck of blood was shed. I checked one last time for any leaks, and then closed up my pet's abdominal incision, making a neat row of external sutures on the outer skin layer.

Dixie recovered uneventfully and I took her home that evening. When I put her into her cage in my bedroom, she immediately drank some water and then curled up to sleep in her bed. The long strenuous day plus a dose of postoperative pain medication had resulted in a tired little girl.

The biggest challenge I had with my furry friend postoperatively was trying to keep her slowed down until she healed. The day after her spay I opened her cage door on returning home from school. Dixie shot out like a rocket and began bounding around the room, clucking and grunting to herself as she did when happy or excited. She seemed oblivious to her naked shaved belly and long line of sutures. I had to chase her down and grab her so that she didn't overdo her exercise and injure herself. When I stuffed her back into her cage, I was rewarded with an hour of noise as she rattled her metal door incessantly to remind me that she should be out playing. I ended up moving to the living room so that I could study in peace.

Some of my other patients I wasn't so sure about. Back at school I continued to see Hans when he came in for recheck evaluations. His owners had taken him home after being taught how to care for him and empty his bladder. They brought him back for regular exams so that we could assess his progress. When they checked in, I would get a brief history of what the family had observed at home. Then I'd perform a neuro exam on the dog and record my findings in the chart. After I was finished, the doctor would evaluate Hans for himself. This gave me a chance to hone my examination skills and see how well I did when compared to the surgeon.

True to his word, the dog's owner had fashioned a small, two-wheeled cart that could be buckled onto Hans, supporting his rear end with the paralyzed legs off the ground. He could then walk using his forelimbs to pull himself along. Hans had quickly discovered that he could move again, and he eagerly anticipated his exercise periods. At the hospital we would put him on the floor to observe his mobility and he would race off down the hall at surprising speed. He panted excitedly and his eyes were alight; I could tell he still had a love of life despite his handicaps. The question was whether his family could deal with him paralyzed and incontinent on a long-term basis. I wasn't sure that they were up to the task, and his fate hung in the balance.

Then one day something astonishing happened. Hans's family came to Tullville for another follow up, but the doctor was involved with another case when they arrived. They decided to drop Hans off and leave to get some lunch. I heard the dog was at the hospital and went to see him in his kennel. It had been weeks since his surgery and I was nearing the end of my time at the hospital.

The Dachshund was lying stretched out in the cage, his wheel cart sitting by the kennel door. He perked up when he saw me, letting out a single yip and dancing anxiously on his front feet. I opened the door and petted his head. As I did so I caught a whiff of feces and sure enough he had smeared excrement on his rear quarters.

I picked the little dog up and took him to the kennel room bathtub, where I washed him off with soap and warm water. After that I grabbed a towel and began to rub him dry, and that's when it happened. I was wiping his right rear leg when he whined and pulled the foot away from my hands. I stopped and stared, unsure of what I had just seen. Reflex activity is common in paralyzed patients; in fact, the reflexes often strengthen when the brain is no longer telling the limbs what to do. Withdrawing the foot when it was stimulated was nothing to get excited about. What had caught my interest was the fact that he had whined when the foot moved. Vocalizing suggested that he had felt something back there. After nearly three weeks of total paralysis, there was virtually no hope of Hans recovering. Yet I knew what I had just seen.

My heart threatened to thump its way out of my chest as I grabbed my hemostats from the pocket where I always carried them. They resembled tiny pointed pliers, and I grabbed one of his toes with the instrument and pinched firmly. Hans whined louder this time and turned to look at me, his foot pulling back harder, twice, before relaxing again. Feeling ever more excited, I repeated the test on his tail and his other rear leg. Each time the pinched extremity wiggled and Hans complained as he looked back to see what was happening. He was feeling the hemostats!

"Yes!!" I exclaimed as I petted the little dog on his head. "That's a good boy! You're healing, and you're going to get even better, aren't you?" The little dog panted and jumped around on his front legs as he picked up on my enthusiasm, and in disbelief I saw his tail wagging weakly back and forth as I patted his head.

The surgeons all came to look at Hans over the next couple of hours. So did the neurologists at the hospital. None had seen a patient recover function after such a long period of total loss. A week earlier there had been no deep pain response when he had been tested. It was almost unheard of that he would improve now, but there was no denying the signs. Hans was healing.

The doctors put Hans on the floor without his wheel harness and clapped their hands, saying in animated tones, "C'mon boy! Come here Hans! You can do it!" When the dog became excited he pulled himself across the floor with his forelimbs, and his back legs also moved! The movements weren't random and spastic; the legs paddled and pushed in a rhythmic manner that was coordinated with the front limb motions. He even lifted his rump briefly off the ground before his legs betrayed him and his rear end collapsed back to earth.

The surgeons were ecstatic. They knew that part of the weakness Hans was experiencing was due to atrophy of the hip and thigh muscles during his paralysis. Now that Hans was moving his legs, he could exercise those muscles and rebuild their strength. His spinal function would likely improve some more as well. Hans showed great promise of walking again in the not too distant future. Even the usually reserved Dr. Brown laughed and gave me a high-five. We all felt exuberant as we watched our little patient's first steps toward recovery.

Charlie the sheep dog was a different story. He came through his surgery and healed rapidly without developing any infection in his jaw. But it became obvious almost immediately that he was going to struggle to eat and drink. Without the front half of his mandibles his lower face was formless and flaccid, and he could not grab hard or soft food with his jaws. His tongue moved, but most of the time it flopped uselessly out the side of his mouth. He struggled to lap up even small amounts of water on his own, making hideous wet slurping and sucking noises as he tried ineffectually to swallow the elusive liquid.

Meeting the caloric needs of a large body wasn't easy under such circumstances. Our patient was ravenous and became excited at the sight and smell of food. We syringe fed him a liquefied gruel, but even then Charlie was unable to hold the meal in his mouth and most came spilling back out through his sagging lower lips. With our best efforts we got maybe half of the feedings down his throat, and he wore the remainder as a soggy mess of food and drool that coated his chin, neck, and chest. His shaggy coat made it a constant battle just to keep him clean and avoid secondary skin infections.

Charlie's family came to visit and they watched somberly as we demonstrated his struggles. On the positive side there was no sign of the mass regrowing, although it was too early to pronounce him cured. But whether or not the tumor reoccurred there were serious practical concerns with caring for Charlie. It would be difficult at best to meet the dog's dietary needs, and he would always be a high maintenance individual to keep clean. Even with students and technicians feeding him four times a day, Charlie had lost significant weight in the two weeks since his surgery. He seemed to feel better with the cancer removed; pain wasn't a significant factor now. Nonetheless he needed to eat and drink. The surgery had impaired his ability to do both, much more so than the surgeons had hoped when they attempted the procedure.

Charlie's family included the parents and three children. The oldest child was in her teens, but the two boys looked quite young, maybe six and eight years old respectively. They were nicely dressed for their hospital visit and the youngsters well mannered. Dr. Brakel talked to them quietly about Charlie's prognosis and I gave them some privacy, busying myself on the other end of the treatment room. I could hear the parents discussing the situation and the children starting to protest. It didn't take much imagination to guess what options were being considered.

Eventually I heard the father say, "It's decided then. We all know that this is what's best for Charlie. He simply isn't happy this way and we can't make him better."

The smallest boy started to wail, stomping his feet. His mom tried to comfort him, but he was having none of it. Through his tears he exclaimed, "No! You said he was better now. This isn't fair! I want Charlie to come home!"

The mother continued to talk quietly to her son, her own eyes wet as she knelt and held him. The older boy stood silently nearby. He looked dazed, not protesting the decision, simply staring at his dog as if he knew this would be the last time he would see Charlie. The teenage daughter was trying to be brave, wiping away tears surreptitiously as she petted Charlie and talked softly to him, her head pressed close to his.

The father stood next to Dr. Brakel, looking unhappy about the decision he had helped make. Now and then he exchanged a few words with the doctor, who nodded and smiled encouragingly. I imagined that Dr. Brakel was telling him that he had made an appropriate decision, that it was a difficult one but humane nonetheless. In situations like these a veterinarian played the role of counselor as much as that of healer. There were no easy choices here, no black and white answers, only a lot of unpleasant grays to deal with. Right then I was very grateful to be just a student, not the person to whom the family looked for cures and for guidance.

After a little while the younger boy quieted down and the father caught the mother's eye. He motioned toward the door and she nodded. Turning to her children she said, "You boys should go for a walk with your father. Melissa, do you want to stay or go with them?"

The teenage girl looked up at her mother, hesitating, then shook her head and said, "I don't want to be here. I've already said good-bye." Her mother nodded, smiling through her tears. She gave her daughter a brief hug and then waited as the father ushered the three children out the door.

When they were gone the woman turned to Dr. Brakel, drying her eyes as she said, "To tell the truth I don't really want to be here either, but I think Charlie would be happier having someone near that he knows. He deserves that. We got him as a puppy eight years ago and he's been a part of our family ever since." As she spoke, her voice caught and tears started running down her cheeks again. The doctor handed her a tissue and she smiled at him gratefully as she dabbed at the moisture. "I'm sorry that I'm making such a fuss," she said, shaking her head. "I didn't think it would be this hard. I just wish things had turned out differently."

Dr. Brakel replied gently, "You don't need to apologize for anything. I wish things had gone better too. I really was hopeful that he could find a way to eat after the surgery. It just doesn't look like it's going to happen."

The mother looked up at him and said, "We're not being selfish by giving up at this point, are we?"

The doctor shook his head. "No, you're not. The simple fact of the matter is we had to take a little too much of his mandibles in order to get rid of the tumor. Now we're faced with a very difficult situation. You might keep him alive awhile with intensive feeding and bathing, but it would be stressful and exhausting for you and for him. Sooner or later you would wind up resenting Charlie, and that's not how he should be remembered."

The woman sighed. "Yes, I agree. I know it's the right decision for everyone. Knowing doesn't make it easy though."

Dr. Brakel nodded sympathetically. "It's not supposed to be an easy decision. If it were, then I'd know you didn't care."

She smiled at that and said, "Thank you for your kind words and all that you've done. You gave Charlie a fighting chance and that's all anyone could ask for with a cancer like his." She paused and took a deep breath, gazing at her dog who sat waiting expectantly nearby. Charlie perked up as she walked over to pet him, his entire rear end wagging back and forth as she stroked his head one last time. For a minute they remained like that, gazing into each other's eyes. Then the woman straightened and turned to Dr. Brakel. In a small voice she said, "All right, I'm ready. You can go ahead whenever you want."

Dr. Brakel nodded silently and motioned me over. I crossed the room to where they waited. The doctor opened the locked cabinet on the wall of the treatment room and found the euthanasia solution. After carefully drawing the required dose into a syringe, he approached and told Charlie's owner, "This is basically an overdose of anesthetic. He'll go to sleep quickly and comfortably, just as if he were going to have a surgery. The only difference is he won't wake back up." The woman nodded, eyes glistening as she petted her dog's head.

Dr. Brakel and I knelt beside the dog on the floor. I helped hold Charlie still as the doctor slid the needle into a vein on the dog's forelimb. The sharp prick elicited only the slightest whine, the dog's rear continuing to wag as his owner spoke gently to him, "It's okay, big boy. I'm with you. You'll be in a better place soon, I promise. No more pain, Charlie. No more ever again."

The dog's gaze was fixed happily on the woman's face as the doctor gave the injection. Nothing seemed to bother him as long as he could feel her fingers scratching his shaggy head. The concentrated pentobarbital flowed from the syringe and sped through Charlie's veins. For just a brief instant a look of surprise passed over his eyes and then he sighed deeply. The massive head lowered to the floor, breaking contact with his owner's fingers as she gave him one last rub. By the time he lay on the ground he was gone.

The woman remained kneeling beside him, her hand frozen in the air where a moment ago it had rested on her dog's head. The words she spoke were meant only for her departed companion, and they were so soft I barely heard them. "Goodbye, Charlie" was all she said. Then she stood and walked quickly from the room.

Dr. Brakel and I looked at each other but neither of us spoke. There was no need to. Both of us understood that this was the harsh reality of our profession. When all our efforts are done, when every bit of skill and knowledge has been used, when we have fought the good long fight to keep our patients happy and healthy, then in the end we will always lose the battle. Such is the way with all practitioners of medicine, and such is the somber truth that tempers our victories. The losses are hardest on those left behind, and that reality too we must face as we deal with the grieving families.

That day I fully comprehended the burden and the responsibility that my chosen calling would lay upon me. It was a sobering realization. The certain knowledge that I would see more cases like Charlie haunted me for a long time thereafter.

CHAPTER FIFTY-FIVE

Thankfully, the final weeks of our time in Tullville were enhanced by some fun and entertaining events. Junior Review was a chance for the students to vent some stress and poke good-natured fun at the lives of veterinary students. Most especially it was a chance to have a few laughs at the expense of our professors.

Both the Washington and Oregon students participated in this stage show presentation. The two junior classes eagerly combined forces in a final cooperative effort before we went our separate ways. After all, we did have something in common: the burdens of heavy class work and often-quirky professors. This was our one chance to get our digs in, and we took full advantage. For several weeks we planned and rehearsed between classes as we prepared for the big event.

The show was held on a Friday night in one of the larger lecture auditoriums at the vet school. This room had a raised stage in front, making it perfect for presenting the skits we had prepared. Students from other classes attended as well, from freshmen to seniors. The faculty were well represented in the audience, although I noted some conspicuous absences. In particular I saw that Drs. Payne and Brisbane were nowhere to be found. As the show progressed through the evening, it became obvious why.

There were a variety of skits presented in the two-hour review. Some were simply oral recitals, such as the poem lamenting the difficulties of staying awake in Dr. Borland's pharmacology lectures. Other productions were more lavish, such as the five-person dance routine featuring Amy Baker (who had danced professionally for a couple of years before pursuing veterinary medicine). Old Dr. Otterman was spoofed in a skit called "The Wizard of Otterman," wherein lost students followed the long road to learn ancient wisdom at his feet.

One of the female professors who was popular with the students also got her share of attention. Dr. Waverly was in her thirties, very fit and attractive, and was a respected internist with a never-give-up attitude and legendary energy. It seemed she never stopped moving, and it was challenging just keeping up with her as she charged down the hospital halls at full speed.

The juniors poked good-natured fun at Dr. Waverly on stage. A female student dressed as the doctor rushed back and forth talking nonstop, and the students who followed her wore roller skates so that they could keep up as they frantically took notes. There were collisions and other mishaps which the doctor blissfully ignored, until finally she turned to ask her students a question and there was no one left behind her. The audience was laughing nonstop, including Dr. Waverly, who sat near the front row. The skit was one of the best portions of the show, but as it turned out the students weren't finished with her yet.

One of the lady doctor's more endearing trademarks (at least to the male students) was that she always wore tight-fitting white slacks in the hospital. The material on some of these was thin enough to be nearly translucent, and on several occasions her underwear showed through when viewed from behind, especially the ones with the bright red hearts scattered over them.

Thus it was that at the end of the skit the students called her up on stage. She sheepishly complied, and as she stood there Stan Hulbert presented her with a gift wrapped box, smiling broadly. He said, "This is a token of our appreciation for working with you this past year." She looked pleased but embarrassed at this unexpected gesture and thanked him profusely. Stan said nothing; he and the other students on the stage simply watched grinning as she opened the package.

The doctor's eyes widened in disbelief as she pulled a pair of women's panties from the box. They were white and embellished with vivid red hearts. Stan said, "We all thought that you could add these to your collection." The gift had the anticipated effect: Dr. Waverly's face instantly matched the color of the hearts. The audience erupted in laughter and applause, and she broke into a wide grin despite herself. She shook her finger at Stan, who leaned over and gave her a big hug. With her gift in hand, she walked back to her seat, still blushing and shaking her head.

Of course, the students had their fun with Dr. Brisbane in his absence. He was just too amusing to leave unscathed. "Special Ed" Martinelli was small enough in stature to make a reasonable facsimile of the ophthalmologist, and when he donned a white lab coat and ocular loupes there was no doubt in anyone's mind who he was supposed to be. Amy Baker had coached Ed on the doctor's mannerisms, and her influence was also evident when the character's name was announced as "Dr. Greeble." Ed did a superb job of emulating the ophthalmologist's speech and movements, and even the other professors in attendance were splitting their sides as they watched.

All of these were memorable skits, but my favorite event that night was when the class roasted Drs. Brown and Payne, the two little Napoleons of the surgery staff. Their large egos and tiny statures made an irresistible combination of traits to exploit.

The surgeon skit employed a pair of male Washington students sitting on stools behind a cardboard screen. The screen had been painted with caricatures of the two doctors' bodies clothed in their surgical garb. The torsos were absurdly short and squat, and holes had been cut out of the pictures for the students' faces, arms, and legs to protrude through from behind. They could move their limbs and talk, bringing the drawn figures to life. In keeping with the small scale of the bodies, only half of each student's arm or leg extended through the cutouts, contributing to the illusion of extremely short gnomes standing on stage.

The two "doctors" had an animated discussion about how no one besides them had achieved surgical perfection. "Dr. Brown" asserted that student admission standards weren't strict enough. "Dr. Payne" agreed, waving his absurdly short arms as he said, "It's enough to make you throw your instruments!" So saying, he tossed a pair of scissors on the floor. "I didn't want scissors anyway!" he continued, shaking his head back and forth as his limbs flailed. "When I hold out my hand, I want hemostats, unless I say otherwise! Why doesn't everyone know that?!"

The two figures continued their cantankerous dialogue while their stubby arms and legs gestured this way and that. Laughs abounded, especially among those students who had had to endure hours of close work with the two domineering surgeons. This was the risk in being an instructor who didn't relate well to his pupils, especially when teaching creative young men and women. I could see why some teachers had chosen not to attend the evening's festivities. Doubtless they had been to one or two reviews in the past, and had decided that it was better to abstain.

At the end of the evening, the main players assembled on stage and gave a heart felt "thank you" to all of the professors and staff at the hospital. Stan Hulbert spoke for the Oregon students, saying, "On behalf of all my classmates, I would like to say that we have enjoyed our stay here. Especially the tropical weather and diverse cultural offerings of the Palouse."

He paused until the laughter had died down, then continued, "We value the education we have gained, and also the people who devoted their time and efforts to pounding the information into our heads, whether we liked it or not." Again the crowd chuckled and Stan grinned before concluding, "I wish to express our sincere gratitude to all the staff and especially the professors for their dedication to the veterinary program. Jokes and skits aside, we learned a lot from every instructor who taught us during our time here. Without you there would be no class of 1986, no future practitioners of this fine profession. Thank you all."

The audience applauded long and loudly, both students and professors standing as the performers on stage waved and filed off one by one into the crowd. Junior Review was officially over.

CHAPTER FIFTY-SIX

My time in Tullville was coming to a close, and I was busy concluding my school work and preparing to travel. Millicent continued to make strides in dealing with her father's illness and her depression. Molly, Miko, and I all talked with her daily, making sure she knew that she had friends and was not alone against the world. She also saw her counselor regularly and I think it helped her cope. Her mood was markedly improved, and she even managed to joke with me on occasion. While she would never possess a bubbly personality, she had regained some of the joy of living that we all took for granted. It was wonderful to see.

School remained as hectic as ever. There were no exams during block rotations, but plenty of cases needed attention. The best part of those final days was seeing Hans coming in one more time before I left. It had only been a week since his previous visit but the doctors had wanted to monitor him regularly. I knew that he was due in that day but when I first saw him far down the hallway I didn't think it was the same Dachshund. The little dog was walking, actually *walking* without his wheels. On closer inspection he wasn't normal yet; his back end swayed and flopped drunkenly as he ambled along, but he was standing on all four feet and they were moving!

The last week of surgery block came to an end, and it was time to say goodbye to the Washington students and professors, and to

Tullville itself. We all had made friends among the faculty and our Washington classmates. I said farewell to a number of students and professors during my last days at school, knowing that I would probably not see them again. Dr. Brakel was my favorite professor at Washington University; I made a point of telling him how much I appreciated his dedication and positive attitude. He seemed genuinely pleased and thanked me, wishing me well on my journey toward becoming a veterinarian.

There were a few Washington classmates I sought out as well. One of those was Jake Levitt, the bird-loving student whose home I had shared the year before. He was still living on the hill by the cemetery. We discussed our plans for the future when we finally graduated. For my part I had found that owning Dixie made me even more curious about ferrets and other small "pocket pets" such as rodents and rabbits. Jake, of course, was interested in pursuing avian medicine. We talked awhile longer and then parted as friends. I have often since wondered how his life and career turned out, and what path he ended up following in private practice.

On my last day in Tullville the vet school held an informal going-away party for the Oregon students. The festivities took place on Friday evening in the main hospital lounge. Many of the professors attended, and those Oregonians who had not already left town were treated to pizza, beer, wine, and other consumables. Small groups of faculty and students sat around on sofas or at tables and chatted about life, school, and all things veterinary. Humor and tall tales ran rampant. For a few hours the professors and their pupils put aside their respective roles and simply were friends without agendas.

The clearest recollection I have of that evening is of listening to the ancient Dr. Otterman reminiscing about the teaching hospital's early days. He had been at the school about as long as animals have been domesticated, so he had accumulated a vast backlog of memories to share. None were more entertaining than the story involving Dr. Payne.

It started when some of my classmates, loosened up by a couple of beers, began discussing the cantankerous surgeon's notorious temper. Amy Baker nodded, her eyes wide as she said, "He threw a pair of thumb forceps one day and they stuck in the wall!"

From a nearby chair Dr. Otterman's raspy laugh abruptly cut through the conversation and we turned to look at him. He grinned at us and said, "You think old Payne is bad now? He was worse when he was younger! Back then he was a real spitfire, high-strung and hot-tempered. He's actually mellowed with age, believe it or not."

I had a hard time envisioning Dr. Payne's current persona as an improved version of any human being. "Oh yes," Dr. Otterman continued, "In his youth he was hell on wheels. Fortunately, Payne was only a junior staff surgeon in those days, so he didn't wield as much clout as now. He had to defer to the senior professors, which didn't always sit well with him.

"There was one older surgeon who took particular delight in baiting the fiery young doctor. Dr. Churchill was a scholarly-looking gentleman, always puffing thoughtfully on a pipe; there weren't restrictions on tobacco in hospitals back in those days. As it turned out, Dr. Payne hated smoke of any kind, and Churchill knew it. If they had a disagreement about how to manage a case (which was common, as Payne was opinionated even then), you could sometimes catch them in the hallway arguing. Payne would be getting worked up and turning red, and as his temper was about to boil over Churchill would smile benignly and blow pipe smoke in his subordinate's face. Often that would end the discussion right there, as Payne would throw up his hands and stomp off while Churchill chuckled at his retreating back."

Dr. Otterman grinned and paused as the students laughed with delight. Mike Callahan raised his beer and declared, "I'd give anything to have seen that."

"Yes, it was most entertaining," the professor replied, adding wistfully, "Ah, those were the days! I remember when Churchill pulled a prank on Payne that really made him blow his top. Do you want to hear that story?"

His question was greeted with a resounding "Yes!" from the rest of us gathered around him.

The old doctor took a long sip of his wine and began, "Well, Dr. Payne was performing surgery one day in the teaching hospital. Back then the surgical suites were toward the front of the building where the reception area is now. He had a particularly difficult pelvic fracture in a dog and was trying to put a bone plate on it. To put it mildly, things were not going well, and he was rapidly becoming more irate. The assisting students were trying their best to be invisible. You could cut the tension with a knife."

My classmates and I laughed as we could envision the scene exactly. Dr. Otterman continued, "Just when it seemed that things couldn't get any worse, enter Professor Churchill. In those days the surgery suite had a small glass window in one wall. It could slide open to allow equipment or supplies to be handed through from the next room. Dr. Payne had his back to this window as he stood at the surgery table. Ol' Doc Churchill peeks through the glass and watches Payne throwing fits in the operatory. The petrified students can see Churchill standing there, puffing his pipe and grinning mischievously. Then he disappears for a moment, and when he returns, he is holding a piece of rubber tubing in his hand, like the type used to drain wounds.

"Dr. Churchill proceeds to open the pass-through window just a smidge, and he slides the end of the rubber tubing into the operatory through the crack. While Payne is sweating and cursing over his surgery, Churchill takes a long draw on his pipe and then blows the smoke through the tube into the operatory. It billows out behind Payne, who is absorbed in his procedure and totally oblivious to what is happening. Churchill keeps puffing his pipe and exhaling into the tube, and the students are all watching wide-eyed over their masks. A small cloud is slowly growing behind Payne's back, and finally when it fills half the room, the odor penetrates the surgeon's awareness.

"Payne abruptly looks up from his patient frowning, and says, 'What's that smell? I smell smoke! Is something on fire? What the hell's happening!?' The students are at a loss for words, and trying very hard not to stare at Churchill's antics behind the glass.

"Payne is frantically looking all around the surgery suite, checking to see if any equipment is on fire. Finally he glances behind him."

Dr. Otterman paused for effect, leisurely taking another drink from his glass. Molly Boyer couldn't stand the suspense and finally asked, "Well, what happened when Payne turned around?"

The old professor chuckled and winked at us. "Let's just say that you could hear the bellowing on the other side of the building." The entire group broke out in laughter, Oregon and Washington students alike. It was a classic "good old days" prank, and one that would have been priceless to witness. Dr. Otterman was full of such stories, and he had a captive audience as he regaled us with tales from the past.

The party lasted into the evening as we continued to converse and enjoy good food and drink. It was a nice note on which to end my stay in Tullville. Although I left town eager to return home, I did so carrying some fond memories as well.

CHAPTER FIFTY-SEVEN

My Washington education was now concluded, and that weekend I packed my things and loaded them into my car. Molly and Miko, of course, were remaining at the house, since their school year was far from over. Millicent hadn't decided whether she would rent my room out when I was gone. I cleaned out the bedroom, filling every nook and cranny of space in my vehicle. When I had wedged the last small items into the car, it was stuffed tight from floor to roof. The only open spaces were my seat and a small line-of-sight for my rearview and side mirrors. Dixie's kennel sat up front, buried under a mountain of my personal effects. Her cage door was accessible, but that was about all that was visible. I could see her pointed little nose poking curiously out between the metal bars as I prepared for travel.

I went back indoors and found Millicent in her usual spot, ensconced in her recliner watching television. Snuggled in her arms was her new friend, a brown tabby cat named Heidi. I told her I was about to depart and she smiled as she wished me a safe trip to Oregon. She hesitated, and then she added, "I know I don't say a lot sometimes. I'm not that comfortable with people, but that doesn't mean I don't appreciate you. I want you to know that I am truly grateful for all that you've done. You have been a wonderful guest in this house. May your life be blessed always."

I felt myself blush at this unexpected show of feeling, and I replied, "I've enjoyed my time here, Millicent. It's not easy being far from home, but having a nice place to live and study makes a big difference. Take care of yourself and be well."

She smiled and said that she would. I left her petting her cat and went upstairs to bid Miko and Molly farewell. I found them chatting in Molly's room, and they looked up when I knocked on the doorsill. "You're leaving now?" Molly asked. I nodded, and she smiled as she said, "We're going to miss you here, you know."

"Aw, you two are always hanging out together. You'll hardly notice I'm gone," I said.

Molly shook her head emphatically. "Don't sell yourself short," she replied. "You've always been someone we could rely on when things got...well, you know, difficult. You've been a stabilizing force as well as a really fun person to talk to. I love your insane sense of humor. It won't be the same here without you."

Miko added, "You are really nice person. I hope you have happy times always."

I was touched by their words and how they valued my friendship. Grinning broadly, I looked from one to the other and said, "I'm going to miss you both too. I've really enjoyed having you here; I can't imagine living in this house these past months without your company."

"Amen to that!" Molly seconded.

We laughed a moment and then I said to them, "Good luck in school and beyond. I know you'll do great. Try to take care of Millicent when I'm gone, okay?"

Molly promised that they would watch out for her, and then there was a moment of uncomfortable silence as we struggled to find the right way to say goodbye. Miko smiled and offered her hand, saying, "Have a good journey. It has been nice to know you, Mark. You are good friend." I took her hand and shook it; her inherent shyness seemed to preclude any further demonstration of affection.

Molly was not so restrained. As I turned to her, she stepped up and gave me a big hug. We embraced for a moment, the physical contact expressing what we could not say with words. Then the moment passed and we stepped apart self-consciously. She smiled at me and said, "Have a good life, my friend. Good luck out there; I know you'll make a great vet."

"Thanks," I said. "I hope so. I've still got a long way to go."

"Don't we all!" Molly groaned, rolling her eyes. "I've got a thesis to write and…well, I won't bore you with the details, but there's a huge amount of work ahead."

"You can handle it," I told her. "You're brilliant and I know you can do anything you put your mind to. Just find a niche in your field where you enjoy what you do."

"I plan on it," she replied, smiling.

I looked at my watch and said, "Well, I guess I should be going. It's a long drive to Portland."

Both of the girls bid me farewell as I headed out of the bedroom. I turned and looked at them from the door. They both sat on the bed grinning at me, and I gave them a parting wave of the hand before I turned and descended the stairs. It was the last time I ever saw either of them.

I paused to leave my house key on the dining room table along with a small thank you note to Millicent. Out then to the car where Dixie was waiting for me, restlessly pawing at her cage door. I slid into my seat and said to her, "Are you ready to head home? I sure am! Let's hit the road…hopefully without bruising our knuckles!"

Dixie just stared at me as if this sparkling bit of wit didn't deserve a reply. I sighed, shrugging my shoulders. "I can tell that you are going to be great company on this ride, aren't you?" I told her, grinning. "I might as well be talking to a tapeworm." She promptly climbed into her litter box and stared at me while she deposited a large stool therein. I shook my head as the aroma reached my nose. Ferrets always had to have the last word.

CHAPTER FIFTY-EIGHT

I drove to Portland in good time. Old man winter had taken a break and the roads were clear of snow and ice. I stopped once to refuel myself and the car. Otherwise I kept my foot on the gas and my eyes fixed on the road ahead. My thoughts swirled with images of Cindy and our apartment in Beaverton. I couldn't wait to see my wife's playful smile and feel her soft touch once again.

I also looked forward to leaving the frozen Palouse behind. It was the end of February and the weather in western Oregon would already be turning toward spring. I knew that even now gentle rains and mild temperatures were coaxing the dormant landscape back to life. Heading west was almost like going south for the winter.

I hit the Portland metropolitan area around five P.M. and navigated the highways taking me toward the west side and Beaverton. I had been on the road for nearly six hours, and was more than ready to be finished. When at last I pulled up in front of my apartment, I parked and killed the engine. Then I took a deep breath and stretched long and slow, smiling as I thought to myself, *That's the last time I'll ever make that trip. I'm back in Oregon for good!"* Dixie heard me stirring and came to the front of her cage, looking out inquisitively. "You're home too," I told her, "and your mom will be happy to see you. Let's go find her!"

I pried her cage out from under the pile of belongings in the passenger seat. With kennel in tow, I ascended the steps to the apartment and knocked on the door. I glimpsed movement to my right and turning I saw Cindy peeking out the kitchen window. When she saw me, her face lit up and she immediately disappeared from sight. I heard running footsteps and then the door was thrown open. Cindy stood there looking lovable in a pair of faded jeans and a red sweater. "You're home!" she exclaimed, and poor Dixie was momentarily forgotten as I put her cage down to properly greet my wife. All was once again right with my world.

I shared several days with Cindy before heading south to Corvine. The day after I arrived was Sunday and we spent every waking (and non-waking) moment together. As always, there was so much catching up to do and very little time in which to do it.

After the weekend Cindy had to work but was home in the evenings. While she was gone I relaxed, did some house chores, and then made dinner for my wife when she returned from her job. My cooking was neither gourmet nor toxic, usually achieving an uninspiring blandness somewhere in between. But it was fairly healthy and as Cindy teasingly put it, "It usually stays down when I eat it." I was glad that her palate had been toughened by the dorm food experience.

Such was our life together in those early days that our reunions were quickly followed by goodbyes. Later in the week I was off again to school, this time heading back to Corvine. I made the drive alone. Cindy had to work and Dixie stayed in Beaverton to keep her company.

The day had dawned grey and rain squalls followed me through the Willamette Valley. Just past noon I arrived in Corvine and checked into a motel near the campus. In the lobby I grabbed a local newspaper, but as I had feared the "roommate wanted" ads were sparse this time of year. The day was still young, so I drove over to the vet school to see if they had any housing listings. As I approached, I could see the familiar bulk of McNairy Hall looming through the mist and it felt like greeting an old friend. I had returned to the place where it had all started. After parking in the guest lot, I ran to the entrance through a steady drizzle.

Pushing through the glass and steel door, I entered the spacious lobby with its red tile floor, seeing once again the sculpture of the lamb in a woman's arms on the wall facing me. It took me back to that moment years before when I had first entered this building. The imposing structure felt much more comfortable now, familiar, like a home away from home. My time in Tullville had made me very glad to be back in Corvine.

I crossed to the reception desk and asked for information on housing opportunities. The lady behind the glass checked and then shook her head apologetically. It was the middle of the school term and no rental vacancies were posted.

Not to be deterred, I wandered the halls upstairs, asking any staff members I met for ideas. Junior students returned to Corvine the same time every year; someone must know how they found housing. Unfortunately no one I spoke to had anything definite to offer. I headed back down into the large animal hospital, strolling through the wide corridors between the stalls. The area was quiet and devoid of people at the moment. A few horses and llamas were hospitalized and I stopped to read their case histories. I was inspecting a dappled grey Arabian horse with a lacerated leg when I heard "Hey there!" from behind me.

I turned and saw Kristina Albright, the classmate who had given me a ride home from Tullville at the end of sophomore year. She was wearing blue coveralls, her long brown curls cascading down the back. With a smile I said, "Hi Kristi! It's nice to see you! Dressed for action already?"

She shrugged and replied, "I had some time to kill so I thought I'd wander through here and see what was going on. Now that we're juniors the staff will be more likely to call on us to help with cases. I dressed accordingly in case I got a chance to pitch in."

I nodded and said, "Well, there's not much happening right now I'm afraid. It's pretty quiet."

"Yeah, so I noticed. I'll probably not stay long. What are you doing here?"

"I came to ask around about finding housing, but I've struck out so far. It's a hard time of year to find a place."

Kristina crossed her arms and flashed a jaunty grin. "Well, today just might be your lucky day. I think I have something for you to check out. You just have to know the right people!" She cockily pointed her thumb at herself, looking very pleased at being able to come to my rescue.

I perked up at this unexpected bit of hope and said eagerly, "C'mon, tell me already! What have you got?"

She smiled and replied, "I'm staying in a townhouse just off of Third Street. There's a half dozen buildings in the development and they're really nice. The guy next door to me is a part-time student, and he told me he was thinking of getting a roommate to help with the rent. I don't think he's advertised yet, but I can ask him if he's still interested." She giggled and added, "I might even put in a good word for you if you pay me enough."

With mock dismay I said, "I'm an impoverished student! I couldn't afford the price."

"You're probably right there," she replied, chuckling. "But I'll see what I can do. Here, I'll give you my number; phone me later and I'll tell you what I found out."

That afternoon I called Kristina from the motel and felt a rush of relief when she said that yes, her neighbor was still planning to find a room mate. His name was Paul Thorne and he wanted to meet me. She gave me his number and I thanked her again. In return she just laughed and said, "You owe me one, mister!"

I called Paul and set up a time that evening to meet. Following his directions, I turned onto a small side road off Third Street, just south of the main downtown area. The road was short and ended in a large cul-de-sac. Two-story white town houses stood in close ranks on both sides of the street. They were attractive and neat, and though their yards were small, they appeared well cared for. The whole development had a nice look to it.

I held my breath as I rang the doorbell. When Paul came to the door, my first impressions of him were positive. He was clean-cut and fit, with a firm handshake and a broad smile framed by a short brown mustache. His attire was casual but stylish, consisting of crisp blue jeans and a bright yellow sport shirt.

The interior of the two story residence was tidy and presentable. The furnishings were nothing fancy, but I saw no dirty laundry or old slices of pizza lying around. One other thing I noticed as Paul gave me a tour: the place smelled clean. There was no reek of old cigarette smoke, no strong pet odors, nothing at all. Sometimes less is more, and I smiled to myself as I headed upstairs behind my host to see the bedroom.

The vacant room was spacious and attractive, furnished simply but adequately in keeping with the rest of the house. I required nothing fancy and this seemed to meet my needs perfectly well. We talked a while and discussed the rent. He was asking a bit more than I had previously paid for housing, but with Cindy employed I could afford it. At the end we shook hands and I had a place to call home.

With that settled, the weekend was mine to relax and unpack my things. The local grocery store was a necessary stop, and then I enjoyed doing nothing for the better part of two days. It was the last relaxation I would know for some time to come.

CHAPTER FIFTY-NINE

The following Monday I was seated in the familiar lecture hall in McNairy, up near the back as I had been my freshman year. *Déjà-vu* struck when I saw our frat boy Ed Martinelli sitting down in the front row and I chuckled to myself. Just then Mike Callahan came in the door, and looking up, he saw me waving from the elevated rear of the hall. He smiled and bounded up the steps to where I sat. When he got to the top, he dropped into the chair to my left and it was as if only days, not years, had passed since we had last occupied these seats. The circle was complete when burly Dr. Lawson walked to the lecture podium and welcomed us back to Corvine, stroking his dark beard as he grinned widely.

There the familiarity ended, however. As juniors we were now taking upper-level courses which made the toils of freshman year pale in comparison. In particular this first term for the returning juniors was legendary among the students. Due to the disparity between Washington's two-semester system and Northern Oregon's three-term schedule, we had arrived back in the middle of what usually would be winter term here. The courses we needed to take before spring would be crammed into half the usual time. The result was a crushing work load that we would have to shoulder for the next six weeks.

To give you a point of reference, an average college student might take twelve to eighteen credit hours a term. Vet school demanded more of its students, and our course load had averaged twenty-two hours a term, all of it difficult, labor-intensive subjects. But our lecture and lab classes this quarter would saddle us with a whopping thirty-two credit hours! The students who had come before us had coined the name "killer quarter." The intimidating title did little to reassure us as we waited to see what was in store.

It didn't take long to find out. The main courses that occupied our time that term were large animal medicine and surgery. Those two general topics spanned a vast amount of material, similar to the small animal courses we had taken in Tullville, but covering even more species. Here we would learn the basics a practitioner would need to treat horses, cattle, sheep, swine, and the like. The burden of new information was worse for those of us lacking prior experience with farm species.

The preceding years had toughened our class, and only that saved us from being overwhelmed during those brutal weeks. Each morning we spent long tiring sessions sitting in lectures and writing until our hands cramped. Sometimes we would take notes for four hours straight, with only ten-minute breaks between classes. Thankfully, we had priority over the freshmen when using the modern lecture hall with its creature comforts; the underclassmen were over in the poultry building on tiny plastic chairs listening to the steam radiators rattle and wheeze. We had paid our dues in the past and now we were reaping the benefits.

In the afternoons there were yet more classes, and two days a week we took large animal surgery lab from three to five P.M. In groups of four or five we took turns performing surgeries with professors overseeing our endeavors, similar to what we had done in the small animal course.

Most of our surgical work was done on small ponies such as Shetlands from nearby stables. The animals had various nicks and wounds, skin masses, and other minor ailments that were within the abilities of junior surgeons. These patients were also small enough not to need the primary surgery suite with its large lifting table; we could easily hoist the ponies onto our smaller operating tables in the student surgery room. Many procedures were, in fact, performed with a local nerve block, numbing an area of skin with the patient standing wide awake. With half a dozen animals able to fit into the huge room at one time, all the juniors could have a chance to learn surgery firsthand. It was large animal practice using not-quite-so-large patients.

A pony still greatly outweighs a human, however, and some of these stout little animals had cantankerous attitudes. We could not afford to get careless. One afternoon in surgery I witnessed just how quickly an injury could occur.

My team had just finished working on our own patient, a bay-colored Shetland named Joey. We had sutured a small laceration on his flank where another pony had kicked him. After we were done, I stretched and glanced slowly around. Across the room from our group stood a roan male pony with his head down. His eyes were squinted in an ill-tempered expression and his stance was tense. I could tell that he was one of the "unhappy campers," as Dr. O'Brien liked to call them.

Behind the horse his team was working to clean up the surgery area. One student, Mary Hackett, stood a short distance from the pony's rump, hands on her hips as she looked around the surgery suite for other items to clean up. I had a split second to realize that she was in the wrong position, neither tight up against the horse nor out of range of his hooves, and then it happened. The pony lashed out with both his back feet, and the left one caught Mary in a glancing blow off her knee. The impact threw her back and she slammed hard against the wall behind her. From there she slid slowly down to the concrete floor, where she sat looking dazed.

Her team rushed to help her, gathering around and asking if she was okay. After a few moments Mary waved them off and stood up shakily. She took a tentative step, then another, and then she winced as her leg buckled and she crumpled back to the ground. I cringed when I saw the unnatural angle her knee had bent in that instant.

Sure enough, Mary had suffered a torn anterior cruciate ligament in her knee. Just like that, the would-be surgeon became a patient herself, and her knee was surgically repaired soon after. Mary's perseverance was admirable; despite being on crutches, she was back in school within two weeks and managed to complete her education on schedule.

Another female student, Alice Brickley, also found herself on the wrong end of a horse's hooves during junior surgery. Alice got kicked right in the face and the blow fractured her lower jaw. As a result she had her mouth wired shut for about six weeks. She was stoic and didn't complain much, though this might have been because it was extremely difficult for her to speak. Although she seemed to take it all in stride, I could imagine that sucking all of her nutrition through a straw for a month and a half must have gotten a bit tedious. Steak and potatoes just doesn't have the same appeal once it's gone through a blender.

In lecture the endless hours of note taking were quickly becoming tiresome. My middle finger sported a heavy callous where the pen rode against it, and I worried that my hand would forever clench into an evil-looking claw shape by the time I graduated. The volume of material was so bad that once I saw Molly Boyer use her class notes as a step stool when reaching for an upper-shelf textbook. It worked quite well.

Molly was one of those people who could make you laugh without trying. Early one morning she was sitting in the lecture auditorium before class started, and I noticed her inspecting her stethoscope. A few weeks earlier she had cracked the thin plastic membrane that covered the head of the scope, the part that you put against the patient to pick up sounds with. She had purchased a replacement but apparently had managed to break the new one already. Looking exasperated she exclaimed, "Damn it! My diaphragm is ruptured again!"

By sheer happenstance, at that moment the background noise in the auditorium subsided, so when she spoke it carried through the room loud and clear. A dozen grinning faces turned to stare at her in surprise, and as she saw the attention focused on her, she realized what she had said. The mortified expression on her face made me laugh so hard that my side ached.

Despite those fun moments that brightened our existence, the struggle to stay afloat dominated every student's waking thoughts. As the six-week mini term sprinted toward its end, the looming certainty of final exams added to the pressure we were all feeling. With lectures and surgery labs taking all our time and energy, when were we supposed to study?

The signs of anxiety were clearly visible for all to see. Normally laid-back individuals grew irritable and short-tempered. The snack machines in the student lounge were being emptied at a hitherto unheard of rate. Stress even made our class look younger, as smooth complexions broke out in that classic teenage affliction known as acne. The veterinary library, which during normal times was avoided like the plague, now harbored students who sequestered themselves in its nooks and crannies with a "do not disturb" look on their faces as they squinted at bloated note binders.

We all found ways to cope as best we could. When I was feeling worn and weary, Cindy's affection proved to be the most potent elixir. The weekends were our time to be together, and after Friday's last class I would pack an overnight bag and head for Beaverton. It was only a ninety-minute commute, but I would drive the entire distance filled with impatient anticipation. When I arrived home, I always raced up the stairs to the door of our apartment. Cindy would answer my knock and then for two short days life would become very simple and very special.

My classmates found other means of handling stress as well. Humor is a great tension breaker, and there was plenty of wit to go around. Sometimes it would just be a comment made in passing, such as Ed Martinelli grumbling about lectures starting each day at the "butt crack of dawn." Or it could be a more formal declaration, like the words scrawled anonymously on the auditorium chalkboard which reflected the prevailing sentiment, "Time to Rest When I Die." Even the old "C=DVM" equation made an appearance, penned in felt tip marker on a large note paper and tacked to the wall of the student lounge.

One of the best inscriptions was left by a student in theriogenology class. Therio is the study of reproduction, including everything from fertility testing to semen collection to maximizing breeding success in livestock. One morning we were met with a large note on the front board of the lecture hall: "Theriogenology—it's all fun and games until someone loses a hymen."

But despite our best efforts, the killer quarter was slowly grinding us down, and adding to the emotional drain was the dreary weather outside. For weeks on end we were greeted each morning with a nonstop grey drizzle. Even at midday the landscape remained gloomy, as if locked in a perpetual twilight. The ground was soggy and waterlogged. It seemed like years since we had seen the sun, and the mood of the students was proportionately dark.

Trina Caldwell had her own unique way of dealing with life's hardships. She was a tall, solidly-built girl with raven black hair and a fiery temper, and as Mike Callahan put it, "No tact filter between her brain and her mouth." What she thought was what she said, and she often said quite a bit. Trina added color to the class, and I liked her candor and her irreverent sense of humor.

One day I was sitting in the main lecture hall waiting for the first class of the day to begin, when I heard an odd sound. It resembled a wet slap, slap, slap coming from beyond the open door to the auditorium, and it was getting louder as I listened. In a few moments Trina's figure filled the doorway and my jaw dropped.

Apparently our outspoken classmate had had enough of the weather. She was dressed in a heavy vinyl rain suit from head to foot, topped off with full-scale scuba gear. This included flippers (which were creating the unusual noise I had heard), a snorkel, and diving mask. When she took a seat in the front row we became aware of the small sign attached to her back which read, "If you can't beat the weather, then adapt!" It was an over-the-top protest of something we were powerless to change, and we understood exactly how she felt.

Humor wasn't the only contribution Trina Caldwell made to our wellbeing during that term. Her outspokenness sometimes paid dividends for her quieter classmates. In mid-April our final exams arrived, and we all were struggling mightily to master the volumes of material we had been given. When pushed to your limits, any perceived unfairness can seem critical. Such was the case in the therio exam, and Trina came to our rescue.

Theriogenology during that term was strictly a classroom subject with no lab section. Our hands-on experience would not come until senior year. Yet the final exam included a short video of a semen sample from a breeding bull, and we were asked to evaluate it. There were a handful of questions regarding sperm quality based on motility, physical anomalies, and so forth. We had covered the basics in lecture, but had never seen a live bovine semen specimen. Not surprisingly, most of us missed several answers due solely to lack of experience. It had a negative impact on our grades and that didn't sit well with Trina. She decided to go on the offensive.

Dr. Lancer was the professor teaching theriogenology that term. Trina marched up to his office the day that we received our exam scores, her test clutched in one hand. The professor was seated at his desk with the door open. She knocked and he looked up, saying, "Yes, what can I do for you Trina?"

She crossed her arms and said, "You can give me a kiss."

Somewhat taken aback, the professor sat up in his chair and said, "I can what?"

"You can give me a kiss," Trina repeated.

Dr. Lancer looked uncertain and said, "I don't understand. Why should I give you a kiss?"

Trina held out her test and said, "Because I expect some loving after I've been screwed."

The professor not only changed her test grade, he also adjusted the scores pertaining to the semen sample questions on all our exams. Sometimes it pays to be just a little crazy.

CHAPTER SIXTY

Despite the trauma and the drama, we all survived killer quarter somehow, and when final exams were finished, I found that my grades were pretty good and my mind still intact. But there was no rest for the indentured servants, and it was on to spring term with only a weekend off in between.

Our classes that spring included continuations of both large animal medicine and surgery. The medicine course began to incorporate a clinical portion called medical rounds. These were where we toured the hospital and evaluated cases in small groups of four or five students, each led by a professor.

In rounds we would look at the patient's chart history which hung on the front of the stall. After discussing the client's entering complaint, the students performed a basic examination on the animal. The professor then would ask us to offer possible diagnoses. The students would talk it over and come up with a differential disease list. Next we would be asked to devise a diagnostic plan, detailing which tests would we want to perform to aid our evaluation.

In the end the doctor would tell us what the hospital staff had diagnosed and how they had come to their conclusions. We could see what tests had actually been done and why, and learn how accurate we had been in our patient assessment. Such exercises gave us a feel for the medicine that lecture notes could never provide.

We also were increasingly called upon to administer treatments to patients. This was where I began to hone large animal skills such as drawing blood samples and giving injections. As usual, these procedures varied between species. Horses had huge jugular veins and we usually drew blood samples there. Pressing on the vein as it ran alongside the neck would make it swell and become visible under the skin. The vessel was easily as wide as my thumb, like a garden hose waiting to be tapped. Even a blindfolded person with palsy could hit it with a needle on the first try. Of course, I missed on my initial attempt.

Cattle jugulars could be used as well, but a popular method of blood draws in the bovines was to hit the caudal vein on the underside of the tail. First you grabbed the tail near the base and jacked it up over the cow's rump. This position exposed the vein, and oddly it also inhibited the cow's ability to kick you while you stood behind her. The needle was inserted into the tail not far from where it met the rump, and a large blood sample could be drawn into the syringe within seconds.

For me the high point of spring term was advanced small animal surgery, an elective class that I had looked forward to for some time. It was the only small animal course offered to the upperclassmen at Corvine, and provided hands-on experience with more challenging surgeries. The procedures covered were ones common to general practice, so many of us signed up. It turned out to be one of the most useful classes I took in veterinary school.

The surgeries varied depending on what cases were available, but they were all practical and valuable to learn. The patient I remember best was a young yellow Labrador Retriever named Bonehead who presented with an intestinal foreign body. He had begun vomiting repeatedly the day before, and his owners had taken him to a local vet. When abdominal palpation and X-rays had confirmed the presence of a blocked bowel, the owners had been unable to afford the needed surgery. As a result they were referred to the teaching hospital. Here they had the option of a lower-cost operation performed by students instead of the staff surgeons. They had given us permission to proceed and the dog became my patient.

Bonehead was only eight months old, adult-sized but still a puppy at heart. At that age dogs often don't have much sense and will swallow objects that they can't possibly digest. When we examined the dog, he carried good weight and had a beautiful gold coat typical of his breed. However he was weak and depressed, and every so often he would retch violently, bringing up traces of greenish yellow bile from his stomach. He looked very unhappy.

We reviewed the radiographs sent by the referring vet, and there was a classic blockage pattern in the bowel: distended, gas-filled intestinal loops in the front of the abdomen, with the dilated portion of bowel coming to an abrupt end. Behind that the intestines looked small and empty. At the area where the swollen bowel stopped, there was a vague grey mass visible. The object didn't look dense enough to be a rock or a bone. We suspected a foreign body made of rubber or something similar, possibly a dog chew toy that had been swallowed.

We took Bonehead to surgery, where I performed an exploratory laparotomy. This involved making a large midline abdominal incision to allow thorough examination of all the organs. I hadn't made an incision this length since my first spay, and I grinned to myself as I realized how far I had come since then.

When I entered the dog, I encountered a bloated stomach filled with fluid. The normally pink loops of bowel were grossly distended and colored an angry red. The intestinal walls were stretched so thin that they were semi-transparent; I could see dark fluid and gas bubbles moving within the gut as I handled it.

I quickly traced the small bowel down from the stomach until I came to the obstruction. Lodged within the intestine was a firm object about the length of my thumb and maybe two and one-half centimeters (one inch) thick. It was wedged tightly in place, acting like a cork and preventing anything from flowing past that point. The bowel was turning dark at the site of the blockage due to pressure and the resulting loss of blood flow; if surgery had been delayed another few hours, the organ might have ruptured.

Dr. Cutler was the supervising surgeon; he took a peek at the gut as I worked and offered some advice. "That darkened area at the obstruction may not be viable; you'll need to relieve the blockage and see if it pinks back up. If it stays dark you are probably going to have to remove that segment of bowel."

I nodded and said, "I should make an incision and remove the object now, right?"

Dr. Cutler replied, "Yes, but don't cut the bowel at the obstructed site. The tissue there is damaged and may not be healthy enough to heal an incision. There's a good chance it would leak. Instead massage the object back up the bowel to a healthier-looking area and make your incision there. Then it will seal more readily when you suture it closed."

Of course! The idea made great sense to me, but I knew I wouldn't have thought of that myself. I worked the foreign body a short distance back up the bowel toward the stomach. Then I packed sterile towels around the intestine where I would make my incision.

The cloth would catch any bowel contents that spilled out, minimizing contamination of the abdomen.

The surgeon nodded as I prepared to open the intestine. "Save the object," he said. "Owners are often curious, and knowing what it was can help prevent a repetition of this problem." So saying, he wandered off to check on the other surgeries being performed at nearby tables.

After toweling off the bowel, I incised it and exposed the object within. It was dark red and coated with gut fluids; I pulled it free and felt its texture. We had guessed right; it was definitely rubber of some type. I tossed it into the sterile bowl on the instrument tray and began suturing the intestine closed. When I was finished, we rinsed and cleaned the incision area before replacing the loop of gut back into the abdomen.

I moved back down to the original obstruction site to check the bowel color there. Already the intestinal wall had turned from nearly black to a brick red, indicating that the tissue was viable. I breathed a sigh of relief, and called Dr. Cutler over to verify my interpretation. He agreed and said, "Good work, Mark. Check the rest of the gut and then get him closed up." I smiled at his encouraging comments, and after verifying that no other foreign bodies were present, I grabbed suture and began the closure.

The story normally would have ended with the completion of the surgery, but there was an amusing bonus to this episode. While I was suturing my patient, one of my team mates took the foreign body and rinsed it off to better visualize what it was. She turned it over in her hands, frowning, and then suddenly said, "Oh, my…!"

The unusual tone of her voice made me look up, and I asked, "What is it, Julie?"

She said, "It's…well, I want a second opinion."

I looked closer at the odd artifact as she turned it this way and that. It was tubular with a slightly flared bulge at one end; I had the feeling I should recognize it, but I couldn't quite determine what it reminded me of. The other end was irregular and appeared to have been chewed off. This meant that it had originally been longer… with a sudden stab of surprise I realized why the object looked familiar. It was fashioned to resemble a portion of male anatomy. *Human* male anatomy. I glanced at Julie, and even though the mask hid most of her face she definitely looked flushed. I couldn't help it then; I started laughing and the other members of my team joined in as they realized what it was that Bonehead had swallowed.

Dr. Cutler sauntered over, attracted by the commotion. "What's up, team?" he asked, grinning behind his mask. "It sounds like you're having fun. If you have a good joke or two, don't be afraid to share. Say, what was the foreign body you took out of this guy? Was it a doggie toy as we thought?"

It fell on me as chief surgeon to summarize our findings, so I said, "Well, it's a toy I guess, but not for doggies. It's more for humans."

"What do you mean?" the doctor asked. "Where is it?"

Julie obligingly produced the piece of rubber and slapped it into the professor's hand. He looked puzzled momentarily, and then his eyes widened. My teammates once again began to giggle as the professor contemplated the object thoughtfully. Finally he cleared his throat and said, "I see. Hmm, well, I'm not sure if the owners will want to know what this was after all. It could be a bit, er, compromising. We'll just say it's an obscure piece of rubber. If they insist on seeing it, we'll bag it and let them view it at their leisure. Preferably with very few people around." He chuckled and rolled his eyes, saying, "Why is it always on my shift?"

"Look at the bright side," Stan Hulbert offered. "At least it was only a replica he ate."

CHAPTER SIXTY-ONE

My roommate Paul turned out to be a truly nice guy, very easy to get along with. He was nearly always in a great mood, so life at the townhouse was stable and predictable. Coming off the ordeal with Millicent, I was thrilled to be able to concentrate on school without major distractions at home.

On the other hand Paul was human, and human beings all have their flaws. Although my housemate was a breath of fresh air emotionally speaking, the opposite was true when it came to his digestive tract. To put it succinctly, Paul suffered from terminally bad flatulence. I'm not sure what vagaries of gastrointestinal dysfunction powered his formidable gas output, but the end result was not good. Most of his accidents were of the silent but deadly variety and could knock down a full-grown mule.

To his credit Paul felt bad about the discomfort his roiling gut visited upon those around him. He did his best to hold in the evil vapors, and if that failed, he'd give me warning of the impending doom awaiting me should I linger. This was always done most discretely. When we were in public he would lean over and quietly utter the code phrase, *"Move on."* Then we would quickly scuttle away from ground zero in the hope of keeping our nasal passages intact.

On several occasions this happened while we were shopping together at a neighborhood supermarket. In each case we hurried further down the aisle, and I would watch out of the corner of my eye as unsuspecting patrons behind us ran headlong into the invisible cloud. The reactions were immediate and startling. Formerly bland expressions twisted into masks of revulsion, and involuntary vocalizations such as "Damn!" or "Oh my!" were not unusual. All the while I stayed busy inspecting goods on the store shelf and trying not to laugh. Despite the inherent hazards, living with Paul kept even the most routine outings from getting dull.

One day in mid-May a strange object appeared in the sky overhead. It careened slowly across the heavens, blinding to the eye and radiating an unusual energy which burned when it touched living flesh. Looking upwards, people pointed in awe and wondered aloud what it could be. Local experts in astronomy were asked to study the phenomenon to help prevent mass panic. Eventually an explanation was found when historical records were consulted. It turned out this event was not without precedent; the same apparition had appeared long ago, and was known as the sun.

With the advent of clear weather the outside temperatures instantly soared. To the non-acclimated denizens of the Willamette Valley, the warmth seemed almost tropical. Shorts and summer shirts were rediscovered, pulled out of mothballs after hibernating in storage for many months. The meadow next to the veterinary building waxed lush with tall emerald grass and colorful wildflowers. Corvine was an idyllic place to live when the weather turned charitable.

Indoors our classes continued to churn out loads of information for us to write down, process and absorb. However, this term the pace was not quite so frenetic, so we kept abreast of the material without feeling as if we were drowning. Some of my classmates even got the silly notion that they had extra time on their hands. These deluded individuals volunteered to be "live-in students" who stayed nights at the hospital, helping to care for patients. It was a thankless job with no pay other than free housing for the duration of their duties. The luxurious accommodations consisted of a small, concrete-floored room little larger than a walk-in closet, furnished with a small folding cot in one corner and a table with a reading lamp.

Mike Callahan had a strong interest in large animal medicine and wanted to see as many cases as he could, so he signed up for the program. That spring he lived at the teaching hospital day and night, helping treat emergencies that came in at odd hours as well as hospitalized animals that needed constant nursing care. With his boundless energy and easy grasp of the curriculum, he seemed an ideal choice for the job. But sleep could be a scarce commodity when living in, and some days I could tell that even he felt the strain.

One morning I arrived for the first lecture of the day, and took my usual seat up in the back of the auditorium. Mike came dragging in at half his usual speed, meaning he was moving at a normal walking pace for the average human being. He stumped slowly up the steps until he reached my aisle and sat down heavily beside me. As I looked him over, I noticed his hair was disheveled and his eyes puffy. The stained coveralls he wore were rumpled as if he had slept in them, and his movements were listless. It was hard to believe what my eyes were telling me, but "living in" had finally accomplished what killer quarter could not. Mike Callahan looked tired.

I grinned at him cheerily and said, "Good morning, Mike! Sleep well last night?"

With a grimace he mumbled, "Sleep?! What's that? I can't seem to remember."

A pang of sympathy made me relent in my teasing and I said, "Tough schedule, eh?"

"Yeah, I spent most of the night nurse-maiding a pygmy horse."

"Wow. We don't see those very often," I said. "Is it really small?"

"Yes, she's only a few months old, no bigger than a dog. Very cute, and very sick."

"What's going on with her?" I asked, intrigued.

Mike rubbed his eyes and answered, "She showed up at the end of the day yesterday, looking bloated and somewhat shocky. Her owners said she wasn't eating very well, especially when it came to solid foods. Her stool output had been scant and inconsistent too. We gave her fluids and supportive care then took some radiographs. It turned out she has megacolon."

"Wow," I said. "Megacolon at such a young age? Do they think it's hereditary?"

"Yep," Mike said, nodding. "The pygmies have lots of congenital problems, and poor gut motility is one of them. She's got a ton of food backed up in her bowel, and the colon is hugely dilated. She's probably going to have problems long term and may not even live to reach adulthood."

"Damn. That's sad," I said. "What a hard way to begin life."

"Sure is," Mike sighed. "In the meantime I get to medicate and syringe feed the little tyke every few hours all night long. It's wonderful fun as long as you don't worry about minor details like sleep. Mae-Mae and I are becoming very bonded. I should just put my cot in her stall. Come to think of it, that would probably be more comfortable than my room."

We shared a laugh at his story, but listening to him, I was glad to have kept myself limited to the standard curriculum. Adding after-hours work to our schedule seemed a choice that bordered on deranged.

The next two months sailed past in a steady routine of lectures, surgery labs, and hospital rounds. Although I had scarcely touched a farm animal prior to vet school, I gradually became more and more comfortable with the horses, cattle, and other livestock that we dealt with daily. When I had spare time, I often stopped to visit the friendlier horses and cows in the hospital, stroking a face or giving a long neck a few affectionate pats before moving on down the corridor. The size and strength of these herbivores could be offset by an incredible gentleness. Feeling a massive head nuzzling my hand as large brown eyes regarded me solemnly, I understood why the owners of these animals were often so devoted to them. Although I eventually ended up in small animal practice, I have always appreciated the opportunity that I had to work with and learn about our largest companion species. Those encounters enriched my life and enhanced my appreciation of the human-animal bond. I truly believe I am a better veterinarian as a result.

There was no summer break between our third and fourth years in vet school, and as a result spring term extended into July. As the days grew longer and hotter, every instinct told us that we should be out of school enjoying the weather. It was harder than ever to keep our noses in our books and our minds on our work.

Final exams arrived in mid-July, just after I celebrated my twenty-fifth birthday. This time the tests signified more than the culmination of months' worth of study. They also marked the end of our junior year and a conclusion to the formal classroom portion of our education. Senior blocks were just around the corner, and from here our education would be mostly clinical work with real patients. Board exams still awaited us, but our days of sitting in the auditorium for countless hours were over. It was a milestone in our path to becoming veterinarians, and that fact was made clear on the final day of our tests.

The large animal medicine final had the honor of being the last regular examination I took in veterinary school. It was a grueling, two-hour marathon befitting the vast sea of material we had covered in the preceding months. When the last pages were completed and the exams handed in, we were instructed to take a short break and then return to the auditorium for a brief meeting.

A little while later my classmates and I sat in the lecture hall, chatting and joking in a carefree manner that contrasted starkly with the mood only hours earlier. The murmur of conversations suddenly grew quiet, and I looked up to see Dr. Hudson, the dean of the veterinary school, walking into the auditorium. His appearance here was unusual, as I had only seen him on a handful of occasions during my entire time at school. He smiled at us and proceeded to the podium where he paused as if gathering his thoughts. I noticed several other professors standing off to the side in attendance, including burly Dr. Lawson and the ever jolly Dr. O'Brien.

After a moment Dr. Hudson cleared his throat and said, "Good afternoon and thank you for being here. I know we would all rather be outside in the sun right about now." A chorus of agreement erupted from the audience and he smiled knowingly.

Looking over the assembled students the dean continued, "First, I want to congratulate you all for completing the third year of your medical training. You are three-quarters of the way to becoming veterinarians, and the hardest portion of your curriculum is now behind you. I know it has not been easy, and yet you persevered and succeeded. We are all proud of your accomplishments."

"Here! Here!" interjected Dr. Lawson from the side of the room, and his applause was joined by the rest of the faculty in attendance. My classmates and I smiled uncertainly at each other. After all, we had simply studied as students are supposed to, and we were unsure of how to respond to this unexpected praise.

When the room had quieted again Dr. Hudson said, "Today is July 19th. It is a significant date because it not only marks your last day as juniors, but also your last day as an intact group. From now on you will be split into block rotations, and your schedules will no longer be synchronized. This is the last time you will sit together as an entire class until graduation day."

My classmates looked around at each other as his words sunk in. We had all known that we would commence blocks after this term, but we had simply been too busy to contemplate what that meant. This group that had weathered the past three years together would not study in its present incarnation ever again. Of course, we would share block courses in small subsets of the whole. Over the next ten months we would spend some time with nearly all our classmates, but it would not be the same. Our class, like our class work, was becoming a thing of the past.

With this realization came a surprising pang of anxiety. Graduation was nearly a year away, but it suddenly seemed like our school days were numbered. All too soon we would be thrust into the working world as veterinarians. I didn't know about the rest of the class, but I felt like I wouldn't possibly be ready when I had to practice medicine on my own. I could only hope that the upcoming months would provide a lot of clinical experience and a dose of assurance to go with it.

The dean concluded his speech to us with the following advice: "All of you are on your way to joining the most rewarding profession in the world. When you graduate you will shoulder the burden of being ethical practitioners, and also of representing our profession to the public. Do not take that responsibility lightly. Each of you will follow your own path, some in small animal practice, some in large animal, perhaps some in research, industrial, or teaching segments of the profession. You will find that veterinary medicine will give back to you in proportion to what you put into it. My fellow professors and I wish you all long, happy, and fulfilling careers. May the best day of your past be the worst day of your future."

When Dr. Hudson finished speaking, Stan Hulbert stood and began clapping. In a moment he was joined by the entire class. The applause was thunderous and must have lasted nearly a minute. The ovation was not simply in response to the doctor's speech. It was our way of showing appreciation for the quality of the education given to us over the past three years. It was also the last action we took as a unified group. When the echoes in the auditorium had faded away, so also passed the junior class. We said our farewells and headed out the door one by one to pursue the final segment of our education as seniors. None of us looked back, for the future was bright ahead of us.

YEAR FOUR

CHAPTER SIXTY-TWO

The first block course on my schedule was large animal surgery. It proved to be a pleasant change from my prior classes; there were no lectures and no exams, just clinical work, almost as if I were a graduate veterinarian.

Most of the cases I saw during those few weeks were horses referred to the hospital for difficult surgeries. I observed an arthroscopic procedure to clean out an arthritic hock joint, and assisted with an exploratory surgery to remove a large mass in a mare's uterus. An eighteen-year-old grey gelding presented with a grapefruit-sized melanoma near his anus; we debulked the bleeding mass to provide some relief for the horse. Unfortunately a cure wasn't in the cards, as the tumor had metastasized to other parts of his body; it was only a matter of time before the aggressive cancer caused his death. His owner knew the end was near, but she was grateful to be able to share a few extra months with her old companion.

Of course, part of the surgical process involved handling patients under chemical restraint. Anesthetizing large bodies that massed 450 kilos (1,000 pounds) or more was a difficult proposition. Patients get dizzy and disoriented during anesthetic induction, that phase where the drugs start to hit the brain and normal awareness begins to fade into unconsciousness. That was fine with a dog; we could hold the animal and provide gentle yet secure restraint. A towering Clydesdale horse was another proposition altogether.

Ingenuity had provided elegant solutions. The bulky surgery table in the main operatory could tilt sideways to a vertical position. When a horse was to be anesthetized it was walked over and lightly strapped to the vertical table surface with heavy leather binders around its belly and chest. A tranquilizer had already been given so that the animal would be relaxed and stand steady.

When the patient was secure in the support harness, an anesthetic drug was given intravenously and the horse would fall asleep still standing in the straps. Then the table was simply flipped to the horizontal position with the animal attached. Surgery could commence with no manual lifting of the heavy body required.

I first saw this process in action when I assisted on a Thoroughbred mare with a mangled forelimb. She had gotten tangled in a fallen barbed-wire fence, suffering two deep wounds plus a score of cuts and abrasions from her fetlock to her elbow. Although she had been treated on the farm, she needed extensive debridement and careful closure of the lacerations to prevent infection and other complications. The extent of the injuries and the mare's level of anxiety had led the doctors to conclude that general anesthesia was needed.

The technicians led the limping mare into surgery and buckled her to the tilted surgery table. She was a rich chestnut color, her sleek coat highlighting smooth contours. Long legs and graceful lines spoke of speed, and her chiseled face was alert and intelligent. I was no expert on equine breeding, but this horse obviously possessed fine bloodlines.

An IV catheter had been previously placed in one of the mare's jugular veins, and now a fluid line was affixed to the catheter's end. The tubing ran to a large glass bottle held in the anesthesiologist's hand. This held a drug cocktail which was a mix of thiamylol sodium (a fast acting barbiturate) and guaifenesin (a muscle relaxant). Once everything was ready, the doctor turned the bottle upside down and held it high in the air, letting the drugs run full speed down the IV line. A bulky equine body required a lot of anesthetic, and the liquid literally poured from the bottle like water from a tap. In less than a minute the mare's eyes rolled and the whites showed as she became excited, struggling just briefly in her restraints before losing consciousness and sagging into the harness.

We all breathed a sigh of relief; despite the precautions, there was always a degree of risk when large patients were going to sleep. Anything could happen, and sometimes did, during that brief delirious stage. But this time all had gone smoothly, and the technicians scrambled to roll the heavy table into its horizontal position. When it was locked in place with our patient atop it, we jacked open the horse's mouth. The anesthesiologist deftly slid an endotracheal tube as fat as my wrist into the open windpipe. The tube was then attached to hoses running to the oversized anesthetic machine standing nearby. The machine was activated and oxygen laced with anesthetic gas began to flow into the mare's lungs.

Next the technicians inserted a small catheter into the facial artery of the horse. The vessel ran just under the skin of her cheek, an easy target to hit once our patient was immobilized. With the catheter hooked to a monitor, we could take real-time readings of her arterial blood pressure while she was under anesthesia.

Meanwhile, I clipped electrical leads to the horse's legs and flipped the switch on the cardiac monitor. Now the slow rhythm of her powerful heart became translated to an audible beep from the machine's speaker. Once we were sure she was breathing steadily and her cardiac rhythm was normal, we shaved and scrubbed the injured areas of the mare's left forelimb.

Viewed more closely the horse's injuries were ghastly to behold. The thick skin had been laid open in two deep gashes longer than my hand could span, revealing the pink and red flesh beneath. Crusted blood was matted into the surrounding hair; we shaved a liberal space around the wounds to create a clean work area. I saw white stripes of exposed tendons running within the darker muscle tissue as I gently scrubbed the region with iodine soap.

When the wounds were cleaned, we began the process of debriding the traumatized skin. This involved cutting or scraping away any unhealthy tissue and creating fresh margins that could heal properly. I worked alongside Dr. Brenda Babick, a short, stocky woman in her mid-forties who was one of several resident surgeons. We were assisted by another student, Karen Thomas, as we cleaned and sutured the wounds. The surgeon delegated much of the skin closure to Karen and me, since it was the simplest task at hand. Meanwhile, the doctor had discovered some deeper trauma and a lacerated extensor tendon that needed repair. As I threw my sutures in the skin, I tried to glance over to watch Dr. Babick work. Her hands sped through the delicate closure as if they had done it a thousand times before, and I felt a touch of envy at her dexterity. When she was finished, the two severed halves of the tendon were perfectly aligned as if they had never been apart.

Meanwhile I had my own work to complete, and I pushed myself to quickly suture the large wound that I had been assigned. Proper skin closure is particularly important in the horse. In most species an injury generates a pink healing tissue known as granulation tissue. This slowly fills in any gaps until the wound surface is smoothed over and no deep craters remain. In horses this healing process sometimes goes awry, especially on the limbs. The granulation tissue can grow out of control, developing into huge pink masses that protrude outward like cancerous growths. This excessive regenerative response is known in horseman's vernacular as "proud flesh." It could be a nightmare to control, and prevention via proper wound closure was the best medicine. We took care to insure that the skin was sutured securely before we let our patient wake up.

When we were finished, the mare looked almost as good as new. I later heard that she healed well and had no lasting effects from her misadventure. We received a large "thank you" card a few weeks later, complete with a photo of our patient standing in her stall at home. The surgeons posted it on the bulletin board in the hospital office alongside other notes from appreciative clients.

Not all cases turned out as well, however. The most memorable incident during my surgery rotation was also one of the most demoralizing. It happened late on a Friday afternoon in my final week of surgery block. The day had been slow, with only a couple of minor procedures scheduled, and I was anticipating leaving the hospital early. Then around four P.M. the reception desk took an urgent call from a local vet. The referring doctor had a mare in late-term pregnancy that was showing signs of acute colic. He wanted to know if the teaching hospital could see the case immediately. At this stage of my education I understood the need for speed in this situation. Digestive upset in the horse could vary from mild cramping to severe distress. The worst cases might progress to shock and death within hours, even without the added burden of pregnancy. From the description of her symptoms this mare appeared to be in trouble. The hospital advised the vet to send the patient as quickly as possible.

While the horse was in transit the clinicians prepared for her arrival. Dr. O'Brien rounded up several senior students, including me, to assist him with the case. He also found one of the surgeons, Dr. Cutler, and advised him of a possible emergency surgery coming in. Dr. Cutler in turn notified the anesthesiologist and had the technicians prepare the surgery suite. The entire process was quick and efficient, and by the time our patient arrived everyone was ready.

The owners pulled up to the rear of the hospital in a four-wheel-drive pickup truck with a shiny red horse trailer in tow. When the rig was backed up to the admitting entrance of the hospital, it was immediately evident that our patient was in severe distress.

Even before the trailer door opened we could hear the animal inside stomping restlessly and groaning. When the owner undid the latch and the portal swung aside, I caught a glimpse of a jet-black rump. At first the mare was reluctant to back out of the trailer, being too absorbed in her own misery to pay heed to our coaxing. When she eventually decided to move, she came down the ramp in a rush and people scattered to get out of her way.

Exposed in full view she was a beautiful animal, a glossy black Arabian with the delicate facial features and flowing lines typical of her breed. At second glance I realized that she was in fact too shiny; her coat was slicked with sweat. In addition her abdomen appeared tense and distended, more than I would have expected from simply carrying a fetus. Even as I watched she turned and looked anxiously at her belly, and her rear foot came up and kicked at her flank as if to swat away the discomfort there. These were classic signs of colic, although dystocia (difficulty giving birth) was another possibility we had to consider.

Dr. O'Brien talked with the horse's owner, a ruddy-faced man in jeans and a white polo shirt who introduced himself as Patrick Carroll. I was standing close enough to take in the conversation. The doctor inquired, "How long has she been showing signs of distress?"

The owner frowned and replied, "I noticed her sweating a little and acting restless maybe six hours ago. She's gotten steadily worse since. I think it's her gut, as she's not due to foal."

"How far out is the pregnancy?" asked the doctor.

Patrick replied, "About 325 days, so she's close to term, but I really expected the foal next week. My vet took a look and thought her bowel was bloated up."

Dr. O'Brien nodded and said, "Let's get her inside and into a chute so I can palpate her. We'll need some quick diagnostic tests too."

"Do what you have to, doc," Mr. Carroll declared. "This little lady is worth a whole bunch, and so is her foal. I'd hate to lose either of them. That's why I came here instead of having my regular vet try to fix her."

"You heard the man," Dr. O'Brien said to us. "Let's go, people!" With that we all moved indoors to work up our patient.

The mare's discomfort made her edgy and uncooperative, but we managed to get her into a chute where the doctor could do a thorough exam. A technician took the mare's pulse and reported it elevated but of low strength. The doctor nodded and donned a palpation glove, basically a clear plastic sleeve with fingers attached that covered his arm from hand to shoulder. After applying some sterile lubricant he slid his hand gently into the horse's vaginal canal. He continued pushing inward until nearly his entire arm was buried in the mare. She whinnied softly and shifted her feet but otherwise offered no protest. Dr. O'Brien palpated for a moment and then pulled his hand free, saying, "Her cervix is closed; she's not in labor. I need to do a rectal exam."

More lube was applied to the glove, and once again the doctor inserted his arm into the horse, this time via the anal opening and up the rectum. He felt around in her abdomen for several minutes, searching for clues to the origins of her illness. He gave a running commentary as he worked. "The fetus is there all right and it's positioned normally. I just felt a little movement when I touched its head. There's no sign of the mare pushing the foal back toward the birth canal. Ah...her small bowel feels distended with fluid, definitely dilated beyond normal diameter. She's tensing up now; the gut is bothering her. Wow, it's really big. I'm worried about a small intestinal accident such as a torsion. I want to auscult her abdomen and see what I can hear."

So saying he pulled his arm free and stripped off the soiled sleeve, then grabbed his stethoscope from his pocket. His frown deepened as he applied it here and there on the mare's belly. Finally he straightened and said, "It's too quiet in there; I don't hear the usual gut sounds. Most likely it's a torsion, but whatever the problem is, it's not good. Draw blood and get me her blood gases as fast as possible. Someone find Dr. Cutler. Meanwhile let's tap her abdomen and see what we get."

The technicians rushed to carry out his instructions, taking blood from the mare in less than a minute and heading off to the lab to evaluate her blood gases. Another tech shaved a spot on the horse's lower abdomen, and after the area was scrubbed Dr. O'Brien inserted a needle and used the syringe to aspirate a small amount of abdominal fluid.

He held the sample up for us to see. There is always a small amount of free fluid in the abdomen, and normally it is a clear straw yellow color. The syringe contents were cloudy and greenish-tinged, and groans went up from the students as they saw the septic-looking material. The doctor handed the fluid off to be run to the lab for microscopic analysis.

In a couple of minutes Dr. Cutler came walking briskly toward us down the hall. He approached and said, "What have you got, Dan?"

Dr. O'Brien replied, "Acute abdomen in a mare who's near term. I suspect a small bowel torsion; we're waiting on her blood gases and abdominocentesis results. But the fluid we pulled looked nasty, and with the way the gut palpates I'd say the bowel's obstructed."

The surgeon rubbed his cheek and asked, "No sign of dystocia?"

"Nope. Her cervix is closed; the foal isn't in the birth canal. I'm pretty sure it's a bad colic."

Dr. Cutler nodded. "Well, you know me, I'm a surgeon. I'd say cut her now before she becomes more unstable. This is one of those situations where you're damned if you do and damned if you don't. Without surgery she'll probably die. Either way she could turn sour on us in a hurry. If you want me to go in there, let's do it fast."

Dr. O'Brien nodded and said, "We'll have lab results shortly. I'll get the owner's approval and then she's all yours." He started back toward the large animal receiving area, while Dr. Cutler hurried off in the opposite direction to advise his surgery staff of the impending procedure.

Within fifteen minutes we had the lab results in hand. The mare's blood gas analysis showed a metabolic acidosis typical of small intestinal obstruction. With the upper bowel blocked, the stomach's acid contents had no way to empty, and as pressure built, the acidity had begun to leak into her bloodstream.

The other telling finding was the analysis of the abdominal fluid. In addition to white blood cells, the sample contained rod bacteria, suggesting that septic material was spreading from the bowel into the abdomen. We didn't have much time before the situation turned deadly.

A short interval later we had the mare in the surgery room and ready to anesthetize. Our patient's condition appeared to be rapidly deteriorating. She was sweating profusely and her breaths came raggedly as she stomped and fidgeted. The techs had placed a jugular catheter in her neck and had started an IV drip. In addition, they had administered boluses of medications to sedate her and reduce her level of discomfort. Although helpful, these treatments were like dousing a forest fire with a bucket of water. If the mare was obstructed, nothing could stop her downward spiral unless we relieved the blockage quickly.

By the time we were ready, the mare's pain had her half-crazed. The doctors and techs worked to strap her against the vertical surgery platform without getting kicked. When at last she was secured in place, we took readings on her pulse rate and strength. "Pulse is one hundred and low amplitude," a technician said as she held her hand to a vein and counted beats on her wristwatch.

"Rapid and weak—she's going into shock," the surgeon interpreted. "No surprise there. Get a cardiac monitor on her now, and increase the IV drip rate. Let's hope that she's strong enough to withstand surgery." He nodded at Dr. Reynolds who held the bottle of anesthetic already attached to the horse's IV line. The anesthesiologist raised the bottle high and the drugs began to rush down the tubing and into the horse.

Things went quietly for about thirty seconds, while the anesthetic took hold and our patient began to relax. As the distress faded from the horse's eyes, I breathed a sigh of relief. It was just about then that all hell broke loose.

The mare suddenly stiffened and began thrashing wildly in the throws of a grand mal seizure. Her restraints kept her in place, but her limbs were dangerous projectiles and we scattered to avoid the flying hooves. One steel-shod foot caught a wheeled supply table and sent it crashing onto its side, strewing catheters and bandaging supplies across the floor. The horse's eyes bulged from their sockets and I saw her pupils roll back in her head as she bucked and heaved. The explosive snorts of her breaths and the heavy clanging of the stressed surgery table filled the confines of the room. Even the two doctors were momentarily paralyzed by the sights and sounds of the giant body gone berserk.

As abruptly as the seizure had begun it ceased. The horse went limp and hung flaccidly in the restraints. For a moment or two a deathly silence blanketed the room, and then the technician monitoring the EKG readings called out, "Her pulse rate is dropping." As he spoke I became aware of the persistent beeping of the cardiac monitor. The tones were slowing, and in addition there was now a disturbing irregularity to the rhythm. The horse's blocked bowel was altering blood electrolytes and pouring toxins and bacteria into the body. The end result was septic shock and the heart was losing function. In a short time it could cease to pump blood altogether.

In an instant Dr. Reynolds the anesthesiologist leapt into action. He lowered the bottle of IV anesthetic to stop its flow into the mare, shoving the half-empty vessel into the hands of a student. "Give me a tracheal tube!" he exclaimed, grabbing the now unconscious animal's mouth and yanking it open. Someone handed him a large tube and he said, "I need light!" A tech was quick at hand beside the doctor, shining a small flashlight down the dark throat. The horse was still in an upright position, held there by her straps.

"Someone grab the jaws," the vet commanded. I quickly stepped forward and obliged. The mare's flesh felt clammy and cool beneath my fingers, her mandibles slick with drool as I struggled to maintain my grip. I pulled the mouth open as wide as I could, straining to support the weight of the bulky head.

My contribution freed up Dr. Reynolds' hands. With his left he grabbed the mare's tongue, pulling it out to better visualize her throat. His right hand then slid the endotracheal tube down her gullet and deep into her windpipe. As soon as it was in place he attached the oxygen hoses and turned on the gas flow.

"She's ventilated," the anesthesiologist called over his shoulder as he monitored his charge.

"Good. Let's get this table flipped quickly," Dr. Cutler answered. The techs and students labored to rotate the table and lock it in its horizontal position. As they did so the EKG monitor suddenly flat-lined and its beeping was replaced by a shrill alarm code.

The anesthesiologist said anxiously, "Are we losing her? We've got no beat!"

Dr. Cutler shook his head as he listened with his stethoscope. "I'm still getting a faint rapid heartbeat here."

I glanced at the EKG leads as we had been taught. Sure enough, one of the alligator clips lay loose on the table, having been dislodged from the skin as we repositioned the animal. I grabbed the metal clamp and reattached it. Immediately I was rewarded with the return of an audible heartbeat from the monitor.

Our reprieve was brief, however. The techs quickly positioned the mare for her surgery, but no sooner had they begun to shave her when the monitor alarm went off again. This time it was for real. Dr. Cutler listened for a moment at the mare's chest, then threw off his stethoscope and shouted, "I've lost the heartbeat! She's going down. Hand me a scalpel NOW!"

A student grabbed the blade from the surgery pack, unconcerned about sterility, and slapped the handle into the surgeon's hand. Jumping atop the table, Dr. Cutler straddled the exposed belly of the dying horse and brought the razor-sharp blade down in a savage motion. The gleaming steel parted fur and flesh as if it were tissue paper. In a scant few seconds he had created an incision the entire length of the mare's abdomen. Blood welled sluggishly from the wound, no longer driven by a beating heart.

Dr. Cutler grabbed the skin margins with both hands and pulled them wide. Subcutaneous fat bulged out of the gaping hole, followed quickly by masses of dark, bloated intestine. But the surgeon had no eyes for the gut; he was after a more important prize. Pawing frantically through the lengths of bowel he exposed a huge pink structure that bulged roundly from the body cavity. It was the gravid uterus of the mare, and it held a tiny life that might yet be saved.

Again the scalpel flashed, albeit with a bit more caution. Dr. Cutler slit the uterus open along its length, then dropped the blade and reached gently inside. His hands emerged with a fully formed foal clutched in his fingers. It was jet black like its mother and covered with shiny membranes. The doctor laid the limp body on the table next to the mare and called for a towel. One was found, and he used it to strip the amnionic sac and fluids away from the newborn animal.

Dr. Cutler opened the foal's mouth and wiped it out, clearing the airway. As techs continued vigorously rubbing the tiny wet body, the doctor put his mouth to the animal's face and blew in its nose. Its thorax expanded just a bit, and then shrank again as the doctor pulled away. He repeated this process once, twice, and then again. Between breaths he called for the techs to bring a small endotracheal tube so that he could intubate the foal.

Meanwhile Dr. Reynolds had his stethoscope out and was listening intently to the infant horse's chest. His expression fell, and after a moment he looked up at the surgeon and shook his head.

Dr. Cutler read what was in the anesthesiologist's eyes and the energy abruptly went out of him. He ceased his attempts to ventilate the foal and rocked back on his heels, his shoulders sagging tiredly as he laid the tiny head gently on the table. One of the techs reached over and switched off the heart monitor, killing its insistent alarm tone.

That was how it ended, with the attending students and technicians standing quietly, gazing at the two doctors slumped in defeat amongst the blood and entrails, nothing to show for their efforts but a dead mare and her dead foal.

CHAPTER SIXTY-THREE

At the end of August I went straight from large animal surgery into the large animal medicine rotation. The medicine block was one of the meatiest in terms of how much I saw. Every day was busy, and there were a lot of opportunities for hands-on involvement.

The five students in the block accompanied the clinicians as they admitted cases to the teaching hospital. There were a handful of veterinarians who practiced internal medicine at the school; the ones I spent the most time with were Dr. Lawson and Dr. O'Brien. Each was rewarding to work with; Dan Lawson's loud voice and imposing stature were offset by a genuine concern for his patients and his students, and he could be surprisingly kind to both. He also knew his medicine and was an accomplished practitioner.

Dr. O'Brien predictably was full of mischief and approached everything with a cheery demeanor. His round cheeks flushed and his Irish accent intensified when he became excited talking about a case, which happened fairly often. Even on busy days he had a twinkle in his eye. I still remembered my first impression of him years earlier during my admission interview. Even with the stress of that day, I had thought he would be a great doctor to learn from because of his comical personality. As a senior student I finally had the chance to work alongside him, and my expectations were more than met; he ended up being my favorite professor that year.

As with large animal surgery, much of the medicine block focused on horses, and much of the horse work revolved around leg and foot problems. Lameness was a constant thorn in our side when treating equines. It could be subtle and hard to localize, but we couldn't ignore it. Left untreated, a small problem often deteriorated into a crippling arthritis. Thus we spent a lot of time diagnosing ailments of bones, tendons and joints in these animals.

Lameness could be caused by acute trauma such as a blow to a leg, or repeated trauma such as the pounding that a race horse's limbs endure during training. Hereditary factors such as poor conformation, husbandry issues such as dirty conditions or poor shoeing, nutritional influences, and systemic diseases all could cause a horse to go lame.

The detection and pinpointing of an equine lameness was in itself an art form. The skill and experience of the practitioner played a pivotal role. One needed to observe the horse at rest and at a trot, and sometimes while being turned sharply or being backed up. Different types of lameness showed up with different tests. Symptoms of pain might worsen with exercise if the animal suffered from sore shins ("bucked shins"). By contrast an arthritic hock joint ("bone spavin") might actually improve when the horse was worked and warm, only to stiffen up again after resting.

There were other odd clues that the average person would not think to look for. A lame forelimb often causes a head bob as the horse walks, with the head raising up as the sore limb bears weight and then dropping back down when the good leg is planted. Some animals lean slightly to one side to take weight off an uncomfortable limb. A trained eye sees much more, and an astute equine vet will note subtle changes that would be missed by most people.

Once the affected leg was identified, we performed manual exams to try to localize where the pain was occurring. This could be anywhere from shoulder or hip down to the foot, and that covers a lot of territory. We would try flexing and extending each joint to assess for pain therein. Palpating (feeling) for heat or swelling along all parts of the leg was essential. We tested the foot for sensitivity by tapping on various spots with a small hammer, and by using a hoof tester. The latter resembled a small pair of fireplace tongs, and was used to squeeze the sole of the foot to see if there was sensitivity to pressure.

When the pain had been localized, we often needed X-rays to identify the exact nature of the problem, as well to determine how severe the damage was. Treatments often included rest, anti-inflammatory medications, and correction of any husbandry problems such as poor diet or housing. Surgical intervention was needed with some lesions such as chip fractures of the bones.

With all the nuances and techniques applied to these problems, it still paid to follow Dr. O'Brien's simple advice, "Start at the beginning." One day a lame Thoroughbred stallion was brought to the hospital's admitting entrance. It was a slow afternoon with little happening, so three different clinicians wandered outside to observe the animal. The lameness was subtle and a handler worked hard to demonstrate it, trotting the stallion this way and that in the parking lot behind the building. Finally the doctors had seen enough, and the horse was walked indoors to be examined by hand.

I was singled out to perform the preliminary examination while the clinicians observed. The lameness had been narrowed to the right forelimb, so I knew where to begin. The three doctors stood in a group just behind me, discussing possible diagnoses. I overheard the deep voice of Dr. Lawson saying, "I suspect it's osselets; the horse is young and he's been worked hard on the track." I nodded to myself; osselets was a horseman's term for an inflamed fetlock joint which was the equivalent of the knuckle on a human. It was common in young horses that were exercised hard.

Behind me Dr. O'Brien's twang responded, "Ay, he's young and all, but I've got a feeling it's bucked shins." Again I couldn't disagree; this was an irritation of the cannon bone which extended between the fetlock and the carpus (similar to the hand bones between a person's knuckle and wrist). Again it was a common problem among youthful equines in heavy training.

The gravelly voice of Dr. Simpson spoke up last. He was the grey-haired senior staff member and had decades of equine experience. "You both make sense, but I'll bet you that it's carpitis. I think he's got a touch of swelling at the carpus (wrist), and it's just not severe enough to be obvious yet."

Dr. Lawson's voice boomed out again, "Do you want to wager a six-pack on it, Henry?"

I suppressed a smile; it sounded like Washington's radiology department all over again.

Dr. Simpson replied, "You're on, young man. I'm feeling thirsty, and you're about to be schooled." I could hear Dr. Lawson snort while Dr. O'Brien chuckled at his colleagues' spirited exchange.

As the debate raged on I methodically felt the leg up and down, and finding nothing untoward I proceeded to the next step, hoof testing. I grabbed the testing tongs and picked up the horse's right front foot. Standing next to his shoulder and facing the rear of the animal, I crouched slightly and used my bent right knee to prop the hoof, freeing my hands. Then I squeezed the foot with the metal tongs, applying one prong to the top of the hoof with the other pushing into the sole. The pressure of the bottom arm was the important part, as it would detect sensitivity in the normally tough sole of the foot.

The stallion stood totally relaxed as I gradually moved around the periphery of the large foot, squeezing each section before moving on. The professors were still wagering on which of their diagnoses were correct when I reached the inner aspect of the hoof and applied the tongs. Abruptly the leg spasmed, jerking the foot violently away from its perch on my knee. The tongs fell to the floor with a harsh clang and the stallion neighed softly, looking around to see what had caused the sudden pain.

The doctors ceased their conversation and glanced over to see what was happening. I looked up at them grinning and said, "He has a foot abscess."

Dr. Simpson raised his eyebrows, then crossed his arms and said, "Show me."

I obligingly picked up the testing tongs and grabbed the hoof, and I squeezed the medial aspect of the sole once more. Again the foot was pulled roughly out of my grip and the horse shifted uncomfortably, appearing most displeased with my efforts. The three clinicians looked at each other, and then Dr. O'Brien burst out laughing. "It just goes to show that you have to start at the beginning," he exclaimed with a broad smile.

"Yeah, yeah, save it for the students," Dr. Simpson muttered as he shuffled away disgruntled. I had to grin at the retreating back of the old vet; I knew he had been looking forward to his cold brews.

Of course, things once again balanced out as it seems they always do in medicine. That same week Dr. O'Brien bustled up to me and said, "Mark, the handlers tell me our girl Annabelle has been favoring one of her rear feet. She has a history of foot infections, and I'd like you to cast her so we can take a look at it." This sounded fairly easy; Annabelle was a nice little Jersey cow that was a resident at the teaching hospital. Having her there provided opportunities for my class to practice our examination and handling skills. Her attractive honey brown color, dainty face and sweet disposition made her a favorite of the staff and students.

Back in Tullville I had learned how to cast a cow, using ropes to topple a patient over. Unlike horses, most bovines resisted having their feet picked up, so if a hoof problem was suspected, it was often easier to put the cow on her side. I reviewed my notes on how to place the ropes on her body. When I was satisfied that I knew what to do, I found an adequate length of strong nylon cord coiled over a hook on the hospital wall. Armed with sure knowledge I headed out into the corral to do battle.

Annabelle was being held in a small fenced area just outside the side entry of the hospital. She stood near one corner of the enclosure contentedly munching hay from a pile on the ground. I trod over bare soil that was wet from recent rain and dotted with fresh cow dung. Looking down I was thankful for my high rubber boots which were as essential as coveralls in large animal work.

I approached the friendly cow and patted her on the neck while she slowly worked a mouthful of food. She stood perfectly still and gazed at me placidly with her large moist eyes, putting up no fuss at all as I passed the nylon cords around her neck, chest, and abdomen. Her cooperative nature made the job easy, and I took my time getting the interlocked loops positioned just right. When I was finished, Annabelle wore a picture perfect example of a casting rope pattern; an expert could not have done a prettier job. Hands on my hips, I smiled to myself. Anyone watching would think that I was an old pro at this, clad in veterinary clothing and moving confidently around the nine-hundred-pound animal. The longer I worked with livestock, the easier it was becoming and I swelled with pride at how far I had come.

Now it was just a simple matter of grabbing the rope's end and pulling her over, so the clinicians could have a peek at her feet. I gripped the cord with both hands. Digging my boots into the moist dirt I leaned into it and gave a hard yank. The rope sprung up from the ground and stretched taut with the force of my pull. Annabelle stiffened slightly and grunted…and then proceeded to casually lower her head and grab another bite of hay.

I was certain this wasn't how the textbooks had described casting. The cow was supposed to crumple neatly over onto her side. Apparently Annabelle hadn't read the same manual, because she showed no hint of crumpling. Feeling peeved, I wrapped more rope around my forearm and really leaned into my next pull.

Annabelle looked up this time as if she actually noticed my efforts. As I applied force to the ropes, she widened her stance a bit and extended her head straight out in front. There she froze like an immovable mountain while I sweated and slipped and cursed to myself. After a minute or two of this I was beginning to tire. The rope loops were cutting into my hands and my attempts to move her were producing no visible results. I could feel my frustration mounting, especially as this was only a petite Jersey cow, not a hefty breed like an Angus or a Holstein. My pride was getting bruised by her casual indifference.

To make matters worse, when I glanced up I found that I now had an audience. Several clinicians and students were lounging in the open hospital doorway observing my demonstration of futility, all of them wearing broad grins. Among them was Kristina Albright, who happened to be one of the designated photographers for our yearbook. Sure enough, when the book came out there was a picture of me desperately pulling on my rope while Annabelle stood defiantly upright. The caption said simply, "Mark Bridges—A Cast of One."

Feeling flustered and self-conscious, I decided to make one more valiant effort to bring Annabelle down. I had been mostly pulling backwards, and in my stress-induced delusional state, the thought occurred that I might be able to pull harder if facing forward. I wrapped the rope several times around my waist and turned away from the cow, digging my feet in and throwing my weight to the front with all my remaining strength. Annabelle stiffened her stance and I leaned further into my pull, until I was angled so far from vertical that I was looking at the ground as my legs churned. The cow's limbs buckled just slightly and for the briefest of moments it seemed that she might topple. Then the moist earth beneath my feet abruptly gave up its traction and I slipped. With the force of my pull and the severe angle of my body there was only one place to go and it was straight down. I had just enough time to see the dung pile before I landed in the midst of it.

I reflexively broke my fall with my hands, and my nose ended up just inches above a fetid pile of goop. The rest of me wasn't so lucky. My forearms were buried in fresh moist cow manure, and I wore a mud-and-muck tuxedo from my chest to my knees.

When I regained my feet, the air was filled with whoops and laughter from the small crowd who had gathered to watch. As I shook the slop from my arms I saw Dr. Simpson, whose wager for a six-pack I had recently spoiled, smiling and nodding with an air of great satisfaction. After a moment he gave a gravelly chuckle and said, "A couple of you students go out there and give him a hand, will ya? I think he's just about had his fill. Ol' Annabelle's been around here long enough to know all the tricks. She'll not easily go down for one person."

Two of the larger members of my class, Stan Hulbert and Robert Reynolds, strode briskly out into the corral, grinning ear to ear as they took in my soiled coveralls and aromatic scent. "Your clothing hardly befits the attire of a medical professional," Stan proclaimed, shaking his head in mock disapproval. "Looks like you need to attend to your personal hygiene."

"Smells like it, too," added Rob, holding his nose dramatically.

"I'd like to see either of you do better," I retorted, breaking into a grin in spite of my condition. "Make yourselves useful at least; your humor stinks worse than I do."

They good-naturedly relented and grabbed the rope, and together the three of us gave a mighty heave. Within a few seconds Annabelle acquiesced as her legs buckled and she tumbled gently to the ground. It was just as described in the veterinary texts.

CHAPTER SIXTY-FOUR

The most memorable case I dealt with in my medicine block was a big roan Quarter Horse named Pete. He had suffered a severe case of choke, getting a large apple stuck in his upper esophagus. The surgeons had removed the obstruction prior to my being involved with his case. Unfortunately, the symptoms of dysphagia (difficulty eating and swallowing) persisted postoperatively, and the doctors were worried about a stricture forming. A traumatized esophagus can easily scar and contract as it heals, narrowing the throat at the site of the injury. This constriction may be severe enough to prevent passage of food or even liquefied gruel.

Pete's surgeons had placed an esophagostomy tube several days after removing the apple. An incision was made in the side of his neck, and a hollow rubber tube thicker than my thumb was inserted into the esophagus below the injured area. After it was sutured in place, the portion of the tube protruding from the skin was wrapped tight to the side of the neck. When a clinician (or more often a student) fed the horse, he or she would undo the bandage to expose the tube's end, attaching a device that looked a lot like a tire pump.

Working the handle would suck liquefied food from a bowl, injecting it into the tube and down the esophagus.

Tube feedings allowed us to provide nutrition to the horse while giving the upper esophagus time to heal. We mixed in medications with the feedings, mainly antibiotics to prevent infection in the damaged throat, along with the anti-inflammatory drug phenylbutazone (commonly known as "bute").

When it was time for Pete's treatments, we would strap on his halter and walk him from his stall into the central treatment room across the hall. There we led him into one of the two restraint chutes in the middle of the floor, closing the gates in front and behind so that he would not wander.

The vast room included a kitchen where we ground alfalfa horse pellets into a gruel. Pete's medication tablets we similarly pulverized using a hand held mortar and pestle. When dosing a horse, we usually would try to mask bad-tasting medications by mixing in a bit of sweet molasses. Here we didn't bother, as the food went straight into our patient's esophagus via the tube, completely avoiding his tongue. Pete never tasted a thing we gave him.

After a few days of doing these treatments, the novelty wore off and it became sheer drudgery. Grinding food in enough volume to satisfy a large horse's requirements was a time-consuming task. The esophagostomy tube proved to be a headache as well. Despite our flushing warm water through it after every feeding, caked food would accumulate and clog the tube's interior. Sometimes we spent a half hour trying to reopen it before we could administer the feeding.

Days followed days with no change to the routine and nothing to excite our interest. The clinicians had a long-term plan of allowing the esophagus to heal and periodically examining Pete's throat. Ed and I primarily did the grunt work of daily maintenance, keeping the horse's weight from dropping too much while he healed. It was an important part of his therapy, but it was far from stimulating.

The object of our attentions wasn't thrilled either. As time went by, Pete became less patient with being restrained in the chute and less tolerant of our handling his tube. After about two weeks of therapy he was downright cantankerous, and once when I was pumping food into him he reached over and bit my shoulder. His teeth didn't break the skin, but it hurt enough for me to drop the food pump. I pushed his head forcefully away, and shouted into his ear, "Knock it off!" He behaved for the rest of the feeding, but it was obvious that he was reaching his limits.

All that changed one day when the doctors ordered a reevaluation of the horse's throat. Dr. O'Brien was heading the team that afternoon and I was his chief assistant. The doctor instructed me to administer xylazine, a sedative used to calm horses for minor procedures. I drew the calculated dose up into a syringe. When I held it out to Dr. O'Brien, he glanced at it to verify the amount, then gestured at the horse and said, "Go ahead and give it."

Now, there is a right way to administer xylazine and a wrong way. The drug is intended to go intravenously, and the jugular vein in the neck is a good target to shoot for. Running just under the skin surface like a big fat snake, it is easy to hit with a needle. The only concern with a jugular injection is that the carotid artery runs just a little deeper along the same path. If xylazine hits the artery it is carried straight to the brain in high concentration, with very unpleasant consequences.

There were precautions we always took to avoid a carotid injection. The first was using a large-gauge needle and inserting it into the vein without a syringe attached. The big bore of the needle would allow us to see how much pressure was in the vessel we hit. Veins carry a low blood pressure, so a needle inserted into the jugular would drip blood steadily but gently. The same needle pushed into the pressurized carotid artery would usually spurt vigorously. It was a quick and easy way to verify which vessel we had entered.

Once a syringe was attached to the needle, we took a second precaution. Before giving the drug, we would draw back on the syringe plunger. This sucked blood into the chamber and we could assess its color. Arterial blood is oxygen rich and bright cherry red; venous blood tends to be a darker hue. If the color was appropriate for a jugular puncture, then we would proceed with the injection.

On this day I hit the vessel easily, slapping the horse's neck several times with my palm and then popping the needle deep with one fluid motion. Pete didn't even notice and I felt good about my technique. Blood dripped rapidly from the large needle bore but no spurting was evident. I attached the syringe filled with xylazine and drew back the plunger. Medium red liquid came welling into the syringe chamber, resembling what I usually saw in jugular venipunctures.

Dr. O'Brien was right behind me, watching over my shoulder. I glanced back and he nodded, saying, "Go ahead, it looks good."

I began to push the plunger and the drug sped smoothly on its way. Things looked great for about five seconds, and then we discovered that the needle was not where we had thought. It was, in fact, in the worst possible place.

My first clue that something was amiss came just as I finished depressing the plunger. The horse's head began to jerk up and down rapidly, and within seconds the tremors progressed to whole body spasms. Out of the corners of my vision I saw the other students around the chute backing away, their eyes like round saucers as they stared at the thrashing animal. Dr. O'Brien shouted, "Get back, he's seizuring! The drug went arterial!"

We all moved back a couple of feet and the doctor pointed at one of the techs, saying, "Get the yohimbine *stat!*" Pete meanwhile continued to seizure, legs and body churning as he violently shook the sturdy metal bars confining him. Although it seemed to go on forever, the spasmodic contortions lasted only a few seconds before his body collapsed limply within the chute. He sprawled awkwardly sideways within the narrow structure, his legs splaying out through the side bars.

"Open the gates and get him out quickly!" Dr. O'Brien commanded, and we helped the doctor untangle the horse's limbs and drag the heavy body carefully through the front entrance of the chute.

We laid Pete on his side on the concrete floor and the doctor checked his jugular pulse. The horse's eyes were wide open and twitching rhythmically. He stared straight ahead unseeing, and I was sure that he was unconscious. The doctor grabbed his stethoscope and listened to Pete's heart, then sighed and said, "Well, his pulse is thready and rapid; he's showing signs of shock."

Just then the tech ran up with a bottle of yohimbine and Dr. O'Brien grabbed a syringe. Yohimbine is a xylazine antagonist or reversing agent, and it can be used to quickly undo the effects of the sedative. It's one reason that xylazine has been popular in large animal medicine; having an available antidote increases the safety margin when problems occur.

The doctor carefully injected the drug into the jugular vein, staying shallow with the needle this time around. Then we waited, watching the horse's respirations and monitoring his heart. The eye twitching subsided, and in a few minutes Pete began lifting his head, trying to sit up. Dr. O'Brien perched on the animal's neck to keep him prone until he had recovered his wits.

I breathed a sigh of relief when it appeared that our patient was going to survive. The doctor must have seen my expression because he said, "It's all right, Mark. I was watching your injection the whole way and it fooled me too. The needle tip must have been up against the arterial wall, which kept the blood flow to a slow drip. It looked just like a jugular stick; this one's not your fault. I bet that next time you'll stay a bit shallower, yes?" I nodded fervently and he chuckled, looking around at the attending students and technicians. "All of you take a lesson from what just happened. It's better to learn from someone else's mistake rather than from your own. I'm sure Mark here would agree."

I felt my face flush, but I was relieved that our patient was okay, and that no one was blaming me for negligence. Right then I was supremely aware of the advantages of being a student, working with a supervising doctor who could step in and take charge if something went awry. Once I graduated, I would be totally responsible for my patients, and liable for all the consequences of my actions.

After about ten minutes we allowed Pete to get up and he stood there shakily, looking wide-eyed and thoroughly cowed. The doctor cancelled the throat exam for the day, proclaiming that our patient had been through quite enough. I led a very passive and cooperative horse slowly back to his stall.

Although I would never wish for anyone to repeat my little mishap, there were two good things that came out of it. One was that the event apparently got Pete's attention, as he never again tried to bite me or get aggressive in any way. Every time we treated him, he just looked straight ahead, waiting quietly for us to finish. He was in fact the perfect gentleman, though I caught a hint of nervousness in his eyes from time to time. Perhaps he was afraid that I would give him another injection if he misbehaved.

The other benefit of the episode was that every detail was burned into my brain. Later when I took the National Board Exams to become a doctor, there was a multiple-choice question that read thusly: "If xylazine is injected into the carotid artery of the horse, which of the following effects will occur? A) Loss of consciousness, B) Seizures, C) Shock, D) All of the above.

As you probably guessed I marked "D" with the utmost confidence.

CHAPTER SIXTY-FIVE

I wasn't the only student who encountered challenges during our senior curriculum. Mary Hackett, my classmate who had been kicked in the knee by a surgery pony, seemed to be a magnet for trauma and misfortune. After her torn cruciate ligament was surgically repaired, she hobbled around on crutches for the first couple of senior blocks. Just as she had begun to walk unaided, she was rolled on by a falling cow and ended up spraining the other knee. Back on crutches she went, and then a couple of weeks after that she was helping tend to a big male llama when it spit in her face and bit her on the arm. Watching her ease gingerly down the halls with one leg braced and her forearm swollen and bruised, I felt relatively good about my own ups and downs thus far.

Not surprisingly, Mary's injuries had dimmed her enthusiasm for large animal practice. One day near the end of medicine block we got together for grand rounds. This was a weekly event in which seniors and professors gathered in the hallway between the animal stalls. Then each of the five students in the block presented a summary of a case he or she had been working with. Other seniors and even freshmen would attend the rounds when they could. Several clinicians were usually present, moderating the proceedings and asking questions.

On this particular day I discussed Pete's case as we all stood outside his stall. We planned to remove the horse's feeding tube the next week, but his prognosis wasn't good, since his esophagus appeared severely constricted at the site of the prior injury. No one knew if he could pass anything substantial through the narrowed area. Surgery to repair the esophagus was considered impractical; all we could do was pull his tube and hope for the best. Pete needed to be able to swallow food, at least a liquefied mash, on his own. His survival depended on it.

One by one each student in our block told the tale of a particular animal in the hospital. The last in line was Mary Hackett. When it was her turn to present a case, old Dr. Simpson turned to her and said, "What do you have for us this morning, Mary?"

She looked the venerable professor straight in the eye, then grinned and shook her head. She said, "You know what, Dr. Simpson? Right about now my idea of 'large animal' is a Great Dane. I'm sorry, but I didn't feel up to preparing a case synopsis. I have nothing to share this morning."

I expected a fiery retort from the senior clinician, as he was not known to be long on patience. Dr. Simpson looked Mary up and down, taking in her crutches, the brace on her knee, and the bruised forearm with bright red bite marks still visible. After a long pause he chuckled and said, "I guess I can't blame you there, my dear." I realized I had been holding my breath and now I let it out in relief. Laughter trickled through the faculty and students as the group dispersed and grand rounds ended.

That was the final week of my medicine block. Friday afternoon I drove north to enjoy the weekend with Cindy. I hadn't been home for two weeks due to covering Pete's treatments. We went out to a movie that evening and slept in late Saturday morning, simple luxuries we had waited too long to enjoy. After sharing a hearty breakfast, we let Dixie out of her cage and watched her bounding happily around the room. The two ends of her long sinuous body seesawed up and down as she frolicked, as if each was on its own pogo stick. Occasionally she would be running while looking backward and careen into a table leg or other obstacle. Then she would dart off in a different direction, hopping and grunting as if offended by the furniture's lack of manners. When she got really excited, her short tail would fluff up like a bottle brush. Her silliness was so captivating that I could amuse myself for an hour just observing her antics.

After awhile my wife came over to sit next to me on the couch. She snuggled close, her head on my shoulder as we watched our happy ferret cavorting. I felt her fingers running randomly through my hair as she gazed at Dixie. Finally Cindy stirred and said, "I've been wondering what's going to happen when you graduate."

I looked over at her in surprise. "What do you mean?"

She started to speak, but was interrupted by a crash as our mischievous pet tipped over a garbage can and began rifling through the papers within. I waited and eventually Cindy said, "Well, you don't know any vets in the Portland area, and it's not likely that I could find work down in Medford where you grew up. What if you can't find a job up here?"

Her voiced concerns were valid but they took me by surprise, and I mulled my answer over before answering. "I'm not too worried about it," I began, meeting her gaze frankly. "This area has the largest population base in the state, and there are a lot of animal clinics to choose from. The local vet association has job listings, and I plan to visit some area vets and introduce myself when the time comes. I can get a good reference from the Medford clinic, too."

"How is the current job market for veterinarians?" Cindy asked.

"I hear it's pretty good. Portland is growing, which means more people moving here—and bringing their pets. I think there will be veterinary clinics looking to hire new doctors as their clientele continues to expand."

After discussing it a bit more, I was able to put my wife's mind at ease, at least for the time being. With business talk concluded, we stretched out on the couch together, enjoying the lazy morning as we held each other close. We quietly watched Dixie play for awhile longer, and then Cindy gave me a rogue's smile and said, "Why don't you put our furry trouble maker to bed; she's looking tired and I have other plans."

I raised my eyebrows and replied, "Oh…what did you have in mind?"

She licked her full lips and purred, "Let's just say that Dixie isn't the only one who enjoys a good frolic."

On closer inspection our little ferret did indeed seem to be exhausted, and I promptly ushered the poor dear into her cage for a nap. Then I allowed myself to be ushered into the next room. A great thing about being in love is that one doesn't need a lot of money or possessions to enjoy life to the fullest.

CHAPTER SIXTY-SIX

The weekend at home passed in a heartbeat, and I found myself back in Corvine much sooner than I wanted. With October arriving, the fading year was giving birth to autumn. For the present an Indian summer held sway and the days outside the teaching hospital were still wonderfully warm. Only the increasingly chilly nights and the rainbow foliage of the deciduous trees told the true tale of the season. The small maples in front of the vet building were dropping their first leaves, the dried skeletons scraping and crunching under my feet as I approached the door of the school.

Life inside McNairy Hall followed its own beat, and when I stepped through the entrance, I was immediately swept back into its energetic rhythm. The current course on my schedule carried the vague title of "clinical services." I soon discovered that this encompassed a wide variety of activities. Students participated in everything from after-hours phone service to filling out paperwork to bottling pathology samples. It was the most eclectic collection of jobs I had encountered in school.

The core of the block turned out to be necropsy duty. This activity took place in a large glass-fronted room with concrete floors that sloped toward a central drain. Farm animals or hospital patients that had died could be dissected here so that we could learn what had caused their demise. The senior students took an active part in the carving of dead flesh. In so doing we learned the proper techniques for necropsy, and were able to see visible lesions caused by various diseases. Though it sounds nasty (and often was), this block provided us with a wealth of valuable experience and knowledge that could not be obtained while working on living patients.

Here scalpel blades were abandoned in favor of large carving knives that could make short work of a thousand-pound carcass. The tough hide and sinews of these animals could dull our instruments in no time; an unexpected perk of the class was being taught how to use a sharpening steel to keep a blade edge honed like a razor. To this day I bear the responsibility of maintaining my home kitchen knives in a state of carving readiness.

Pathology had colorful terminology as well. I found it ironic that the most nauseating pursuit in veterinary medicine utilized food terms as descriptive aids. Clear serum that had gelled after death was termed a "chicken fat clot," whereas a red blob of coagulated blood became a "currant jelly clot." Of course, the written reports used nomenclature that was more formal and scientific. Sticky soft exudate resembling tan colored paste was dubbed "fibrinous." Liquid pus was "purulent," whereas the solid chunky variety was "caseous." These various textures of dead nastiness were enough to challenge even the hardened stomach on occasion, especially in the quantities we encountered in large animals. But that was nothing compared to the assault on our sense of smell.

I remember one afternoon early in the course of the block. The weather had waxed hot for several days, giving us a last tantalizing taste of the summer that had passed. Returning from lunch, I walked from the steaming parking lot toward the teaching hospital, my brow beading sweat under the hard sun. Once inside the blissfully cool building, I wound my way through the hallways, eventually pushing through the wide doors that opened onto the necropsy floor. When I got a good look at the animal lying there I wished that I had stayed outside.

The bloated carcass of a large, black-and-white Holstein cow filled the middle of the room. One whiff told me she was not a fresh specimen; whatever had caused her death had done so some time ago. Dr. Brent Coulson, one of the pathologists, stood at the big sink on the opposite wall. He was slight of build, with sandy hair and eyes matching his baby blue coveralls. He turned as I walked in and said, "Oh, good, you're just in time for the festivities. This lovely lady passed away three days ago and has been lying out in the hot sun ever since. The farmer finally got around to hoisting her into his truck and brought her here for a necropsy. Lucky us! She's plenty ripe and I don't know how much we'll find. Decomposition is pretty advanced here." I nodded with a grimace as my nose strongly agreed.

I walked to the clothing closet and pulled a pair of necropsy coveralls off a hanger. After donning them and refastening my boots, I grabbed a pair of rubber gloves and a face mask. The latter was a weak attempt to deflect the odor of the carcass. Fully dressed for combat, I joined Dr. Coulson next to the cow. He pulled on his own gloves and then grinned fiendishly as he brandished his knife. Striking a dramatic pose he declared, "Here we go...no guts, no glory!" In fact it was the guts part that I was worried about.

He stabbed the sharp blade through the cow's abdomen near the midline and drew it down to enlarge the hole. When the knife entered the bloated animal an audible hiss erupted as noxious gases vented from the pressurized belly. I could see the animal's sides slowly collapsing as what was inside came out. The stink was incredible, and my eyes watered as I gulped repeatedly, fighting a wave of nausea.

The pathologist continued to saw with his blade, extending the incision all the way to the pelvis. Meanwhile, I steadied myself and stepped forward to assist. With my knife I enlarged the opening forward until I ran into the ribcage. Then I used an instrument like a tree branch lopper to cut each rib along the left side of the chest. When all the ribs had been cracked in two places, we could reflect them back and expose the chest cavity.

With the carcass opened, we waded through miles of distended bowel and bucketfuls of greasy, rancid fat as we looked for clues inside. When Dr. Coulson prepared to open the gut I stood back, wary of the four swollen stomachs. Just as I'd feared the fumes released from these viscera made the previous stink seem like perfume.

Unfortunately, there was no escaping the work to be done. The cause of death was not immediately apparent, so we had to biopsy everything. The size of the carcass magnified our difficulties and our discomfort. At times we were half inside the animal, hemmed in by rotting flesh on all sides as we took tissue samples. To call it memorable was an understatement; to say it was enjoyable in any sense of the word was just plain wrong.

Even after stripping off the coveralls and gloves, I carried the essence of that dead cow with me the rest of the day. On arriving home I entered the front door of the townhouse and found Paul lounging on the couch watching the news. He started to greet me, then his smile faded and his nose wrinkled. "What the heck is that smell!?" he exclaimed, looking appalled. "Did you eat something dead? You really reek!"

At this stage my nose was accustomed to the odor of decayed bovine, so I was impervious. I grinned at his discomfort; for once the tables were turned and he was on the receiving end of the stink. "Technically we all eat dead things, even vegetarians," I pointed out.

"Yeah but they aren't rotten at the time!" my roommate retorted, unimpressed by my attempt at humor. "What the heck happened?"

I related the story of the afternoon's activities and he interrupted me part way though, holding up his hand and saying, "Okay, I get the idea! The last thing I need is nasty visual images to go with the smell. Please, go bathe in lemon juice or something!" I was quite willing to oblige and I headed upstairs to wash away the remains of the day.

As I lathered my hair under hot water, I concluded that now I had seen the most unsavory side of veterinary medicine. I had come, I had smelled, and I had survived. If I could handle necropsies like that, then there was nothing else that could bother me.

As fate would have it, less than a week passed before I found that carcass dissection might not be the pinnacle of nastiness. Exactly six days after my decayed cow extravaganza, I saw Kristina Albright in the hospital hallway. She was currently in surgery block, so we encountered each other only occasionally. Just a few days earlier she had laughed heartily at my necropsy story, showing not a trace of sympathy when I had described my stomach-churning experience. Perhaps there is such a thing as karma, because on this particular morning I caught a whiff of something decidedly unpleasant as Kristina passed by. Surprised, I stopped and turned back toward her.

"Kristi!" I called out, and she turned and looked at me quizzically. I beckoned her with my hand as I approached her.

"Yes?" she replied, walking slowly back toward me. We stopped a few feet apart and once again the faint stench of decay reached my nostrils.

"What is that wonderful aroma you carry with you?" I asked, smiling broadly.

Kristina grimaced and said, "Oh great, do I still stink? I can't smell it any more after bathing three times and using half a bottle of shampoo. How bad is it?"

"Not too bad, if you have a taste for carrion," I teased, enjoying her discomfort. "It would hardly be noticeable outdoors in a strong wind."

She looked aghast, and then she saw the smirk on my face and scowled. "You're having fun with me, aren't you? How strong do I smell? Tell the truth!"

I gave up the jesting then and assured her that the odor was barely evident. Still, I was curious as to how she had come by such a fragrance outside of necropsy block.

Kristina groaned and said, "Oh, it was a wonderful case. A Belgian mare from the Seattle area came in yesterday. She was in late stage pregnancy and the owner had noticed her straining a week ago but then she had stopped. He thought nothing more of it until she started to smell real bad several days later."

I whistled and said, "Oh-oh."

She nodded. "Yes, exactly. Their local vet took a look at the mare and discovered that she had a dead foal inside of her; the feet were all he could feel on vaginal palpation as the baby was in a breech presentation. That's why the mare couldn't give birth and the foal died during the contractions."

I shook my head at the unpleasant image and she continued, "The horse was sent down to us, and the trip took awhile so she didn't arrive until early evening. By the time she was evaluated and into surgery, it was ten P.M."

"Wow, a late start," I remarked.

"Tell me about it. The darned surgery took all night, and we weren't done until six A.M. Dr. Cutler opened the uterus and we did a Caesarian section on the foal; it was nasty and putrefied, practically falling apart in our hands as we removed it. The body was more liquid than solid. It smelled incredibly bad and I wanted to vomit, but with a surgery mask on that would have been even more disgusting!"

Now it was my turn to laugh at her tale of woe, and she ruefully said, "I'm not going to get much sympathy from you, am I?" I shook my head gleefully. Kristina nodded, saying, "Well, I guess I deserve that. Anyway, by the time we were done the smell had permeated my clothes, my skin, my hair, everything. When I went home my two cats wouldn't come anywhere near me; they just hissed and backed away! Five years I've had them and they acted like I was some sort of monster. Come to think of it, my husband's reaction wasn't all that different...."

At this point in her story I was laughing so hard that Kristina joined in despite herself. She added, "I washed over and over trying to get rid of that smell. I thought I had succeeded."

I grinned and shook my head, no. She shrugged resignedly. "Oh well, I didn't have time to do more anyway. I only got a few hours' sleep before I had to be back at school. I've got another surgery soon."

I wished her luck and walked away chuckling. On reflection it seemed that even when I had it bad, I didn't have it so bad. Kristina had been stuck in one of the worst procedures imaginable, and it had been an all-nighter as well. On top of that, she still had necropsy rounds to look forward to next month. No matter how difficult you think things are, there is always someone less fortunate to make you feel better.

Two days later the necropsy floor received another animal to examine. This time it was a large roan horse that had been euthanatized due to incurable illness. I stood over the animal, sharpening my knife against a honing steel in preparation for the dissection. The rhythmic rasping sound of metal on metal echoed hollowly off the walls and floor of the room. As I worked I glanced down at the animal lying on its side at my feet and I did a double-take. It was Pete, the horse with choke that I had spent so much time treating during my medicine block.

My hands stopped their movement and I gazed at him for a moment in silence. I had grown fond of the big gelding during my time working with him. Though his problem had been serious, I had hoped that he would find a way through his illness. Instead he had ended up here. Disease and death weren't charitable or kind, they simply happened. I was learning that in this line of work I would see both on a regular basis. It wasn't always pleasant to deal with.

When the pathologist and I opened Pete's throat, it was easy to see why he had failed to recover. His esophagus was a large muscular pink tube, about as wide as three of my fingers. But when we followed it down from the mouth we found the spot where the apple had been lodged weeks before. The injury and resulting scar tissue had severely constricted the esophageal diameter; I could barely squeeze my pinky finger through the passage that remained. The poor horse had had no chance of ever swallowing food again.

It was clear that euthanasia had been the only alternative to a slow death by starvation. Pete's suffering had at least seen a merciful end. Sometimes that was all that we could provide for our patients, when there was nothing else left to try.

CHAPTER SIXTY-SEVEN

The remaining weeks of clinical services block kept me busy. During the days I was working on the necropsy floor or processing lab paperwork. On selected nights I sat alone in the vacant vet building, reviewing my medicine notes and ordering pizza for dinner while I monitored the phones for emergency calls.

Some of the work that month was boring, some was fascinating, and some was downright funny. Even in the world of necropsies and pathology, humor still managed to find its way into the mix on a regular basis. Perhaps it was needed most here, where appalling sights and smells were encountered daily. Or maybe people in the medical professions simply have an irrepressible joy of life.

Dr. Coulson turned out to be quite a character himself, albeit with a rather disturbing sense of humor. A great example of this occurred one day when a large bottle came through the pathology lab for analysis. The glass container held nearly a pint of pale tan liquid, thick and creamy-looking. The doctor took the specimen and entered the item on his paperwork. I asked him what it was and he read the label on the bottle. "Aspirate of an abscess on the brisket of a dairy cow," he announced. "In other words, a prime vintage of pus. Goes great on sesame wheat crackers!"

I curled my lip in distaste and he laughed, opening the bottle and smearing a small sample of the liquid onto a microscope slide. "Let's see what this looks like," he commented. "I'll bet you that this is from a sterile abscess; do you know why I think that?"

I shook my head and he said, "Because there's no odor to it. I suspect the cow bumped up against a fence or something and ran a splinter into her brisket."

The area of the cow's body that he referred to was the leading portion of the chest between the front legs, so that type of injury made sense. The doctor continued talking as he worked, "A foreign body can cause an abscess without the presence of bacteria. The body will try to reject the unfamiliar material and send white blood cells to fight it, producing pus. But infection is usually what yields a foul smell; without bugs the sample can be fairly bland."

I added this information to my mental list of useful minutia as the doctor examined the liquid under the microscope. After a minute he straightened with a smile and said, "Boy, it's hell to be so good!

There are no visible bacteria on the slide, only white blood cells and debris. Essentially, it's pus without infection, just as suspected."

Right about then Trina Caldwell and another student walked into the necropsy room. When they approached, Trina spotted the jar of pus sitting near Dr. Coulson. She gestured curiously at the container and asked, "What's that stuff?"

Dr. Coulson said perfectly straight-faced, "It's a milkshake. Do you want some?"

Being a prankster herself, Trina was cynical by nature. I doubt she'd have trusted a bottle found in the necropsy ward even if her own mother had vouched for it. So she simply cocked an eyebrow and replied, "Is that so? Let's see you have a sip, then, and tell us if it's good."

The doctor grinned and said, "Actually this is from a sterile abscess, so it would be perfectly safe to drink."

Trina crossed her arms challengingly and replied, "Oh, really? If you are so sure, then put your money where your mouth is and take a drink. Show us how confident you are in your diagnosis!"

Dr. Coulson hesitated for only a moment, then he shrugged and unscrewed the lid of the bottle. Holding the glass high he said, "Bottoms up!" and proceeded to take a long swallow of the viscous contents.

Trina's face went pale and she looked like she was going to die. Despite my own gag reflex kicking in, I burst out laughing at her shocked expression. She in no way had imagined that the doctor would call her bluff. As he finished his slurp of cow sludge, she gulped and said weakly, "Umm, you have a little pus mustache on your lip, there." She pointed at the doctor's upper lip and he wiped his mouth with his sleeve. She nodded numbly when he had gotten it all and he chuckled.

"Never make the mistake of thinking that you can outdo me in here," he advised, shaking his finger at her. Trina didn't look like she would ever try again. It was the one time I saw my outrageous classmate totally defeated.

Trina was a tough lady, though. On the last week of necropsy duty she got the chance to redeem herself and show her fortitude. When I first heard about the case coming in I thought it was a hoax, but the worried look in the clinicians' eyes made me realize it was for real. The Corvine police department was bringing in two adult female African lions that had been secretly living in a local man's house. They had been discovered when the man had not turned up at work nor answered his phone for over a week. When his boss had reported him missing, the sheriff's department had dispatched a patrol car to the residence.

Upon entering the house the officers had been confronted by two huge predators stalking toward them, deep rumbling growls emanating from between their bared fangs. The surprised men had beaten a quick retreat and called for help.

The lionesses had aggressively defended their territory and would not allow anyone to enter the dwelling, eventually forcing authorities to shoot them dead. Inside the house a grisly sight had confronted the police: the main living room was covered in blood and the homeowner's head was found lying on the carpet. That was all that was left of him; the rest of his body was presumably inside his pets.

The authorities were bringing the lions to the teaching hospital for necropsies. The purpose was to see if human body parts could be found within the animals' stomachs, and to determine if any signs of foul play were present. The police wanted to rule out the possibility that the man had died or been killed by other means prior to the lions dining on him. Dr. Coulson was skeptical that we would be able to tell anything from partly-digested remains, but we had to try.

The pathologist needed assistants to help with the dissections, but he told us that any student contribution would be strictly voluntary. He looked around at the five of us who were in the clinical services block, and at first no one came forward. Finally Trina squared her shoulders and said, "I'll do it." The doctor smiled gratefully and said, "If you are up to it, I'd be much obliged." She nodded and Dr. Coulson turned back to the rest of us. "Anyone else?" he asked.

I thought about it for a moment, and then I raised my hand as well. The doctor smiled and pointed at me, saying, "There's our second volunteer. That should be enough; the rest of you can go. Mark and Trina, I'll let you know when the lions arrive."

The animal control vehicle carrying the two giant cats pulled up to the vet school around one P.M. Handlers used wheeled gurneys to move the heavy carcasses from the admitting entrance to the necropsy floor. On the way they stopped at the scales to weigh the bodies; each cat massed nearly 135 kilograms (300 pounds) and measured around 2.4 meters (eight feet) in length. They were incredible specimens. Their heavily-muscled frames, long curved teeth, and razor claws provided silent testament to their design as killing machines.

Crouching next to one of the cats, I ran my hand through the coarse fur on its massive head, awestruck at seeing and touching such an exotic creature. Even in death these animals were things of beauty, but I couldn't imagine living with them. Apparently their owner hadn't envisioned dying with them either.

Once the lions were deposited on the floor of the necropsy room, we got to work. Dr. Coulson performed the main dissection, due to the grisly nature of the case and the need for expert examination. Trina and I took notes of the proceedings and provided occasional assistance, retracting tissues for the doctor and handing him instruments.

The lions appeared to be in good condition, other than several blood-matted wounds marking bullet entry points on the bodies. As Dr. Coulson worked on the first cat, Trina and I waited anxiously for the pathologist to examine the digestive system. When at last he incised the stomach I steeled myself for the worst. Holding a large specimen bag wide open, I stepped in close so that the doctor could deposit the stomach contents of the lion therein.

The pathologist's gloved hand fished around inside the open organ, pulling out bits of unrecognizable meat which looked typical for any carnivore's gut. Then something more substantial appeared. It was flat and pale, with multiple cylindrical projections coming off a central structure. I frowned in puzzlement before I saw it clearly, and then the doctor held it up for us to see. I suddenly felt dizzy and lightheaded, a loud rushing sound filling my ears and the acid taste of bile spilling into my mouth. In the background I was dimly aware of Trina bent over retching. The object Dr. Coulson had pulled from the stomach was a human hand.

The remainder of the necropsies was a horror show filled with bits and pieces of the unfortunate owner-turned-prey. A foot joined the hand in the specimen bag, and a number of crushed and shattered bones were found as well. No evidence of previous foul play was discovered, although it would have been difficult to say with certainty. Toxicology studies of the tissues found no evidence of drugs or poison. As Dr. Coulson concluded, things were probably just as they appeared. The lions had simply eaten their owner. It was the most disturbing thing I have ever encountered in all the years of my veterinary career.

I was talking with the pathologist a couple of days later, and I asked him why the animals would have attacked someone they had grown up with. Purchase records found at the house showed that the big cats had been obtained as cubs. I thought that they would have been bonded to their owner and therefore tame with him.

Dr. Coulson nodded, saying, "They probably were. But you have to remember, 'tame' is not in any way 'domesticated.' Dogs and housecats are truly domesticated animals, bred for many generations to reduce the normal aggression of their wild ancestors. Even then they still have many of the instincts of a predator, which is why dog bite incidents are common. But you take a wild species and raise it in captivity, and you still have a wild animal. It is tame, meaning it is accustomed to people, but it still retains all of its wild instincts. That makes such an animal dangerous and unpredictable, especially when it reaches adulthood."

"But why would the lions suddenly attack their owner after living with him peacefully for so long?" I asked him.

"Who knows? Those animals take an incredible amount of food to keep satisfied. Maybe they got a little too hungry. More likely they simply had a trigger response and jumped him."

"What do you mean?" I said.

"Predators such as cats have attack responses that can be triggered by visual cues," the doctor answered. "Have you ever thrown a small toy on the floor and watched a house cat pounce on it? The motion triggers a reflex that makes the cat attack without thinking. The same thing can happen with larger predators. The owner might have been playing or wrestling with one of them and gotten knocked over. Heck, even tripping and falling could do it. Once he went down the animal would have pounced, probably going for his neck. His struggles would have only made matters worse. I suspect his life ended very quickly, although the cats may have taken their time eating him."

I shuddered at the image. Living with animals that could kill you the moment you showed weakness was a terrifying prospect, and not one I would willingly embrace. Although I have since worked with dangerous wildlife as part of my veterinary practice, I have always made sure that the animals were safely controlled with all precautions taken. It doesn't pay to take chances. Getting a hand mauled can end a veterinary career, even if the appendage doesn't end up in the patient's stomach.

CHAPTER SIXTY-EIGHT

When my clinical services rotation concluded a few days later, I made a beeline for Beaverton. There my wife awaited me with open arms and an open heart. A weekend's rest enveloped in her warmth allowed me to focus on something positive, and helped to put recent events behind me. I have always found that life's darker side is balanced by the light, if one is willing to open up and see it. Cindy's love reaffirmed my joy in living, and while I benefited from her presence, I made sure to give back as well as I got. We shared each other's energy for two days, then reluctantly we said goodbye and I headed back to Corvine on Sunday night.

November had a tumultuous beginning, with a major storm front blowing through the Willamette Valley. After parking my car at school Monday morning, I ran to the front door of the veterinary building with my head bowed against a cold driving rain. Inside the lobby I shook off the chill and headed back into the maze of the hospital.

Radiology was my next block course, and compared to what I had just experienced, it was refreshingly low-key. To my delight Mike Callahan, Molly Boyer, and two other students joined me in this block. I had missed Mike and Molly, and we spent time between cases sharing our experiences and reminiscing about the past four years. Some days there were only a handful of films to take, so we had plenty of time to relax as well as debate the finer points of radiography.

Dr. Denise Wright was the chief radiologist at the veterinary teaching hospital. She looked to be in her mid-thirties, surprisingly youthful for someone in her position of responsibility. Her appearance struck a balance between casual and professional; she wore her light brown hair straight and long, but usually donned a white smock when working on patients. The distinctive *click clack, click clack* of her hard-soled black shoes echoed down the halls whenever she approached.

Face to face the radiologist's eyes were intense and focused during a conversation. Of all the doctors on staff she was one of the most generous with her time, and I never saw her turn away a student who needed assistance. She would challenge us in the process, often answering a question with a question and forcing us to think. But she was never demeaning, and despite her driven personality she could break out laughing at the slightest provocation.

The radiology duties were divided up between the doctors, techs, and students. The head technician in the department took most of the X-rays. Dick Maynard was a flamboyant character unlike any other medical staff at the hospital. He wore his wavy red hair long in the back, undaunted by the fact that it was steadily receding in front. Ignoring dress codes, Dick usually wore street clothes, since he had minimal contact with clients. When sequestered in the bowels of the radiology department, he could often be found clad in a funky sweatshirt and baseball cap. On those occasions when he did interact with the public, he would don a lab coat and deftly cover his wardrobe deficiencies.

Dick reminded me a little of Dr. Brakel back in Tullville, in that he possessed an endless collection of jokes which he dropped on the students at every opportunity. Some were real groaners and elicited gut spasms in his captive audience. Once while we were struggling to position a horse for radiographs, he unexpectedly looked up from the patient and asked us, "Have you heard about the zoo vet who specialized in elephant circumcisions?"

We all stared at him in bewilderment and shook our heads, at which he spread his hands and said, "Well, the work was hard but the tips were big." A chorus of boos and catcalls greeted this comedic masterpiece. Dick feigned offense as if this were the first time he had ever received such a response. His hurt expression garnered more laughs than the joke had done.

One of the lasting impressions I have of Dick Maynard was when he was immortalized in the class yearbook. The photo showed him standing dressed in nothing but sneakers and a white lab coat. He was facing the X-ray machine with the coat pulled open in his best imitation of a flasher. Of course, the picture was taken from behind but you got the idea. The caption read, "Our beloved Dick— catching some rays." When we got our yearbooks, the best comment came from "special" Ed Martinelli, who squinted at the photo dubiously and offered, "I'm sure glad they capitalized his name."

Though eccentric, Dick was a capable radiology technician. Apart from the doctors, only he was entrusted with using the expensive equipment around patients who could disable the machine with one well-placed kick. We students would mostly observe and assist. Our duties included helping to restrain the animals, fetching fresh X-ray film, and then taking the exposed plates to the developing room for processing.

Most of the radiographs we took were studies of legs in lame horses. We were looking for fractures or arthritic changes, especially in the foot and ankle regions. Arthritis was a common finding secondary to injuries or due to stress on the joints from heavy exercise. On film it could manifest as increased joint fluid or thickened irregular bone. Sometimes the X-rays would detect small chips off the leg bones as well.

When the images were completed, we would hang the films on the light box on the radiology room wall. There the students would examine the pictures and try to visualize what pathology, if any, was illustrated therein. Dr. Wright would eventually come along and listen to our conclusions. After she examined the pictures, she would then render an opinion on the case.

This was our last formal exposure to radiology before graduation, and there were a couple of skills that the course was intended to hone. Students needed to learn how to position the animals and the X-ray beam to get the best pictures, and then interpret what we saw to make an accurate diagnosis. We had evaluated large animal films before, but this was our first experience with actually taking views on horses. The imaging techniques were entirely different than with dogs.

The five seniors in my block were gratified to find that our X-ray interpretations agreed with Dr. Wright's about eighty percent of the time. A pessimist would point out that we totally missed the diagnosis in one out of five cases. That was true enough, but we also remembered our monumental struggles in radiology back in Tullville. When you start out at the "haven't got a clue" stage, any progress is encouraging. We finally began to see that practice could make perfect, or at least it had us headed in the right direction.

Despite the more relaxed pace in radiology, we did have some exciting moments. The biggest example, literally, during my block was when a Shire mare and her foal were admitted to the hospital. Shires are large draft horses, similar to Clydesdales but even taller. They are distant descendents of old English war horses. Over the centuries these gentle giants have been bred to a size and strength that is unsurpassed by any other breed.

The mare was a wondrous animal to behold, massing more than nine hundred kilos or two thousand pounds. She stood well over seventeen hands at the withers. In layman's terms, this meant that her height measured at the shoulders was nearly six feet or 180 centimeters, just about even with the top of my head. Needless to say, her neck and head towered considerably higher. She was beautifully marked in black and white, with long, silky feathering on her feet that made her look as if she wore white furred boots. Each time I passed by her stall I would stop and stare awhile.

The owners of this behemoth had saddled her with the cute name of Nunu. Typical of her breed, she was friendly and possessed an even disposition. We could enter the stall and handle her with no problem. Like most mothers she was moderately protective of her offspring, and would occasionally whinny anxiously as we examined her baby. One handler remained with the mare while others worked on the foal, but if she had wanted to be boisterous, the restraining hand on her halter would have proven no more deterrent than a bit of sewing thread around her neck.

The male foal in turn was young, still nursing and very dependent on his mother. He had a persistent lameness which was the reason the pair were at the hospital. The situation between the two
horses and their human handlers seemed fine, but maternal instincts
can be powerful and volatile. This is always a cause for concern
when the mother in question is built like an army tank.

Our initial examinations had narrowed the foal's lameness to
the left rear leg. Beyond that the doctors could not isolate the source
of pain, and predictably they had decided that radiographs were in
order. That afternoon we walked the foal down the hallway to the X-
ray room. As we headed away from the stall I heard the mare neigh-
ing loudly as she watched her progeny being taken. Then we were
through the wide doors at the end of the hall and entering radiology.

The cavernous X-ray room with its grey concrete floor and high
walls dwarfed its human occupants. It was mostly empty except for
supply carts along the periphery. Near the room's center floated the
large X-ray imaging head, suspended by a telescoping metal arm
from the ceiling. I had never gotten used to the dimensions of the
place, although one glance at this foal's mother was enough to explain why the designers had been generous in their space allotment.

Mike Callahan and I were assisting Dick that day. We donned
lead-lined gowns and positioned the foal in front of the X-ray head.
The young horse was nervous and timid without his mother, and we
had to hold him in place while he fidgeted. Several times he whinnied in his small reedy voice, and once I thought I heard an answering call from the mare up the hall.

The radiology tech used calipers to measure the thickness of the
foal's leg at the fetlock, at the level where the first picture would be
taken. He then strode over to the control panel on the near wall and
adjusted the machine settings. The exact strength and duration of the
X-ray pulse needed to be specified, and after years of practice Dick
was a maestro with his machine. Rarely did a second picture need
taking unless the patient moved during the exposure.

With the settings adjusted, we slipped a blank film cassette into
the vertical holder and positioned it next to the horse's leg, opposite
the machine's imaging head. We all made sure that our bodies were
not in the path of the X-ray beam and Dick punched the hand-held
remote switch. A high-pitched beep sounded and the room lights
dimmed for an instant as the machine fired. The cathode shot an invisible beam of radiation horizontally through the horse's limb and
into the film plate on the other side.

Dick nodded with satisfaction; the little foal hadn't moved during the exposure. He grabbed the film cassette and set it aside.

Things were going quite smoothly so far, but as we measured the leg in preparation for the next X-ray, an abrupt noise intruded from the hallway. In a second it was gone but it had been loud enough to draw our attention. Dick froze and listened with a puzzled expression on his face.

In a few moments we heard it again, a deep rumbling boom that seemed to vibrate the very foundations of the building. Its echoes had scarcely died away when a third percussion assailed our ears. Throwing down his calipers, Dick ran to the doorway to look up the hall. Curiosity dragged Mike and I close behind.

The stall that housed the Shire mare was a fair distance down the corridor from radiology. We could just see the barred front of the enclosure at an angle from where we stood. As we watched, a shadow darkened the stall front and a massive body threw itself against the retaining bars. The impact sent a shudder through the floor, and another thunderous crash echoed down the hall.

We looked at each other in disbelief. The mare was frantic from the loss of her foal, and was doing her best to beat down the enclosure and escape. Having seen those steel bars up close I expected that they would hold, but you couldn't have paid me enough to stand next to them right then.

Hospital staff came running toward the stall from both ends of the hall, drawn by the commotion. Dick looked at us and said, "We've got to get this foal back to its mom before she hurts herself. C'mon! As quickly as he can walk."

I gulped and glanced at Mike, who shrugged fatalistically and said, "This is what we paid good money for." We headed out the radiology room door and down the hallway. Dick led the way and we came behind him walking the foal. The din got louder as we approached the mare's stall, then abruptly it ceased. A moment later an odd scrambling noise ensued. As we came abreast of the enclosure, I looked inside and stopped dead in my tracks.

The concrete walls between adjacent stalls were as thick as my waist and nearly three meters (nine feet) tall. At that moment the mare had her forelegs clear over the top of one wall and was struggling to heave herself over. I didn't want to contemplate what would happen if she succeeded. That heavy body crashing down off balance was a prime recipe for a severe injury. We had to halt her efforts to scale the barrier.

Just how that would be accomplished I wasn't sure. Dick ran forward waving his arms and shouting, "Hay! Hay! Nunu!" In her aggravated state of mind the mare was having none of it, and Dick's voice fell on deaf ears. The animal's huge rear hooves scraped and gouged the wall as she strained to reach the top. Several doctors were also arriving on the scene, but no one looked eager to enter the stall right then. The situation was critical with no quick solution in sight.

Surprisingly, the cause of the entire ruckus also ended up coming to our rescue. The little foal saw his mother and whinnied frantically at her. His shrill voice cut through the mare's distress like no other could; she immediately whipped her head around and called back to her offspring. The foal pushed toward the stall and we let him approach. As he did so, the mare dropped her forefeet back to the ground and strode forward to meet him. Dr. Lawson quickly opened the stall door and shooed the foal in.

The two animals came together and the mare nuzzled her offspring, investigating every inch of his small body. She whickered contentedly as his familiar smell filled her nostrils. The foal pushed close against her, seeking the reassurance that only a mother can give. His fear assuaged, hunger quickly took over and before long he was reaching under the mare's abdomen and suckling insistently.

After the two were settled down, Dr. Lawson secured the stall door and turned to the rest of us, rubbing his beard thoughtfully. Then he clasped his hands together and said dryly, "We may have to adjust our protocol for dealing with these two. Does everyone agree?"

Not one dissenting opinion was voiced.

Naturally the diagnosis and treatment of the foal's problem would require that we handle him repeatedly. Exactly how to do that safely was a subject of much head scratching and debate among the vets. The foal was nursing, so his mother had to be housed with him. No one wanted to heavily sedate her, but we couldn't have a repeat of the previous episode either.

The final solution to our conundrum proved unexpectedly easy. The foal remained in the same stall as his mother and no sedatives were used. When the staff needed to work on their little patient they simply took steps to avoid provoking the mare's protective instincts. This was accomplished via the straightforward expedient of distracting her, turning her gaze away from the foal as he was led out of the stall. If she didn't see him leave she apparently didn't miss him, at least not enough to become agitated. I couldn't believe that it worked, but the results were hard to argue with.

We eventually diagnosed a hairline fracture of the cannon bone in the foal's lame leg. The injury may have been self-inflicted or could have stemmed from his mother accidentally traumatizing him. The little guy ended up wearing a cast for over a month, with several recheck exams along the way. His leg healed nicely and both horses eventually went home happy and healthy.

CHAPTER SIXTY-NINE

Thanksgiving that year was a simple affair due to the fact that I had only one day off. There was no time to visit either Cindy's family or mine, so I drove to Beaverton Wednesday night and shared Thanksgiving Day with Cindy at our apartment. We baked a nice small turkey and had an intimate candlelit meal, just the two of us. Although we could not include our families, we enjoyed the chance to be together and share the holiday. I stayed as late as I could that evening, and drove back to Corvine with a stomach stuffed decadently full of dinner and pumpkin pie. By the time I arrived at my townhouse and crawled into bed it was nearly one A.M. I barely had time to register the lateness of the hour before I was sound asleep.

Six hours later the alarm clock on my nightstand jarred me from a pleasant dream. I dragged myself fuzzily out of bed and managed to get to school on time. Fortunately I was fully awake by then, because when I arrived I landed straight in the middle of a rush of cases at the hospital. Just a handful of days remained in my radiology block and they were the busiest I had seen yet. I was loaded with work from morning until evening.

As the month's end approached, we were sinking into a cold wet winter and I was thankful to be indoors the majority of the time. The good thing about staying busy is that time flies by quickly. The last Friday of the block was upon us before I knew it, and I bid adieu to my classmates who had shared those four weeks with me. Mike and Molly were off to rural vet practice. I wished them luck as they tackled cases outdoors in the inclement weather. With radiology behind me, I set my sights on a new block that began the following Monday.

My December course was theriogenology, which covered various aspects of farm animal reproduction. Taking this block in the cold season yielded a lot of down time, since most species prefer to have babies in the spring or summer. I remember afternoons where the hours dragged and I was crammed into a small conference room with the other therio students, yawning as we watched educational films on pig reproduction and horse semen quality.

It got a little more entertaining when we obtained a real live semen sample via masturbating Hogie the hospital horse. That was good for a couple hours of fun watching thousands of sperm swimming under the microscope. We played semen critics, tallying the percentage of dead versus live sperm, and noting defects such as double-headed or double-tailed individuals.

Even more exciting—and dangerous—was assisting in the breeding of two Standardbred horses behind the vet building. The female was cooperative and held perfectly still when a twitch was applied to her lip. The stallion was the one we had to watch. He was excited and inexperienced, which made him a handful to control. We lined him up behind the mare and he eventually got the job done, but not without rearing up and balking once or twice. A telling sign of the risks involved was the fact that everyone had to wear crash helmets in case we got clipped in the head by a flying hoof.

What made the biggest impression on me during that block was the time spent palpating the school's dairy cow herd. Across the railroad tracks from McNairy Hall, just beyond the old poultry building where we had languished as freshmen, nestled a red barn with a large pasture behind it. Inside the building stood a long row of stanchions where cows could be restrained head-first, their faces buried in feeding buckets while the rear quarters were presented for us to work on.

Before we could practice palpation, we needed to round up some cattle. Several students in the block went out into the pasture accompanied by Dr. O'Brien. Waving their hands and shouting, they separated six cows from the herd and flushed them toward the barn where I waited. Despite greatly outweighing their human handlers, the timid animals easily allowed themselves to be herded through the open pasture gate and into the dirt barnyard.

Once out of the pasture the cows came charging right at me, lured by the sight of open space beyond. I stood my ground, waving my hands and yelling, *"Hiya!"* The stampeding animals came to a screeching halt as if I were a brick wall. The barnyard fence barred their way to the left, so they veered right and headed straight through the open barn doors, disappearing inside. Dr. O'Brien and my classmates came through the pasture gate and closed it behind them. Then we all headed into the barn to find the cows.

I was wondering how we would get the skittish creatures restrained for exams, but I need not have worried. The cows knew the routine. When we entered they were already standing in the stanchions gobbling up grain from the buckets hung low on the wall. All we had to do was walk up and lower the restraining bar where each cow's neck protruded through the front of the device. This locked the animal's head in place so it couldn't back out. The cows never even looked up from their feast.

With our patients in position, my classmates and I each donned a long plastic sleeve and lubed it well. Then we slid our hands slowly into the cows' rectums to attempt palpation of the reproductive organs. This was my first experience at feeling an animal from the inside. The cow's anal muscles were surprisingly relaxed and my hand went in almost effortlessly. Once inside, I felt my arm encased by soft warmth which pressed in gently from all sides. It felt like being stuck in a deep bowl of thick oatmeal.

I moved my fingers against the wall of the cow's bowel, grabbing upwards and out to the side. First I tried to snag the broad ligament of the uterus to pull the reproductive organs into position for easy palpation. The ovaries sat just beyond the rectal wall to the left and right, and it was my job to catch one between my thumb and fingers. Once that was done, I could run the tip of my thumb over the walnut-sized structure, feeling for lumps or depressions in the surface.

An astounding amount could be determined by ovarian palpation. A cow that was ready to ovulate would have an egg follicle which felt like a soft fluid blister on the surface of the ovary. If she had recently ovulated, then the follicle would have ruptured and released its egg; we could feel a sunken cavity on the ovarian surface in its place. If she was pregnant, we would feel the corpus luteum, a thickened, firm lump which formed where the follicle had previously been. This structure produced hormones such as progesterone to maintain the pregnancy.

Of course, if the cow was pregnant, we might also feel enlargement of a uterine horn where the fetus was developing; this could be detected as early as forty-five days into the pregnancy. In late term pregnancies, the bulky head of the calf felt like a hard melon sitting near the rim of the pelvis.

I have to admit that I never developed much facility for finding the ovaries on livestock. Some of my classmates had a knack for it even on our very first day in the barn. These palpation prodigies would routinely determine the stage of their patients' estrus cycles with annoying ease. They went from cow to cow, their arms in each animal for only a heartbeat before they would have an answer. The professor would palpate the animals and verify their findings with a smile and high praise for their proficiency.

Not so with me; I could struggle the entire afternoon just trying to grab an ovary on my first patient. If I couldn't find it in reasonable time, I'd eventually move on to the next cow in line and hope for better luck. Sometimes my prayers were answered, and after rooting around helplessly for ten minutes or so I'd feel the elusive structure suddenly pop into my hand. The problem was that I didn't have a clue as to how I had accomplished the feat.

Other aspects of bovine palpation proved aggravating as well. The loose anal tone that permitted easy entry also allowed what was inside the bowel to exit. Sometimes this took the form of a large burst of flatulence which blew past one's face in a warm odorous rush. The student on the receiving end would invariably have a pained expression, eyes squinted and nose wrinkled as he or she tried to face away from the cow's rump.

Other times a gurgling noise would be followed by a gush of hot liquid stool which erupted forth around the inserted arm, spilling down the front of one's coveralls like a brown mudslide. When Dr. O'Brien observed this, he would point at the unfortunate student and say, "Ay, he's got a pocketful of poo!"

Since my school days, the methods of reproductive exams in cattle have advanced. The advent of ultrasound represented a big step forward in the accuracy of evaluating a cow's estrus cycle and pregnancy status. Had I chosen livestock medicine as my area of work, I would have adopted these newer methods as they became available. Even all these years later, I find it reassuring to know that my lack of ability to grab a bovine ovary probably wouldn't have made that much difference in the long run.

CHAPTER SEVENTY

Therio block ended early because of Christmas break; I had the last week of December off and gratefully headed out of town for the holidays. First Cindy and I drove to Bend to visit her family. Precipitation there had been scarce, but the light painting of snow on the ground was a perfect fit with the holiday season. The rural setting of the high desert made for a restful break from the stress and bustle of home.

As had become our holiday routine, on the Twenty-Sixth we headed south to Medford for a Christmas encore with my parents. Cindy and I thoroughly enjoyed both halves of the vacation, seeing loved ones and updating our always curious families on the progress of my wife's career and my education.

When the whirlwind trip was over, we returned home to Beaverton for some extended time together. We were tired from traveling so many miles in a mere handful of days, but the weather was benevolent and the roads passable, so we made it home with no delays. This was an exciting time for Cindy and me, since January was scheduled to be my vacation block. Some students preferred to take time off in a warmer month, but I had deliberately scheduled this block for winter. The reason was simple: both the State and National Board Exams were coming up at the end of January, and I wanted a month of uninterrupted study time. Well, I should say mostly uninterrupted, as Cindy saw to it that I took a well-earned break every now and then.

Throughout my school career, I had been a quick learner and had rarely reviewed notes more than a day or two ahead of an exam. But now I was faced with the biggest and most important tests of my life. The board exams were the profession's attempt to evaluate a student's overall competency to practice veterinary medicine. If we failed, then we could not become licensed doctors.

The good news, I kept telling myself, was that I only needed a passing grade. Any score over seventy-five percent was enough to earn my doctorate. As this was below my usual test marks, I felt confident that I would do fine if I studied the materials well. So study I did, for three and a half straight weeks, morning until night.

I had laid out my notebooks at the beginning and decided which subjects warranted attention. Large and small animal medicine topped the list, along with surgery. Parasitology and radiology were close behind, and microbiology got some attention as well. Some subjects like freshman histology and gross anatomy I left mostly untouched; the relevant portions had been covered repeatedly in later courses.

Once I had selected which subjects to study, I settled down to the formidable task of reading and reviewing hundreds of pages of notes. It would not have been possible to absorb such a large volume of material, even in three weeks, if I hadn't already learned it before. Page after page turned before my tired eyes in a seemingly endless procession, but the progress I made was encouraging. Much of it I knew by heart, and even little details I had forgotten came back to me quickly once I saw them again. Reviewing was a heck of a lot easier than first-time learning. Days passed and my spirits rose as I plowed steadily through the shrinking pile of material.

The subjects I saved for last were large animal medicine and surgery. Farm animals, I knew, would be my weak point if I had one. I reviewed those courses last so that they would be freshest in my mind when I sat for the exams.

After two solid weeks of studying I needed a break, and we drove to the coast that weekend for a quick day trip. A short distance west of Portland sat Canon Beach, a cute little coastal town with long sandy beaches, a plethora of small shops and restaurants, and plenty of outdoor activities. One could hike, bike, fly kites in the ever-present coastal winds, or simply walk the beach looking for shells. We sat on the sand and watched the waves breaking in long curls of white under the dark grey sky. The perpetual roar of the surf and the salt smell of the ocean filled our senses, and it seemed that out here time slowed to keep pace with the ocean's vast rhythms. We topped off the day with a seafood dinner at a cozy restaurant and drove home relaxed and refreshed. Later that night as we lay in bed, Cindy's head cradled on my shoulder, I could still hear the calls of sea gulls echoing in my ears as I drifted off to a peaceful sleep.

CHAPTER SEVENTY-ONE

After my brief respite from studying, I returned to my notebooks with renewed energy. Cindy was a gem, bringing me dinner while I worked in the evenings, and trying her best not to be a distraction. She was eager to spend time with me during my break from school, and I hated having to focus my attention elsewhere when she was so close by. Despite the sense of urgency surrounding my studies, I tried to find moments in each day when I could show her that she was not forgotten.

The fateful weekend quickly approached when I would determine my destiny. This was the end point of nearly four years of learning. The day before the National Board Exam, I reviewed my large animal notes one last time, and quickly glanced through parasitology and radiology as well. It was ten P.M. when I closed the final book and dropped it on the bed. Gazing at the pile of folders scattered around me, I relaxed for a moment and inhaled deeply. If the exams went as planned, then I had just done my last formal studying as a veterinary student. It was time to get a good night's sleep.

The tests were held at a local college campus in downtown Portland. I followed the directions I had been given, and eventually found the brick five-story that I was looking for. I parked in a garage across the street and walked over to enter the building. Once inside,

I was directed down a long hallway to an open doorway near the end.

The examination room turned out to be a large auditorium brightly lit from the glare of overhead fluorescent lights. The main floor had been furnished with a hundred or so portable desks loosely arranged in rows. To the front of the room sat a long wooden table with a half-dozen examiners seated behind it. Several stacks of tests stood on the table top waiting to be handed out.

I found a desk toward the back and waited for everyone to show up. Students straggled in gradually, most of them classmates from Oregon. Some I hadn't seen since blocks started, but we kept our greetings brief as the weight of the moment bore down on us.

A number of Washington students also made their way into the auditorium, along with a handful of faces that were totally unfamiliar. The latter had to be out-of-state students from California or elsewhere. Apparently they wanted to practice in Oregon upon graduation or they would have not bothered to come this far. The National Board Exams were the same everywhere, but the state tests varied. To practice in a given area you had to pass that state's particular exam.

As I fidgeted restlessly, I looked across the faces of the examiners at the front table, and one suddenly jumped out at me. It was Douglas Strom, the doctor I had observed with before entering vet school! Seeing him now, I recalled that he had been appointed to the state examining board years earlier. Despite my nerves I felt a smile come to my face. It was great to see a familiar figure up there, and I thought it fitting that the person who had helped me get into veterinary school would be here to see it all come to fruition.

I stood and made my way to the table where Dr. Strom sat. He was busy looking at paperwork, but after a moment he glanced up. When he saw me standing there, his face split in a huge grin. "Why, look who's here!" he exclaimed. "How have you been, Mark? You're taking the boards today then?"

"Yes, the time has arrived at last," I answered with a smile.

"That's great! I always knew you'd do well. It seems like only yesterday that you were observing at my practice. You know that I wrote one of the sections on the state board exam?"

I told him that I was aware of his involvement, and he shook a finger at me teasingly, saying, "You'd better make me proud and not flunk it!"

I laughed and said, "I'll do my best. I had a good teacher, you know."

Dr. Strom smiled and replied, "I only gave you a leg up at the start; everything you've accomplished has been through your own hard work and smarts. Give yourself credit where it's due." I thanked him and he wished me well with the tests. Then I returned to my seat as the exams were being handed out.

An assistant came down my row distributing tests to the left and right. When he dropped one on my desk, I quickly looked it over. The pale yellow cover was plain and unpretentious. Its only adornment was the veterinary logo, the now familiar snake curled around a staff with the letter "V" superimposed over it. Below that were the words, "National Board Exam in Veterinary Medicine, 1986."

I wasn't fooled by the bland exterior. As I held the letter-sized booklet, I could feel its weight and the substantial thickness of the pages between my fingers. There was a lot of content to be met and conquered before the day was through. Just then a loud voice asked for the students' attention and I looked up from my desk.

One of the examiners stood at the front of the room, hands clasped in front of him as he looked out over the assembled group. He was a tall, distinguished individual clad dapperly in a dark blue suit. His brown wavy hair was tinged with silver at the temples and crow's feet crinkled his eyes as he smiled out at us.

"Hello and good morning," he said. "My name is Dr. Cahill and I'm happy to welcome you to the National Board Exam for Veterinarians. I wish all of you the best in your efforts today. Please do not open your booklets until told to do so, and listen carefully to my instructions.

"Each of you has been given a number two pencil. Use this, and only this, to mark your answers. This test is multiple-choice. Please choose a single answer for each question and fill in the appropriate box completely with the pencil. If you change your answer, be sure to erase the incorrect response completely so there is no confusion. The test is eight hours long…."

He paused as a chorus of groans erupted from the class at this revelation. Smiling he continued, "Every hour there will be a ten-minute break before resuming. There are eight sections to the test, each intended to be completed within the hour allotted. If you do not finish a section within the time permitted, you can go back to it if you complete a later section ahead of schedule. Do not go forward to new sections until asked to do so. Are there any questions?"

Dr. Cahill looked around the silent room and spotted one hand raised. He nodded and said, "Yes, what is your question?"

Molly Boyer's voice called out, "When do we get our test scores?"

"Ah, yes, I meant to mention that," the doctor replied. "You should receive your results in the mail by March 15th. Any other questions?" Looking around he saw no further hands so he said, "All right then, please open your booklets to the first section and begin."

I flipped the cover back and looked at the first page of the National Board Exam. The sheet was covered with a long list of multiple choice questions, each offering five possible answers. My heart was pounding, but I found reassurance in the familiar format. I had tackled questions like these since I was an undergraduate. The only difference here was the length of the exam and the magnitude of its importance. Best to not concentrate on the big picture, I told myself. Start at the beginning and keep moving forward, and with a little persistence you can conquer the world.

I gripped my pencil and scanned the first question. "An abdominal aspirate in a patient with congestive heart failure would most likely yield which type of fluid? A) a modified transudate, B) an exudate, C) a transudate, D) either A or C, E) none of the above. With a grin I marked "D" and moved to the next question. It too was straightforward and my pencil flashed down to mark the box. On then through the page I moved as quickly as I could manage. Speed had to be balanced with care, as I misread a couple of the answers on first glance, and twice I nearly marked the wrong one.

Time lost all meaning as I became immersed in the exam, completing each question in turn, only to be confronted with another. Turning a page revealed yet more challenges, more chances to show the examiners the extent of my knowledge or ignorance, with no end in sight. A few questions left me unsure of the correct response, and I hesitated momentarily over those before taking my best guess. There simply wasn't time to linger if I wanted to finish the section.

After an intense forty-five minutes that seemed like twenty, I reached the bottom of a page and read the words, "End of Section 1." I had finished in time.

With a sigh I put down my pencil and sat back, looking around for the first time since the test began. A handful of other students also had closed their exams and were lounging in their seats, with more finishing as I watched. Not surprisingly, I saw Mike Callahan leaning back with his hands laced behind his neck, grinning as he stared up into space. He had probably breezed through in half the allotted time. Mike caught my gaze and waved at me; I smiled and waved back. He gave me a thumbs-up sign and I nodded. We both were doing fine so far.

The moderator abruptly announced, "Okay, the time is up. Put down your pencils and close your books." I could hear sighs and groans from the students still struggling to finish, but they complied and grudgingly closed their exams. Dr. Cahill continued, "You have a ten-minute break; feel free to get up and stretch. There is a drinking fountain in the hallway if you are thirsty. Restrooms are a bit further down the hall for those who drink too much." Weak laughter greeted the doctor's jest, and chair legs scraped as people got up to move around.

Out in the hallway I stood in line for a quick sip of ice-cold water from the fountain. After that I walked about aimlessly for a few minutes. I saw Stan Hulbert lounging nearby and glimpsed a flash of blonde hair over his shoulder; it turned out to belong to Amy Baker, who was barely visible behind Stan's bulk. I was happy to see both of them and strolled over for a quick chat. Stan and Amy greeted me warmly, and then asked me how I was doing on the test so far.

"Not bad," I answered. "I know I didn't ace it, but I don't think I missed many questions either. How about you two?"

Amy looked pensive and said, "I don't know. I think I did alright, but I'm worried. Some parts seemed almost too easy; maybe I'm missing something or they were trick questions."

Stan nodded, frowning as he said, "I'm sure I missed a handful of answers, and the ones I thought I knew may have fooled me, like Amy said. What do you think? You're always good on exams."

I chuckled as I shook my head. "Look, the exams aren't tricky. They simply want to know what you know, and they aren't trying to fool you. I only saw one question where the wording was a bit misleading. The rest were straightforward: what you saw was what they meant. So just read them carefully and give the answer you think is right."

Stan said doubtfully, "You sound pretty sure about all this stuff."

"I am. You'll do fine; you don't need an 'A' to pass this. If you miss one out of every four you'll still make it!"

Stan's expression brightened as he absorbed my words; he hadn't thought of it quite that way. "Thanks, Mark," he said, giving me a grateful smile. "You've always helped me, even back in our freshman year. I don't know if I'd have made it through school on my own."

"Oh, bull!" I retorted. "You've always had what it takes or you wouldn't have gotten into the program. The admissions committee members aren't a bunch of slackers; they chose you for a reason. You've proven them right all the way along, and you'll do it again today."

Stan nodded and thanked me again. When he walked back to the testing room, he did so wearing a smile. Watching his back I saw that his posture was straight and he had a confident energy in his stride. I had a good feeling that he would pass this test.

Amy saw it too, and she sidled up next to me, saying, "That was kind of you! You'd never know it to look at him, but Stan always doubts his own abilities. He's too humble and doesn't give himself enough credit."

"You're right about that," I said.

Amy added, "You seem to know the right things to say to give him a boost. Thank you for taking the time; I know you must be preoccupied with your own efforts today."

"You and Stan have been good friends to me these past four years; I'd do the same for either of you," I told her.

She smiled and looked at the floor, saying quietly, "It's been fun knowing you, and I've missed seeing you and Stan during blocks. Before long school will be over." Her gaze came back to meet mine as she added, "I hope we can stay in touch when we're out in the world, all of us."

"I hope so, too," I answered. "But first let's go kick butt in this test so they'll let us out. Fun or not, I don't want to be a student forever!"

"Ain't that the truth!" Amy declared, and we shared a smile as we walked back into the testing room.

We waded through three more grueling hours of examinations that morning. At noon we had reached the halfway point and we took a well-deserved meal break. I had sixty minutes to relax and enjoy the sack lunch I had brought. I hadn't expected to have an appetite until after the exam was over, but hours of concentration and adrenaline had burned a lot of calories, and hunger was gnawing at my belly.

Mike Callahan came over to join me, sitting at the desk to my right as I munched on my sandwich. The auditorium was surprisingly empty as most students had gone off to find a cafeteria or nearby restaurant. Only a handful of desks were occupied and our voices echoed hollowly in the silent room.

"Hey, it's nice to see you again, Mike," I said as he opened his lunch sack. "X-rayed any Shire foals lately?"

He chuckled and shook his head, saying, "That's one episode I hope to not repeat."

"Yep. Never let them tell you that radiology is boring!" I replied with a grin.

"Never let anyone tell you that two-thousand-pound animals are boring," he answered. "The moment you relax is when they'll kick your fanny."

"Most definitely," I agreed, nodding. For a moment we fell silent, lost in our thoughts as we ate our meals. After finishing the first half of my sandwich, I took a swallow of water and asked him, "So how are you doing on the test?"

He shrugged and said, "Oh, all right I guess. The questions aren't that bad, there's just a lot of them." In the silence after he spoke I heard a faint sound coming from under the table. It was familiar, but it took a minute for me to place its origins. When I recognized the soft *pat, pat, pat* of Mike's foot tapping the floor, I smiled inwardly; some things never changed.

I took another bite of my sandwich and then a thought struck me. "Say, there were a couple of questions about legal issues on that last section. I didn't study the regulations much. Is scabies a reportable disease in cattle?"

He nodded emphatically. "Yes it is. The correct answer on that one was "E—all of the above. Foot-and-mouth disease, scabies, tuberculosis and brucellosis are all reportable."

I smiled with relief. "Good, I thought so but I wasn't sure. One answer included all those diseases except scabies and I almost marked that one."

"Well, you got it right, that's the important thing," Mike said as he tipped back a soda. Watching him it occurred to me that Mike wired on sugar and caffeine could be an amusing sight; if he overdid it he'd end up jogging in place while taking his exam.

When lunch hour ended, all the students filed back into the room and we launched into another four hours of examinations. The brief breaks between sections were barely enough to catch a breath. By the time the last test was completed, my head was spinning and I was exhausted. The time was five P.M. and we had been sitting at our desks the entire day.

Despite my fatigue, I was flying high with relief. I had completed all the sections on time, and had left no questions unmarked. In addition, I was confident about most of my answers. The few that I hadn't known would not comprise much of my score. Either way, it was done!

Now I could get a good night's sleep and look forward to the relatively quick and easy Oregon State Board Exam the following day. It was "only" four hours long, practically a picnic compared to what I had just completed. It's funny how perspective changes everything; at no other time in my life would a four-hour marathon of questions have seemed friendly.

When I arrived home, Cindy wanted to hear all about my day and I filled her in as best I could. In truth I could clearly recall only a smattering of questions, since the exam had already become a blur. She rubbed my back as I talked, and I felt the last remnants of the day's tension fading away beneath her magical fingers. Later we had a relaxed dinner without a notebook in sight. My exam preparations were completed for the duration, and I only had eyes for my wife. When the evening grew late, we snuggled close and for once I got to study something other than veterinary medicine.

The next morning in the auditorium I saw Dr. Strom again. He asked how I had done on the national exam and I told him I thought it had gone well. He nodded and said, "Well, I expected no less from you, Mark. You've got a sharp mind and you apply yourself well. Good luck on today's exam."

I gave him a cocky smile and said, "Luck has nothing to do with it."

He laughed and answered, "That's the spirit. Show me what you can do!"

"I'll give it my best shot," I promised as I headed off to find a seat. I settled again into a vacant desk near the rear of the room and waited for the test to be handed out.

There were four sections to the state exam, each lasting an hour, and each written by a different Oregon practitioner who held a position on the examining board. This test was similar to the national exam in form and content, but it paid special attention to diseases endemic to our region. For instance I discovered that "salmon disease" of dogs was the focus of several questions. This was a rickettsial infection obtained via eating uncooked salmon, steelhead, or rainbow trout. The illness was specific to the Pacific Northwest, occurring nowhere else in the world. Many veterinary schools paid it only passing notice, but practitioners in Oregon needed to be aware of it, since the infection was common here. If not treated promptly with tetracycline, the feverish canine would nearly always die.

The local flavor of the exam made it seem somehow more comfortable, like an old acquaintance. Maybe part of that feeling came from knowing that my mentor had written one section. Regardless of why, the pages seemed to fly by, and before I knew it I was handing my exam in at the front table. Dr. Strom took my completed test and winked as he said, "Did you ace it?"

I chuckled and shook my head. "Not quite. But I think I did well. Hopefully in a few months I'll be a DVM just like you."

He looked at me seriously then and said, "I hope so too, Mark. You'll be a fine addition to our veterinary community." He shook my hand and congratulated me on having come so far, and I thanked him again for all his help along the way. We chatted awhile longer and then I took my leave, walking across the room and out the auditorium door. As I exited, it felt as if a huge burden had been lifted from my shoulders. My veterinary board exams were behind me.

CHAPTER SEVENTY-TWO

February began with the Willamette Valley still locked in the clammy embrace of winter. The sodden landscape huddled under brooding skies, the trees in the meadow blurred into indistinct shapes by rain mist and ghostly grey fog. We even had a couple of mornings where snowflakes fell briefly, causing people to point excitedly out the vet school windows. As usual, none if it managed to stick on the ground.

In the midst of this alluring weather came my rural animal medicine block. Here the students accompanied doctors on house calls to local farms. Eight seniors attended the course that month, including my good friends Stan Hulbert, Amy Baker and Ed Martinelli.

Dr. James Fayer headed up the hospital's mobile service. In my eyes he personified the large animal veterinarian. His full head of brown hair was perpetually disheveled and I never saw him wear a tie. Coveralls comprised his entire wardrobe as far as anyone knew; I would not have been surprised if he had worn them to his wedding as well. Within his pockets resided every instrument that one might need while working in the field. Lean and wiry with corded forearms and a weathered face, he looked a spry fifty years old. I was later shocked to learn that my guess was ten years shy of reality.

On days when there were farm calls to handle, the students on rural block would pile in a school van along with the good doctor and we'd head out on the road. Weather aside, I found myself enjoying the leisurely drives through the farming country around Corvine. The fertile land possessed a picturesque beauty that never grew old. Cultivated fields and farm pastures were interspersed with stands of firs, cedars, and maples that had once blanketed the region before the arrival of settlers. An occasional low hill rose up from the valley floor, fog often shrouding the dark forested slopes. Life out here moved at a different pace than in the teaching hospital, more relaxed, more in touch with the earth and things that grew from it.

Dr. Fayer had been practicing medicine in the valley for a long time. As a result he had an encyclopedic memory of the region's inhabitants and history. He would often provide a running travelogue as we meandered along country roads, pointing out this farm or that, and telling of the families past and present who had made their lives on that acreage. Despite practicing at a modern teaching facility, he reminded me of an old-time vet who was part of the community, dispensing his knowledge and skills with a personal touch.

The medicine I observed on these farm visits also called to mind the simpler days of veterinary practice. Farmers worked hard for a living, but they had a narrow margin of profit. Although their livestock were their bread and butter, they could ill afford high medical bills on a given animal. If the cost of treatment exceeded the value of the patient, then euthanasia was a serious possibility. A pet horse or a prized breeding bull might warrant special consideration, but typical herd medicine was, as Dr. Fayer termed it, "quick and dirty." It was a real eye-opener to discover just how quick, and how dirty, field work could be.

The good news was that livestock, in particular cattle, were hardy beasts and would often survive if given even half a chance. One of the first procedures I witnessed in rural practice was correction of a displaced abomasum in a Guernsey cow. We arrived on the farm in response to a call about a milker who was "ADR." I asked Dr. Fayer what that acronym stood for, since I did not recall it from my medicine notes. He snorted and said, "Ain't Doin' Right."

"Ah-ha," I replied, for there wasn't much else I could say to that.

When we talked to the amiable farmer, he described a gradual progression of decreased appetite and poor milk output. The cow ate hay fairly well, but was off her grain. Her stools were scant and pasty.

The doctor nodded and asked, "Had she been on increased grain intake before she took ill?"

"Yep, she's pregnant, so I've been pushin' the grain and silage to her," the farmer answered. "She was gaining well for awhile, but I'm worried about her now. She's turnin' to skin and bones."

"Okay then. Let's take a look at her, shall we?" Dr. Fayer said. The farmer nodded and led the way down a rutted dirt lane to a modern-looking brown barn. In front of the building a fawn and white cow was tethered to a fence post, mouthing hay from a small bale placed in front of her. We approached and began our initial assessment of our patient.

Even at first glance I could tell that something was wrong with this animal. Although her size and conformation bespoke good stock, she was far from her prime. Her pelvic bones protruded alarmingly above her rump, and her shrunken udder hung limply between her legs. I thought she seemed listless, and her attack on the hay bale lacked enthusiasm.

Dr. Fayer contemplated the cow and then turned to the rest of us, saying, "Is there anything peculiar about her build, other than being thin?"

Now that he mentioned it, the cow's abdomen did seem to be disproportionately distended considering her overall weight loss. Some of that could be due to her pregnancy, but her belly was asymmetrical, being pushed out more on the left. I mentioned this to the professor and he nodded. "Any idea what the problem might be?" he asked.

"A displaced abomasum?" Amy Baker piped up.

"Very likely," the doctor answered, nodding. "Any way to verify that?"

Amy had a strong interest in farm animals and she responded without hesitation, "Ballottement of the abdomen with auscultation should yield a ping."

In plain English, the abomasum was one of the four stomachs in a bovine. In certain situations it could move left from its normal position, becoming stuck on the flank alongside the rumen. Thusly positioned, it failed to empty properly and would build up gas, becoming swollen and tight as the pressure built. One could detect the distended organ via tapping sharply on the bulging left flank while a stethoscope was placed there. A characteristic high-pitched "ping" would be heard, sounding remarkably similar to tapping on a pressurized metal air tank.

The doctor had each of the students listen to the ailing cow. When my turn came I put my stethoscope on the furred belly and flicked my finger against the thick hide. Instead of the dull thud one would usually expect I heard a high, bell-like note resonating in my ears. I felt a flutter of excitement as I listened several more times; this was right out of a textbook! Nothing was better than seeing the words on the pages come to life.

Harking back to quick and dirty field work, this simple exam gave us our "quick" diagnosis; now came time for the "dirty" treatment. We had to open the cow's abdomen, move its abomasum back to where it belonged, and suture it in place so the problem would not reoccur. The cow was walked into the barn and tethered at a stanchion along the wall. We used portable battery-powered clippers to shave an area on the cow's flank, and then scrubbed the skin liberally with iodine soap.

That's as clean as the procedure got. After the surgical site was prepped, Dr. Fayer donned a plastic sleeve, the same non-sterile type we used in rectal palpation. Amy Baker leaned over and whispered to me, "At least he's using a fresh one!" I chuckled under my breath and watched as the doctor gave an injection of local anesthetic to numb the area he would incise. After a few minutes he took a scalpel and made a long incision in the animal's flank, deep enough to enter the body cavity. Blood gushed out of the wound in what would have been an alarming torrent for a small animal. For a Guernsey it was a mere drop in the bucket. I say that literally because the doctor kicked a large steel one underneath the cow to catch the crimson liquid dripping on the ground.

Our patient took minimal notice of the whole affair and continued picking at the hay bale set in front of her nose. Dr. Fayer proceeded to slide his entire arm through the incision into the cow's body cavity and began rooting around. While he was doing this I was watching in amazement at the total non-sterility of it all. The sleeve that was shoved inside the animal wasn't even close to aseptic; neither was the dusty barn with flakes of dirt falling from the rafters every time the cow bumped the wall. I watched as debris landed directly on the incision. At one point the doctor's arm was so far inside that his coveralls were pushed up against the open wound. Bits of the animal's shaved hair were also stuck into the raw flesh. If this had been a horse or a human, then a nasty peritonitis would have surely resulted.

But cattle were a different story altogether; a surgical procedure could be frankly contaminated and they would still heal. All you had to do was rinse off any heavy soiling and suture it closed. Antibiotic injections might be given on occasion, but really the cow did most of the work of healing. They truly were amazing creatures.

Our patient proved to be true to her heritage. After Dr. Fayer had repositioned the swollen abomasum into its normal location, the incision ended up healing routinely. On a follow-up phone call, the farmer reported that his cow had begun eating aggressively within twelve hours of the procedure. Quick and dirty had done the trick.

Of course, cattle were not impervious to disease, and when an infection did occur it could grow to startling proportions. A week later we visited a large dairy farm south of Corvine to treat a cow with a swelling on its left rear leg. The property was large and modern, with acres of lush fields bordered by gleaming white fences. I spotted sizable Holstein and Jersey herds grazing in the distance as we drove down the long private road off the highway. Ahead of us loomed two barns and a handful of outbuildings, all sturdy with clean straight lines and looking very well maintained.

We pulled into a parking area in front of the buildings and met up with the dairy herd manager. He led us into the nearest barn, where a long row of black and white cattle stood tethered awaiting their morning milking. At one end away from the other animals stood a nice-sized brown Jersey cow, her face buried in a bucket of grain. She carried good weight and her udder hung full and turgid with milk. At first glance nothing seemed to be wrong with her. Then I moved around to where I could get a good view of her rear quarters, and I decided that maybe she had a small problem after all.

Protruding from the back of the left rear leg was a huge rounded mass the size of a basketball or maybe a large watermelon. The skin overlying this monstrosity was stretched tight, parting the fur to reveal an angry red tinge beneath. My classmates and I stood staring at the lesion while Dr. Fayer talked with the manager.

"Looks like a large abscess," the vet pronounced.

"Yep, that's kinda what I thought as well," the farm man replied. "How did it happen, do ya think?"

"Mmm, dunno for sure," the doctor said, chin in his hand as he contemplated the cow. "Probably got a small wound there and it festered. The fur hides a lot of nicks and scratches so you might not see anything until it swells up. By then the skin has healed over."

"Gotta drain it then," the manager stated.

"Yep," Dr. Fayer replied. "No way around that. You'll need to give her antibiotics for awhile; she'll be off the milking line until the drug residues clear out of her body."

"Yeah, I know," said the farmhand in a resigned voice. "Lost production, but it's better than culling her. She's a good milker for us and she's a nice little gal too. We'd best get it done."

The doctor nodded and looked over to us. "Are you ready for some fun, class?" he said.

We nodded and Mike Callahan answered, "Let's open it up!"

"Exactly what I had in mind," the vet replied. "We'll get some supplies from the van and get to work."

A few minutes later we gathered behind the cow once again, loaded down with the bizarre implements of field surgery. We set the items on a plastic tarp to keep them off the dirty ground, and then turned to our patient. First we tied the animal's tail up over her back to keep it out of the way and reduce her tendency to kick. Then the doctor took a long pole resembling a broom handle and fastened a large wad of clean cloth to one end. After dipping this in a bucket of liquid iodine soap, he handed the pole to Mike Callahan and said, "Why don't you scrub that leg up for us, Mike."

Mike took the implement and said, "We're not going to shave the hair around there?"

Dr. Fayer grinned and shook his head. "Nope, we'll just wash it and cut. What's inside is worse than what's on the skin."

"All right, then…," Mike said with a shrug. He extended the pole with the soapy cloth, rubbing it up and down vigorously over the swollen portion of the leg. The length of the tool kept him out of range of the cow's hooves should she decide to throw a kick his way. When the area was suitably saturated with the yellow-brown lather, he lowered the pole and said, "Okay boss, what's next?"

Dr. Fayer looked over to Amy Baker and said, "Do you want to cut that open?"

She nodded with a big grin and said, "Sure! I'm willing to take a shot at it."

The doctor took a sharp carving knife with a long gleaming blade and strapped it firmly to another pole that had been adapted for that purpose. He handed it to Amy, saying, "Just stab deep into the center of the mass, and then pull the blade down to lengthen your incision. We want a large drainage opening. Don't forget to stay back from those feet!"

Amy hefted the pole knife experimentally, gauging its weight and balance. Then she stepped up behind the cow and extended the blade until it hovered just over the ripe bulge of the abscess. She took a deep breath and then plunged the gleaming steel deep into the yielding flesh.

The cow looked up and gave one half-hearted kick backwards in annoyance at the sting. Then her head turned back to continue plundering her grain bucket. As the sharp blade pierced the abscess wall, a rivulet of pea green pus erupted from the wound. It thickened into a torrent as Amy pulled the knife edge down the leg, opening an incision the length of a grown man's hand. Cups of viscous liquid cascaded down the limb, mixed with large chunks of thicker exudate that appeared semi-solid. A couple more kicks came Amy's way as she worked, but she was safely positioned out of reach. The cow didn't even bother to look up from her meal. As for me, food was quite low on my list of interests right at that moment. At least the open air environment helped dilute the odor wafting from the steaming pile on the ground.

Finally the infection stopped pouring from the open wound, but we weren't done yet. Dr. Fayer and Cindy used pole handles to push in from opposite sides, squeezing additional pus from the abscess. More chunky goodness erupted from the incision; it was sort of like popping a titanic pimple. The rest of us watched mesmerized. Whatever nasties a small animal could generate, livestock surely did it bigger and better.

When the collapsed abscess seemed totally drained, the doctor wrapped another piece of cloth around the end of a pole. This time he dipped it in iodine solution, not scrub soap. Then he rammed the cloth into the abscess cavity, twisting it all around inside to debride and disinfect the wound. When he was done, the incision was left open to allow further drainage in upcoming days; it would close soon enough on its own.

The dairy manager thanked us for our efforts, and the doctor gave him an invoice for services rendered, along with some injectable antibiotic to administer until the cow healed. We returned to the school with lingering images in our heads, and a lingering odor in the van from the soiled instruments in back. It had been quite an outing, enough so that the day found a permanent place among my memories. Though that afternoon is now ancient history, I have never forgotten the little Jersey cow with the monstrous leg.

CHAPTER SEVENTY-THREE

Not all the facilities we serviced were as modern or as large-scale as the dairy we visited that day. Some were modest family ranches with a handful of herd animals on a couple of peaceful acres. It was at one of these smaller farms that I made my first acquaintance with equine rectal palpation.

The horse in question was a Percheron mare, a jet-black draft horse nearly as big as a Shire. She was to be bred, and the owner wanted an assessment of where she was in her estrus cycle. That meant finding those elusive ovaries and feeling for follicle development.

Percherons lack fetlock feathers but are heavy and muscular, far outsizing the more common riding animals. When we arrived at the farmhouse, I saw the hulking mare tethered to a fence post and I swallowed reflexively; we were supposed to palpate *that*?

The owner was a tall, stooped fellow who moved with the slow deliberation of one who didn't care to be hurried. To my eyes he looked as if he had led a long hard life. Dr. Fayer knew the man's history well. On the drive out the doctor had told us that Thomas Michaels had been a successful farmer in the area for decades. But times had slowly changed, and age and economics had taken their toll. Over the years he had reluctantly sold much of his property to home developers to reduce his work load and help pay bills. He was down to a fraction of the magnificent lands he had once commanded, and housing subdivisions now bordered his northern fields. He persisted nonetheless, managing a small herd of beef cattle and raising a corn crop every summer. In addition, he kept a few prized breeding horses, the big draft animals that he had always had a soft spot for.

Tom shuffled slowly down the front steps of his two-story wood frame home, waving to us as we piled out of the van. He made his leisurely way down the stone path that cut through his front yard, then out through the gate in the white picket fence, turning to close it carefully behind him. When he trod across the gravel parking lot to meet us, I got my first good look at our client.

The aging farmer wore denim coveralls with suspenders and a red cotton shirt beneath. Like most men who had spent their lives outdoors, he eschewed style in favor of sensible protection from the elements. His salt-and-pepper head was topped with a plain, wide-brimmed hat, while sturdy work boots capped off his wardrobe below.

He ambled over to where we stood and Dr. Fayer made introductions. The worn skin of Tom's face resembled cured leather stretched over his strong cheek bones. Time and care had etched their signatures in a myriad of fine creases, but he still gave the impression of residual strength and vigor. Slate grey eyes frankly sized me up as I shook his hand. The calloused palm he offered felt like warm sandpaper, and his grip was steely firm. After pleasantries were concluded, our host led the way as we walked slowly down the dirt driveway to where the mare awaited.

From a closer vantage point the horse seemed larger than life, a black monolith boldly set against the pastel colors of the fields behind. She shifted anxiously at the approach of so many strangers, and her young handler reached up to rub her neck, talking to her in low tones. I glanced over at Tom Michaels, and saw his expression soften as he gazed at his horse.

It's a funny thing about old-time rural farmers. Many possess only a minimal formal education, but living close to the earth has taught them a simple wisdom that gives them a wonderful perspective. They often look at life from a slightly different angle than most of us city dwellers. That afternoon I encountered an amusing example of this. While the doctor went back to the van to grab supplies, I made small talk with Mr. Michaels, and we chatted about the farm and days past. In the course of the conversation I casually asked, "So, have you lived here all your life then?"

The old farmer scratched his stubbled chin thoughtfully, looking off to the distance, and after a moment he replied, "Not yet."

It was about then that Dr. Fayer returned with the needed equipment. He sized up the situation and pronounced, "Let's move the mare out into the middle of the road where she can't hurt herself if she gets antsy."

The handler looked to Tom Michaels, who nodded. Undoing the hitching rope from the fence, the young man led the mare over to stand in the open. "Now we can palpate her and see if she's ovulating," the vet said, looking around as he rubbed his hands together. "Who wants to give it a try?" Before anyone could respond his eyes settled on me and he said, "Mark, you've not had a go at a horse before, have you? Let's see what you can do."

With a sinking feeling, I grabbed a plastic sleeve and slid it onto my right arm, after which I took the tube of gel and applied it liberally. Right then I was feeling very charitable, and if there was any way that I could minimize the mare's unhappiness during palpation, then I was all for it. By the time I was done my entire arm glistened and the tube looked appreciably shrunken.

I stepped forward with my arm extended and asked, "How will we restrain her out here?"

Dr. Fayer replied, "Oh, we'll put a twitch on her; that should do the trick." As he spoke, the handler looped a rope around the mare's upper lip and tightened it down. "There you go; she's all yours," the doctor announced. I looked dubiously at the small man holding the small twitch on the very large horse. Then I mentally shrugged; at least if I died it would be quick.

I moved up next to the massive rump of the animal, making sure to stay very close where it was safer. With my left hand I cranked the heavy tail upwards to expose the anus. My target was so far above the ground that I had to stand on my toes to slide my arm in. I pointed my lubed hand and pushed, and slowly it disappeared inside.

As I probed further and further in, trying to reach the ovaries on this huge mare, I became aware of a significant difference between palpating a horse and a cow. The good news was that horses had firm stools and would not decorate your front in chocolate syrup.

Unfortunately, this animal also had sphincter tone from hell, and when she tightened up around my arm it felt like being caught in a vice. If the owner had fed her a lump of coal every so often he could have remained financially solvent via collecting the diamonds she passed.

I eventually had my arm inside of the mare up to my shoulder and as I struggled to find each ovary, I was quickly losing the ability to feel my hand. When I pushed a bit harder I felt the mare shift her weight in protest and I happened to glance down. The rear feet were visible below and just in front of me, and I contemplated the huge black hooves, each the size of a large dinner plate. If the mare decided to lash out and kick me with one of those, I would probably fly twenty feet and end up draped over the fence on the far side of the road. Or perhaps not, as my arm was anchored firmly in the animal's derriere.

An image flashed through my mind then: I was riding in an ambulance, flat on my back, struggling to breathe with the large imprint of a hoof imbedded in my chest. My right shoulder hurt and as I turned my head, I beheld my detached arm sitting alongside me on a metal tray. "We found you stuck on the fence," said the paramedic hovering nearby. "Your arm we had to extract from the horse's butt."

I shook off the thought and redoubled my efforts to palpate the mare, fighting a battle against time as the circulation in my arm was being progressively pinched off. I was giving up hope and about to pull out when I finally succeeded in grabbing one of the ovaries. Clinging desperately to the walnut-sized lump, I ran the tip of my thumb over the surface and thought I felt a soft mass protruding from one side. It felt like a follicle; if I was correct, then it meant she was close to ovulating. Breeding time was near at hand.

I pulled my arm out and briefly stated my findings. When Dr. Fayer palpated her, he agreed with my assessment. "Good job, Mark!" he said when we were walking back to the van. I sighed with relief as I worked the feeling back into my tingling fingers. I had survived the episode with body and limbs intact, and had somehow managed to make an accurate diagnosis in the process. Sometimes it's better to be lucky than good.

The next week or so passed uneventfully like the calm before the storm. The tempest in this case was the overnight arrival of a myriad new faces in the teaching hospital, as mid-February marked the return of the junior class from Tullville. Suddenly the hallways seemed full of activity while the school absorbed an additional thirty-five students. The juniors would be mostly in lectures until summer, but they visited the hospital ward whenever possible, so I encountered them from time to time. I noted with amusement that they often had a dazed look about them, perhaps due to killer quarter commencing.

In general I had little time to pay heed to the class behind us, as my own schedule remained busy. One of our more unusual activities during that block was visiting the prison farm. The Oregon correctional system operated a small dairy near Corvine, and inmates who were deemed lower risk could spend time working there. This allowed them to learn job skills while getting some fresh air outside their cells. The veterinary school provided medical care for the facility's animals. Thus it was that on a cold day in late February we drove out to the rather unique farm for routine examinations of the dairy cows.

While en route the doctor briefed us on policies and procedures at the facility. "How safe is it for us to be there?" asked Amy Baker.

"It's pretty safe," Dr. Fayer told her. "The farm doesn't house violent criminals. Nonetheless, it pays to be prudent. Stay in groups always, and if you need help for any reason, then approach one of the guards."

"There are guards there?" Stan Hulbert asked.

"Of course," the doctor said. "There are inmates, after all; someone's got to keep an eye on them so they don't leave. They don't wear uniforms on the farm, but guards are there all the same."

"If there are no uniforms, how do we know who the guards are?" Amy asked.

"Good question," replied Dr. Fayer. "The guards wear red caps, and the prisoners wear blue. If you need help, find a red cap."

We all nodded as we committed this to memory. The doctor drove along in silence for a minute, looking thoughtful, and then he added, "Oh, and you students with two X-chromosomes, don't go wandering off by yourselves." Amy and Trina looked at each other askance, and we made the rest of the trip in silence.

On arriving at the farm, we met with one of the guards. He gave us a similar orientation speech to that we had heard from Dr. Fayer. Then we moved as a group through a couple of locked gates and into the main dairy barn. It sat atop a low rise overlooking rolling fields of pasture below. The building was large and housed scores of stanchions for cattle to stand at as they were milked. To our dismay we found that the barn had no real walls, only a metal roof supported by large timbers on all sides. The exposed location combined with the building's design made for minimal protection from the weather.

We were out of the rain, but a wickedly chill wind whipped through the barn unimpeded.

We glanced around uncertainly as we walked down the wide corridor. Approximately a dozen men clad in coveralls and blue-billed hats moved here and there, attending to various chores with the animals. Along the periphery of the building's interior stood a handful of other men similarly dressed. They made no attempt to join in the work, but simply watched with hands clasped behind their backs. I noted that these individuals each wore a bright red cap.

Dr. Fayer observed our wandering stares and said quietly, "Just ignore them and go about your business as usual." Following his advice we hunkered down against the cold and began our work. Rows of cattle stood along the two main corridors within the barn. There were several items on our agenda for the day, including Brucellosis testing and examining mammary glands for signs of mastitis. We moved down the ranks of animals, pushing each cow's tail up high and inserting a needle in the caudal vein to obtain the blood sample. Brucellosis is a bacterial disease that can be shed in the milk of affected animals, and it can lead to abortions in many species, including cattle and humans. Although Pasteurization of milk should kill any hidden pathogens before consumption, testing the cows periodically was another safeguard for the human population and also helped reduce herd losses.

As the afternoon wore on, we completely forgot about the prisoners, since another concern demanded our attention. The bitter cold was slowly but certainly taking its toll on all of us. By the time we had sampled the entire herd and palpated dozens of teats, we were shivering uncontrollably and hugging our bodies. The short-sleeved coveralls provided little protection from the freezing gusts blowing through the barn. Icy fingers caressed our faces and found their way inside the loose-fitting garments. I thrust my bare arms beneath the thin cotton in a vain attempt to warm them. The problem was that we couldn't dress heavily; jackets would have made it impossible to perform rectal palpations and also would have been severely soiled by day's end.

There was one way to warm up though. As our last chore we had to palpate some of the cows to determine if they were pregnant. The students eagerly grabbed sleeves and lube and rushed to find animals. An audible "Ahhh" was heard from multiple throats as frozen arms plunged deep into warm bovine bodies. My hand was numb but I didn't even care if I could feel an ovary; it felt so good to have my arm bathed in soothing heat that I could have stayed there all afternoon. When I went to the next cow I switched arms, ignoring the fact that I had never palpated anything left-handed before. After four or five animals I was beginning to revive, and by the time we loaded back into the van the students were all smiles. Even the streaks of liquid cow manure down our fronts couldn't darken our mood. After all, what's a little odor compared to hypothermia?

It is fun to look back and smile at my adventures now, but they had a positive impact on me aside from their amusement value. With every new experience I gained some knowledge and insight into the practice of veterinary medicine. I could draw a blood sample on nearly any species of farm animal without hesitation, and could herd cattle into squeeze chutes like an old pro. I knew how to calm a wild-eyed equine and avoid getting kicked or bitten in the process. Lameness evaluations were no longer a thing of mystery. It happened so slowly that I was barely aware if it, but I was becoming more confident and competent as my senior year rolled along.

One afternoon I was strolling through the hospital ward, having just returned from palpating another herd of cattle at a nearby farm. My blue coveralls were stained and smeared with dirt and dung. I had my stethoscope slung around my neck due to more of the same goop coating my front pockets. As I walked down the wide corridor, I saw someone emerge from a horse stall just ahead of me on the left. She too was clad in coveralls and carried a syringe in one hand, her light brown hair pulled back in a ponytail. Her youthful appearance and garb identified her as a student, but she was not from the senior class and I didn't recognize her face. That pegged her almost certainly as a junior, because freshmen weren't usually seen alone working on patients. She caught sight of me and hurried over, a relieved look on her face.

"Would you be willing to give me some help, please?" she asked breathlessly. "I'm supposed to give this injection to that foal in the stall, but he's moving all over the place and I can't get the needle in. I don't know what to do!" She looked up at me hopefully, and I realized that to her I must seem the epitome of age and experience.

I nodded and said, "Sure, I can give you a hand." She smiled at me gratefully as we walked to the stall door. The animal in question was very young, still smaller than a full-sized Shetland pony. As we walked into the stall I reflected on how much I had learned in these past months. At this point I could do a foal injection with my eyes closed, yet this junior student seemed to find it a daunting task. Had I really been that tentative only a year ago? Thinking back on it, I was forced to admit that indeed I had.

I grinned as I approached the foal from the side and quickly wrapped my left arm under its neck, pulling it tight into me. Simultaneously I grabbed the base of the tail with my right hand, jacking it up in the air. Then I drove my legs forward until I had the small horse pinned against the back wall of the stall. With restraining grips to the front and back, the foal was helpless to resist and I said to the student, "Go ahead, you can give the shot."

She stepped forward and put the injection smoothly into the hip muscles. The animal didn't even twitch. When she pulled the needle out, I released the little foal and it scampered off to the corner where it stood watching us warily. I laughed and dusted off my hands, saying, "There you go. Sometimes it helps to have a second person."

Eyes slightly wide, she nodded and said, "That was fantastic. You really knew how to handle him. I wasn't raised on a farm and I'm still learning to deal with these big animals. I hope that someday I can do it as well as you."

"Oh, you will," I laughingly assured her with a nod. "I had no prior large animal experience at all, but after four years I'm getting the hang of it. Just keep working and you'll surprise yourself. It does get easier, I promise."

She thanked me again and I smiled as I walked leisurely away down the hall.

CHAPTER SEVENTY-FOUR

March brought enjoyable changes both in curriculum and weather. The long-awaited spring made its first appearance as sun and milder temperatures greeted us at last. My block that month covered zoo and laboratory animal medicine, an elective course that highly interested me. Up to that point I'd received nearly four years of training in dogs, cats, horses, cattle, and other farm animals. Unfortunately, this had left a void when it came to ferrets, rabbits, guinea pigs, hamsters, and other "pocket pets." Reptiles and wildlife hadn't even rated a passing glance.

This block was the school's attempt to pay at least small homage to the exotic species. Of course it was not nearly enough for us to become competent with these animals, but it was better than nothing. I had a great time the entire month as the course threw a variety of activities at us. First we spent a week in the lecture hall covering diseases of birds, small rodents, and the like. Then we tackled zoo animal medicine, and that's where things really got interesting.

One day the course instructor, Dr. Katrina Madsen, took us on a field trip to a wildlife park just southwest of Corvine. This was an outdoor preserve with extensive acreage and beautiful facilities. A meandering road carried visitors on a safari-like tour where they could see everything from ostriches to elephants to Bengal tigers roaming the land uncaged. Of course the public had to stay in their cars at all times, but as veterinary students we were treated to a behind-the-scenes look.

Much of the senior class attended this trip, since the wildlife facility couldn't hold multiple tours for individual block courses. We arrived in separate cars and gathered in the parking lot out front of the main office. Students who hadn't seen each other for months chatted animatedly as they caught up on events in each other's lives. I joined Mike, Amy, Stan, and Molly as we waited for the show to begin.

The weather that day was overcast but dry, with temperatures mild enough that a light jacket was quite comfortable. Our tour guide was Dr. Jean Foster, one of the vets employed full-time at the park. She gave us a brief talk, discussing the facility and the day's agenda. We learned that we would not walk through the African section due to animals like lions and elephants that could be slightly hazardous to our health. None of us protested much at this lost opportunity.

After fielding a few questions, Dr. Foster started walking toward the main gate, waving for us to follow. We moved en masse behind her, and slowly headed into the wild animal park.

The first animals we encountered were a group of adult ostriches. They showed no fear at our numbers and stalked straight for us. The vet was prepared and handed out long wooden poles, telling us, "Use these to keep the birds at a safe distance. Ostriches can be aggressive and peck or kick you. The kick is what's dangerous; their rear claw can slit your belly open and disembowel you with a single stroke. If you ever are face-to-face with an aggressive ostrich, it's best to lie down; they can peck and stomp on you, but you'll live."

We thought it best not to let it come to that, so we used the poles to push away the inquisitive flock as they crowded in. The animals were imposing in their height and bulk, and it was disconcerting to see brown bird eyes peering down at me from above. The intimidating aura of the giant birds was only slightly diminished by the ludicrously small size of the heads topping their long necks.

Their beaks were still big enough to do damage, and I saw a few choice pecks doled out when students allowed them too near.

We moved slowly through the ostriches' territory as a tightly packed mass of humanity bristling with poles. Eventually the birds stopped following us and we spread out, hiking freely over rolling grass-covered terrain. After a while the vet cautioned us to slow down, and I wondered what was ahead. As we crept forward I craned my neck and finally saw a flash of yellow hidden amongst the low vegetation. Lying casually not ten strides from our group was a pack of five or six cheetahs!

The vet instructed us to approach very carefully and we inched ahead, poles at the ready. We got to within four or five strides before the animals began to protest our presence. I heard a low rumbling growl emanating from multiple throats as they bared their fangs at us. Dr. Foster said, "That's far enough; these guys are used to people, but I wouldn't push it." We all took turns coming to the front of the group so we could see the animals up close. Their sleek, spotted forms were beautiful to behold even at rest. They seemed to know we were not a threat, and made no attempt to attack or move away. After a few minutes we slowly backed off and headed up the slope in a different direction.

In an open field we encountered a pair of emus, large flightless birds, but much smaller and less dangerous than ostriches. The pair pranced up to us eagerly and Dr. Foster explained that they were looking for treats. Although they were not your garden variety songbirds, they appeared more cute than intimidating as their fluffy round bodies came only up to my waist.

Regarding the birds thoughtfully, the vet said, "These two need health exams and I'm thinking this is a good time to do it, since I've got a lot of helpers today." At her instruction two of my larger classmates grabbed and tackled the surprised birds. Small brown feathers flew everywhere as the emus squawked their offense at the handling. But they were easily overpowered and we did thorough examinations, checking for external parasites, evaluating body condition and other health indicators. When we were finished, we released the birds, watching them jump to their feet and stalk off indignantly. Dr. Foster called fondly after them, "Oh, don't get your feathers ruffled!"

Soon after we passed by a large pond where several hippos lolled partly submerged in the murky water. They paid us no heed, but one of the larger animals began to defecate as we watched. Normally this would be of no great interest to veterinary students, who had seen all variety of stools large and small. But in this case we did a collective double-take, pointing and staring at the unexpected show.

It turns out hippos have their own unique style when it comes to bathroom duties. As the animal in question began to pass wastes, its tail spun furiously like an airplane propeller. When the semi-soft feces struck the tail they sprayed everywhere like a detonating fecal bomb, scattering the noxious blobs for many meters to the left and right. My classmates and I burst out laughing at the bizarre sight. I now knew what it would look like to actually see the proverbial "shit hit the fan."

There was a logical reason for this unusual behavior, as Dr. Foster explained, "Hippos spend much of their time in the water, in part to reduce the weight that their legs have to carry. They also produce a lot of fecal material which can soil their habitat. Spreading the feces far and wide dilutes the effect on the water quality, especially the standing water directly around the animal." It made sense, I guess, but I was glad that I didn't have to defecate in my own drinking water, whether it was diluted or not.

One of the last items on our tour that day was visiting the rehab facility at the park. This was a concrete building off limits to the public where injured or ill animals received veterinary care. Here they could recuperate protected from the elements and from other animals, until they were fit to rejoin the general population.

A veterinarian named Stan Winslow joined us on this portion of the tour. He guided us through the modern treatment and surgery rooms, and eventually ushered us past a reinforced steel door to see the inpatient housing. The ward consisted of two rows of heavily constructed concrete cells, looming close on each side of a long narrow hallway. Most of the rooms were empty, but the second one on the left was occupied. I stepped up and peered through the small barred window that offered the only visual access into the cell. On the opposite side of the enclosure, maybe three or four strides from me, reclined a large male African lion. His maned head was raised and his intense gaze was fixed directly on me. Looking into those amber eyes I was transfixed; I could only imagine how it would be to stare down that predator with no wall between us. The other students slowly crowded in behind me, filling the constricted hallway as I stood there.

The last to come through the door was Dr. Winslow. As the vet worked his way through the press of students, he came up alongside me. For an instant his face was visible to the lion through the window, and in that instant everything changed. With a mighty roar the animal leaped, covering the distance to us in a split second. His snarling visage hit the barred window, slavering and baring his huge fangs. In the confines of the small hallway the sound was deafening and all of us reflexively jumped back, plastering ourselves on the opposite wall. Unfortunately, the walkway was very narrow and we were still way too close for comfort.

In a few seconds the lion fell silent but he remained tight against the small window, staring at Dr. Winslow with a ferocity that was frightening. My ears were still ringing from the animal's roar when the doctor chuckled wryly into the hushed silence and said, "Leon doesn't like me very much. He had an abscessed wound that we had to treat repeatedly under sedation, and since then he has held a grudge. You'll have to pardon his manners."

I was willing to pardon Leon for anything as long as he didn't become angry with me. Seeing the huge carnivore in action gave me a new appreciation for the raw speed and power he possessed. I also gained even more respect for the vets who made a living tending to animals like this. It took a rare combination of courage and caring that few people possessed. Wild species benefited from the treatments they received, but they would not reward their caretakers with a tail wag or a friendly swipe of a tongue. The work itself had to be the reward, and the dedication to helping these difficult patients had to come from within. I could sense Dr. Winslow's passion for his job; he loved nothing more than making his charges well again. Based on Leon's impressive display, I estimated that the good doctor was close to completing yet another cure.

CHAPTER SEVENTY-FIVE

One student activity that occurred outside of the block courses was the writing and presentation of our senior papers. We could cover any medical or surgical topic within veterinary medicine, although we had to get approval before proceeding. I chose Dr. Katrina Madsen as my advisor because she had an interest in exotic species; the topic I wanted to write about was "the pet ferret."

Once Dr. Madsen had approved my proposal, I researched all the relevant journal articles I could find in the veterinary library. In addition, I bought a couple of books on ferret care for the pet owner. My own experience with my pets provided some personalized input as well. When I was done writing, I had a fourteen-page paper that covered virtually everything known about ferret medicine and diseases. That goes to show how much knowledge we have gained about exotic pets over the past twenty-plus years. Nowadays fourteen pages might cover a single disease topic in ferret medicine.

I presented my paper in the same lecture hall I had sat in for so many of my veterinary classes. To my delight a fair percentage of my classmates attended, as well as a few junior students and staff members. I reviewed the basics of ferret care, including diet and vaccinations, and covered the few diseases that were known in this species at the time. Back then most people had never seen a ferret, so the highlight of the talk was when I showed off my pet to demonstrate proper handling and restraint. When I finished my presentation, the audience erupted in a loud round of applause, and a mix of gratitude and relief washed over me as I walked smiling from the podium.

Having my senior paper behind me freed up my evenings, and I looked forward to playing a bit more. It was mid-April and I drove to Beaverton, bringing Dixie home with me to share the weekend with Cindy. When I arrived, she showed me two envelopes that had come in the mail that week. She hadn't opened them as they were addressed to me and in her words "looked official." When I saw the logos on the fronts, my heart began pounding. With trembling hands I eagerly ripped them both open and sure enough they were my test scores from the board exams.

First I looked at the National Board score; to my great relief it was eighty-six percent, more than a passing grade. Cindy was leaning over my shoulder as I sat at the dining room table and she squealed with delight. "You passed, hon!" she exclaimed. "Let's see the other one!"

I unfolded the sheet from the Oregon Board of Veterinary Examiners, and it told me that I had scored ninety-two percent on the State Board Exam. As the meaning of it sunk in, I heard Cindy next to me saying, "That's my guy! You did it! You did it!" I stared at the papers for a moment longer, then I slowly lowered them and looked up at my wife with a big grin. She was smiling back at me as she reached out her arms for a hug. I granted her request, and as I held her close I said in her ear, "The hardest part is over now. There's no longer any question about it, I'm going to be a doctor come June."

She shook her head as it rested on my shoulder and replied, "There was never any doubt, you silly man. Not for me. I always knew."

And for the rest of the weekend we celebrated as only two people in love can do, because our future was full of promise, and our present was wonderful beyond compare.

Senior papers did not preclude the vet students' regular work, and the month of April was also the time of my anesthesiology block. This reminded me of my surgery rotation in many ways, in that I spent much of my time in the operatory watching and assisting the doctors. But this month I was concentrating on the drug protocols used for anesthesia and pain control, and I spent hours monitoring the patients' vital signs instead of suturing incisions. By now everything was starting to feel pretty routine, since I had been exposed to most of it before. But medicine can always throw a new surprise your way, as I was about to discover.

One of my duties during this block was helping to move the unconscious animals to the recovery room after surgery. On my very first tour of the vet school, I had seen the padded cell just off the operatory and had wondered about its purpose. Now I knew, and on numerous occasions we had left an unconscious horse lying in the middle of the room with Dr. Reynolds sitting on its neck. A horse can't come to its feet unless its head rises first; keeping the neck pinned prevents a disoriented animal from trying to stand too soon.

Once the anesthesiologist was situated, the rest of us would leave. There was nothing anyone could do to help, and horses recovered best if the room was quiet. Besides, more bodies meant more chances for someone to get hit with a flailing leg. The students would file out one by one, with the last to leave closing the door tightly. The doctor would be left alone in near total darkness with his half-conscious and often delirious patient.

I didn't envy Dr. Reynolds that portion of his job. Although being a student wasn't always easy, at least I could take solace in knowing that I was exempt from some of the more nerve-wracking tasks in the hospital. So I thought until that day we handled a large bay Quarter Horse having eye surgery.

The animal was brought in with an ugly, apricot-sized mass growing from its right upper eyelid. The surgical procedure went smoothly enough, and the doctors were able to excise the tumor with minimal deformity to the eye. When they were finished, we used a heavy-duty steel gurney to wheel our patient into the recovery room. After the mobile platform was lowered, we pushed the bulky body off it onto the middle of the cushioned floor pads. Two of my classmates rolled the empty gurney out through the door. Dr. Reynolds and I stayed behind, positioning the horse with legs out straight and its neck at a good angle for breathing.

The doctor said, "It looks like we're all set. The tracheal tube will need to be pulled when he starts chewing on it. Otherwise you just need to sit on his neck and keep him calm."

I nodded and then did a double take. "Did you say…I'm doing it?" I croaked in surprise.

Dr. Reynolds nodded. "I've got some things I need to attend to. You're experienced enough now to do a routine horse recovery; just pull his tube when he's awake and don't let him stand. I'll come around in awhile and see how you're doing."

I felt my level of anxiety rising as he stood and walked to the exit, and when he closed the door the light disappeared with him. I could barely make out the dim bulk of the animal beneath me as I sat perched on its muscular neck. With the heavy padding on the walls, I heard nothing of the outside world as the minutes ticked slowly by. In the stillness the harsh puffs of the horse's exhaled breath sounded like a steam locomotive in slow motion. I felt tremors rippling through the muscles beneath me as the recovering body shivered to warm itself.

After an indeterminate period of time my patient began to move, pawing weakly at the floor and trying to raise its head. Several times the horse's strong neck tensed and lifted me several inches before collapsing back to the floor. I did my best to think heavy as I used all my weight to pin the animal down.

Eventually the horse began mouthing the endotracheal tube as it became more aware of the foreign object inserted in its throat. I reached over and grabbed the stiff plastic cylinder, pulling it carefully out between the large incisors. The tube was dripping with viscous saliva and I tossed it quickly aside. When it was removed, the horse coughed spasmodically five or six times as its trachea protested the irritation. The animal's movements were becoming more vigorous now, more coordinated, and it began trying to sit up in earnest. I wondered how long I could hold it down, and what would happen if it succeeded in getting to its feet.

Time slows to a crawl when you are alone and confronting the unknown. Sitting in that darkened room with a disoriented half-ton animal under my thighs, the minutes stretched interminably. At times there was no movement from my patient and I would begin to relax, then the animal would buck its head upward, legs flailing, and my heart would once again be in my throat as I struggled to maintain my position. It seemed like I was in there for hours, but when the door cracked open and poured blinding light into the room, only forty-five minutes had ticked off my watch.

Dr. Reynolds walked quietly over as I squinted up at him. Squatting next to me, he said in a low voice, "How's he doing?"

I was slightly offended that he hadn't asked how I was doing, but I answered, "He's been mostly quiet so far, but he tries to raise his head every now and then."

"Okay, let's allow him to sit up now," the doctor said, and I stood and backed away so the horse could roll to an upright position. In a few moments he did so, looking around calmly at his surroundings. His movements were steady, with no head bobbing or swaying that I could discern.

Dr. Reynolds nodded with a satisfied look and said, "He's coming along well; I'll stay with him until he decides to stand. He may still be a bit dizzy, so I'm not going to rush him. You can grab some lunch if you want; we have another surgery coming up at two P.M. Thanks for your help; you did great."

I thanked the doctor and headed for the student lounge feeling a strong sense of relief and accomplishment. Another challenge had been met, another hurdle leaped, and I was inching ever closer to graduation.

CHAPTER SEVENTY-SIX

With board exams and senior papers in our rear-view mirrors, my classmates and I all felt the need to unwind and have some fun. Amy Baker was hosting a senior party at her place on the last weekend of April and nearly everyone was coming. Cindy had a conference to attend in California that Saturday, so she wouldn't be home; it was a perfect time to stay in Corvine and attend the festivities.

Trina Caldwell said that she would pick me up on her way to Amy's Saturday night. She was carpooling with Kristina Albright, and since I lived in the same cul-de-sac as Kristi, it was easy to take both of us. Around six P.M. the doorbell of the townhouse rang and I hurried down the stairs to answer it. The two women stood on the porch grinning at me when I opened the door. I almost didn't recognize them with coveralls off and makeup on.

"Hi Mark," Trina said, looking past me into the living room. "I've never seen where you live; it looks nice! Can you give us a quick tour?"

"Sure," I said, stepping aside to let them enter. "My roommate isn't here right now, so I've got the place all to myself." I took them on a brief excursion through the townhouse, glad that Paul and I had cleaned house recently.

Trina nodded with approval, saying, "It's a pretty nice setup you have here. The layout is almost identical to your place, isn't it Kristi?"

"Yes, I think these buildings are all stamped from the same mold, more or less," Kristina answered. "But they're pretty nice so I can't complain at all. I've enjoyed living here this year."

I seconded her opinion, and we made small talk for a few more minutes before heading out to Trina's car. She owned an old green station wagon, and when we got to the vehicle, I could see the large head of an Airedale Terrier peeking out at us through the window. "Is that your dog, Trina?" I asked while she unlocked the door.

"Yeah, that's Bessie. Don't mind her, she likes everyone," she said, and when she opened the driver's door, the dog shot out and began bouncing excitedly among us, licking everything within reach. "Down! Down!" Trina scolded, and finally Bessie paid heed and sat with a guilty look, though her short tail continued to beat furiously side to side.

"In you go then," Trina commanded us with a wave of her hand. "Sit in the back; Kristi's potato salad is on the front seat." We obediently piled in the back seat while Trina opened the rear of the vehicle, putting the dog in the cargo area behind us. After Bessie was situated, Trina came around front and got in on the driver's side.

I had turned to say something to Kristina when our chauffeur let out an ear-splitting screech. "Holy crap!" Trina yelled, and she twisted to look back over her shoulder. "You are in trouble, Bessie! Bad dog! Very bad!"

"What's wrong?" Kristina and I said simultaneously.

"I'll tell you what's wrong. That little pig got into the potato salad! The lid's off and there is a big gouge in one side where she licked it. I'm sorry, Kristi. Everyone was looking forward to your famous recipe, too," she finished disgustedly.

"Let me see," Kristina said, and Trina passed the bowl back to us. Sure enough there was a deep depression in one portion of the salad where a large tongue had eagerly lapped up the tasty treat. Kristina frowned in thought for a moment, then she took the serving spoon and stirred the bowl's contents vigorously. When she was finished, the surface was smooth and unmarred. "There we go, no harm done!" she pronounced proudly. We just stared at her, and she looked back at us innocently, saying, "What?" After a moment we all started to giggle, and we were still laughing when we arrived at the party carrying our little secret.

Amy Baker was renting a small house with two other students in a quiet residential area in west Corvine. We parked on the street just down from her place, and strolled up the sidewalk until we found the narrow two-story home with the correct address over the door. Amy answered the doorbell and happily invited us in; half our classmates were there already, and the living room was full of life and merriment. People milled around with drinks and hors d'oeuvres in hand or sat chatting in small groups. Several hailed us as we walked in, and I broke off from my companions to talk with Ed Martinelli and Molly Boyer who were standing nearby.

As we shared stories of our block rotations and board exams, I glanced around the room at the assembled students. More arrived by the minute until nearly everyone from our class was in attendance. Some juniors had crashed the party as well, and hung out in a small group in one corner of the room. Music was blaring from the stereo, and tasty smells wafted from the kitchen where pot luck contributions from guests were accumulating. I felt my stomach rumbling as the aromas hit my senses and I followed my nose to their source. Soon I was back in the living room carrying a plate loaded with wheat crackers, spinach dip, lasagna, fruit salad, and home-baked brownies.

As I ate, I watched my classmates and smiled at the familiar mix of personalities brought together once again. Most everyone was dressed casually in jeans or corduroys topped by cotton shirts and sweaters. But there was Vincent Studebaker, wearing slacks and a button down dress shirt as he expounded on the nuances of acid-base balance in equine intestinal upsets. To his left I saw Stan Hulbert laughing and talking with a small crowd of shorter students, mostly female, who were clustered around him. Kristina had joined Molly and Ed, who were listening with wide grins as she told a funny story about losing her thermometer up a cow's rear end.

Toward the other end of the room Trina sat drinking beer with some of the farm boy contingent, including "Cowboy" Bob Welsh and "Country" Carl Hewitt. The always amusing Joe Wrobel was there as well, and sure enough he was making people cringe with tales of his rodeo days again.

The scene took me back to that party long ago when a younger version of this group had gathered at Molly's house and we had begun to know each other outside of school. The passage of time and events since then had certainly wrought their changes. Some of us sported different hair styles (and in some cases less hair altogether) and waistlines had gradually expanded. The faces around me looked more mature than that hopeful group of freshmen I remembered, with laugh lines and crow's feet having crept furtively onto formerly smooth visages. Most of us were now in our mid to late twenties and some were well over thirty; I hoped that this would help us gain respect as new doctors out in the world.

Despite our added years, there was still plenty of silliness to go around, and I was reminded of this when Ed Martinelli returned from the kitchen carrying a plate of Kristina's potato salad. "This stuff is awesome!" he gushed as he gulped a big forkful. "It's even better than usual. Did you change the recipe? I can't quite place the flavoring, but it's really good!"

Just then I choked on the wheat cracker I was eating and Amy thumped me on the back. Vincent Studebaker chimed in with, "Yes Kristi, it's a very good dish. I don't like a lot of potato salads, but yours is wonderfully smooth and creamy, different from other recipes I've tried. You've got to tell me your secret."

I managed to keep from laughing out loud as I watched Kristina and Trina fighting to maintain straight faces. Fortunately no one seemed to notice that the three people who had brought the dish had abstained from sampling it. To Kristina's credit, she had great self-control and gave nothing away as she calmly said, "Thank you guys, it's nothing really, just the same recipe I've always made. You all must be really hungry tonight." Her appearance of modesty brought on even more compliments from our classmates, and I had to turn away to hide my face.

We all had a great time for the remainder of the evening. It was refreshing seeing everyone under one roof again, and it would be the last time we would do so in a social setting. Graduation would provide one more opportunity for our class to gather, but it would be under entirely different circumstances. This night was one to relax and enjoy, with no agenda other than friendship. The party brought closure to a long and eventful four years together, and it added to my storehouse of fond memories. As a side note, even decades later Kristina's special recipe remains the subject of much amusement whenever I encounter a classmate.

CHAPTER SEVENTY-SEVEN

The month of May proved to be a really enjoyable time for me. The weather waxed warm and sunny, and I headed up to the Portland area for my externship block. An externship or preceptorship is where a student gets to observe at a medical facility outside of school. It was a fun and exciting opportunity to put our hard-earned knowledge to use in authentic practice situations. In other words, we got to treat real patients with real owners. Exhilarating to be sure—and a bit scary.

As Cindy and I were planning to remain in Beaverton after I graduated, it made sense for me to take my externship there. I'd have a place to live while working, and I also might be able to make contacts that would lead to job opportunities. The metropolitan area had little farm animal work. Any practices I would visit in the city would be treating small pet species. I had to decide ahead of time where to spend my block, and I chose a facility with a good reputation. It was a large, busy practice, and rated highly in evaluations given by previous years' students. Even better, it was conveniently located within a few miles of our apartment.

On the first day of my externship, I dressed in nice work slacks and a short sleeved dress shirt. Then I went to the hall closet and grabbed the light blue medical smock that I had purchased the week before. After I shrugged it on and zipped the front, Cindy gave me an approving look and said, "You look very doctorly! I love a man in uniform!"

I laughed and posed for her, and when I was done, she gave me a long hug and told me, "Good luck, hon. Go save some lives!" I told her I'd try my best and set out for the clinic.

Hampton Heights Veterinary Hospital was one of the largest and most respected practices in Oregon in the 1980s. In addition to three general practitioners, the clinic boasted a board-certified surgeon and a neurologist. The presence of the specialists enhanced the expertise the hospital could offer its patients. Being big and prosperous also paid dividends, since the doctors were able to afford the best equipment. It was a great place to observe and learn good medical habits.

What helped me choose Hampton Heights was that it was the only practice in the area with an emphasis on exotic pets. Dogs and cats still made up the bulk of the case load, but ferrets, rabbits, rodents, and reptiles made regular appearances during the time I observed there.

On my first day in the clinic, I met all three of the general practitioners. The oldest was the hospital owner Dr. Dan Benner, a stout, heavy-jowled man with graying hair and a deep voice. He had been working in the Portland area for several decades, and had built the practice from scratch with a combination of good bedside manner and strong business acumen.

The other two vets were considerably younger, probably in their late thirties. They were also more fun to be around, since they were constantly jesting while they worked. Tyler Johnson was a rural boy turned city doctor, and still had a strong touch of country in his speech and mannerisms. He was tall and lean, with a stout mustache and medium-length, brown hair combed carelessly straight back from his forehead. The randomly swept locks made him look like he had just driven a high-speed motorbike without a helmet. .

Darin Longley was Tyler's antithesis both socially and physically. Short and stocky with a soft pale complexion, he looked like he spent as much time indoors as possible. His nails were manicured and his oiled dark hair neatly styled. He originally hailed from Los Angeles, and was a hardcore urbanite through and through. One of his favorite pastimes was poking good-natured fun at Tyler Johnson's small town origins and (lack of) style sense.

Despite their contrasting backgrounds and habits, each doctor had a healthy sense of humor and a commitment to practicing a high standard of medicine. Like Drs. Thurman and Strom back in Medford, these positives seemed to outweigh their differences, and they shared an excellent camaraderie. Watching them I learned a lot about medicine and even more about how to mesh as a team.

Of course, there was the business of veterinary practice to attend to, and I saw a lot of cases while I was there. In general I spent little time with clients, mostly observing and assisting the doctors as they tended to patients. They were good about letting me participate in the treatments. I received plenty of practice drawing blood samples, squeezing bladders for urine specimens, flushing infected dog ears, and expressing anal sacs. While doing so I got quizzed about everything imaginable, from the possible causes of pale gums in a cat to the most common skin masses seen in dogs.

One day a young man brought in his Siamese cat as an emergency appointment, with the complaint of profuse diarrhea "that is getting splattered everywhere." At first I couldn't fathom why an intestinal upset would warrant an emergency exam. Then I opened the jar containing the fecal sample, and one whiff of the contents told me why the owner had decided not to wait.

Back in the laboratory I smeared a bit of the foul liquid on a glass slide. Then I peered through the microscope to examine the sample. What met my eyes caused me to sit back in surprise. The entire visual field was packed with swimming protozoa, resembling oval balloons with flailing strings attached. The threadlike appendages were flagella which propelled the tiny parasites through their liquid environment. The slide was filled with nonstop motion as the tiny creatures jiggled and jostled for position.

I grinned with delight as I watched the unusual display. The organism was known as Giardia, a common inhabitant of ponds and streams where wildlife deposit it via defecating in the water. Animals or humans drinking from such sources could easily become infected unless the water was boiled first. The surprising thing was seeing the active "trophozoite" form of the parasite. Most animals with Giardia only shed cysts in their stool, which were like a dormant egg stage of the infection. The cysts were usually few and hard to identify, since they were tiny and resembled other debris found in feces.

Knowing that, I was not surprised when my confident assertion of "she has Giardia" was met with skepticism from Dr. Longley. "Let me see that slide," he huffed as he walked over to the microscope and switched on its lamp. I watched him peer through the oculars at the sample. It only took one second before his eyebrows shot up in surprise and he turned off the scope. Glancing over at me, he said, "I guess she does have Giardia!"—and without another word he walked out of the room to talk to the cat's owner. In truth it was a fortuitous finding on my part, but Dr. Longley never openly questioned any of my diagnoses after that.

As the staff gradually came to trust in my abilities, I was allowed to perform some minor surgeries. One morning I treated a tomcat with a large abscess on his face, courtesy of a rival male who had raked his head with needle claws. As he lay on the table anesthetized, I lanced his swollen cheek to drain the infection. Yellow green fluid gushed out and I mopped it up with gauze sponges, thankful that cats couldn't match cows when it came to volume of exudate.

After flushing the hollow pocket where the pus had resided, I packed some thick antibiotic ointment into the space, leaving the incision open to allow drainage. An injection of penicillin into his thigh muscles completed the treatment, and I placed the wounded feline in a kennel to recover. The owners would have the joy of giving their kitty oral amoxicillin until he healed. I hoped that they didn't end up wearing the medication.

Hampton Heights was also where I gained my first experience handling many exotic pet species. In the course of those few quick weeks, I learned how to safely pry a stubborn box turtle out of its shell for an examination, and how to restrain a flighty rabbit so that its powerful rear legs didn't cause injury to itself or its handler. I wrestled a Burmese python that stretched twice my length, and gingerly juggled a pygmy hedgehog that rolled itself into a prickly ball of spines. Most importantly, I had fun with the animals and the staff as I learned valuable lessons every day. After four years in school, I couldn't believe how much there still was to know.

Dr. Benner told me as much while we chatted in his office one afternoon. Although a bit aloof at first, he had warmed to me as we had gotten to know each other. When I wasn't busy I would sometimes seek him out, mainly to ask his advice about finding work. With his history he knew most of the local clinics and who had good reputations as employers and as doctors.

The subject of learning after graduation came up one day, and he leaned back in his leather chair, spreading his hands as he said, "You get the theory in school, Mark, but the practical knowledge takes time and experience. One has to see cases, a lot of cases, to really get a handle on clinical medicine. The first year out of school is a steep learning curve. After that you'll begin to get comfortable with being a doctor. In a couple of years you'll be up to full speed and productivity. It takes a good while, there's no way around that."

"So I'll still have a lot of learning to do even once school is through. Not an encouraging thought," I replied.

"You'll never stop learning, at least if you want to be a good practitioner," Dr. Benner said, pointing a thick finger at me. "There is always something more to know, and new information bombards us constantly. Of course, it gets easier to keep up once you have grasped the basics, but you can never become stagnant and cease to grow. If you do, then it's time to retire."

I took his words to heart, and to this day I have found them to be true. To do our best as medical practitioners, we have to keep improving. In the time since I graduated, there have been amazing advances in companion animal medicine and surgery. This is particularly true with the exotic pet species, where diseases unheard of twenty years ago are now commonplace diagnoses. For that matter, some of the animals I treat today were themselves virtually unknown to veterinarians when I began my career.

But I have also found that the lure of the unknown and the thrill of discovery are driving forces that keep me interested and excited about my work. Every day offers the possibility of encountering something new. I wouldn't have it any other way.

CHAPTER SEVENTY-EIGHT

During my externship I received a phone call from my room-mate Paul in Corvine. He was planning to visit the Portland area to do some shopping, and he wanted to know if he could stay the weekend with me and Cindy. After asking Cindy, I told him that he was welcome if he didn't mind sleeping on the floor or the sofa. He agreed, and told me to expect him on Friday evening.

Cindy and I were already home from work when Paul arrived. I helped my wife fix dinner in our cramped little kitchen, and the three of us ate together at the apartment. The conversation at the table was lively, as our guest was his usual talkative self. We had a good time trading stories about school and the work place while the food and drink disappeared. I had anticipated that entertaining a houseguest would be a nuisance, but I found it surprisingly fun having company for a change. Cindy seemed to enjoy herself as well.

On Saturday Paul drove into Portland to shop for clothes. I accompanied him, since I needed some new dress shirts and slacks for job interviews. We tried a couple of men's stores in the downtown area, and I quickly found what I needed, buying two pairs of pants and three shirts. When I was done, Paul was still looking for a suit that met his tastes. A clerk suggested a well-known clothier located on the fourteenth floor of a high-rise building. Since it was only a short distance away, we set out on foot to find the store.

When we arrived at our destination, we passed through the main entry into the concrete and glass tower. The elevator was located against the back wall of the lobby, and we waited there for a ride. It was three P.M. and the building bustled with people; when the door opened, we allowed the packed car to empty and then squeezed in along with a handful of others. The last to board was a delivery man with a hand cart full of office supplies. We all shifted back to make room for him and the door was just able to close.

I had punched the button for the fourteenth floor as we had entered, and now the delivery man selected the eighth floor. Apparently, the clothing store was a popular choice, because none of the remaining six people chose a different destination. The elevator lurched and we began our slow ascent. The car stopped once at the third floor, and one more person managed to wedge herself into the pack. When the doors had closed and the car resumed moving, Paul glanced over at me. We stood together near the back wall and after a moment he leaned in to speak quietly into my ear. I felt my heart sink as he whispered three little words: *"Can't move on."*

I barely had time to register their meaning before his noiseless expulsion hit my nose. Even for Paul this one was horrifically offensive, and inside the confined space its effects were magnified beyond reason. In mere seconds the bland recirculated air was transformed into something reminiscent of a backed-up sewer; my eyes watered and I tried my best to breathe without inhaling. At that instant I longed to be back at school dissecting bloated cow cadavers—they would have smelled considerably better.

The effect this unseen assault had on the elevator's inhabitants would have been hilarious if I hadn't been one of them. Not a word was spoken, but expressions tensed and bodies began shifting uncomfortably as the group of total strangers shared the silent torture. Throats were cleared repeatedly, desperate eyes glancing up at the agonizingly slow progression of the floor numbers flashing by on the display.

After a lifetime or two the elevator ground to a halt on the eighth floor. This was the delivery man's stop, and the door opened onto what appeared to be a mostly deserted warehouse level. The man practically flung his handcart into the corridor and scrambled headlong after it. Before the door could slide shut again the entire complement of passengers followed him out, leaving only Paul and me standing guiltily in the back of the elevator.

After exiting the impromptu gas chamber, the group turned as one and stared back at us accusingly. I pasted a weak grin on my face and pointed a clandestine finger in Paul's direction. Then the door slid shut, and the scowling faces were thankfully cut off from sight.

We managed to make it through the rest of the day without any further toxic incidents. The next day Paul headed home to Corvine. Cindy and I had Sunday night alone together before work resumed the next day. It was a chance to focus on each other and take time to smell the roses—or at least some decent untainted air.

On Monday morning I drove to the clinic eager for a few more days of observation. That week was my last at Hampton Hills, and also the last of my veterinary curriculum. I wanted to pick up as many pointers as possible before I would be thrown out into the profession as a graduate vet.

As I had gotten to know the doctors and staff, I had come to appreciate the relaxed atmosphere and friendly banter that characterized their interaction. There were times when the workload was hectic and critical cases demanded serious attention. In those situations the staff was all business, with everyone focused on the tasks at hand. But when things eased up a bit, humor made a quick resurgence and the mood became light and playful once again. Between the high-quality medicine, the focus on exotic pets, and the friendly staff, I had to admit I really liked it there.

One of the last cases I treated during my stay was a perky little Cairn terrier who had been in a dog fight; she was crisscrossed with lacerations and smeared head to tail with blood. Despite her horrific appearance, she appeared unfazed and her tail wagged nonstop. She was pronounced stable enough for surgery, so we anesthetized her and the technicians shaved her numerous wounds. By the time they were through clipping and scrubbing, there was scant hair remaining on the poor little dog. I stepped up close to assess the damage. There appeared to be about six major lacerations with skin flaps hanging loose, and a dozen or so smaller cuts and punctures. Blood still oozed sluggishly from several of the deeper wounds.

Taking a deep breath, I grabbed a pair of thumb forceps and a needle and got to work. As I sat at the treatment table painstakingly suturing the wounds, I was suddenly struck with a flash of *déjà-vu*. An eternity ago in Southern California, I had watched wide-eyed while a young vet named Dr. Harding had patched together a small poodle. My experiences that night had set me on the path to becoming a veterinarian. Now here I was near the end of my education, performing exactly the same procedure on another small dog in need. My life had come full circle, and I was about to complete one journey, only to begin another. I couldn't wait to see where it would lead.

On my final day Dr. Johnson asked me if I had time to chat for a moment. I said sure and followed him upstairs. Here he and Darin Longley had side-by-side desks against one wall of a small office. I followed Tyler Johnson into the room, and he gestured for me to take a seat in his associate's vacant chair. As I sat down, my attention was drawn by a sign on the wall over the doctor's desk. It was boldly printed in black letters against a yellow background, and it listed prices for services rendered. The wording was as follows:

Dog Spays—$25.00
While You Wait—$35.00
If You Watch—$55.00
If You Help—$75.00

I chuckled out loud, and Dr. Johnson grinned, saying, "I always liked that one too. It pays to have a sense of humor no matter what your profession." He regarded me thoughtfully for a moment as he twirled his mustache. When he spoke again, the subject abruptly changed. "How are things going with you? Do you have any job prospects yet? It's not long until you'll be done with school."

"No, I haven't had any time to pursue employment," I answered with a sigh. "I'll have to start visiting practices in the area soon. Dr. Benner gave me a few ideas of places to try, so I've got somewhere to begin at least. I hope it won't take too long to find a job."

Dr. Johnson nodded and said, "I wanted to talk to you about that. Darin and I have enjoyed having you here these past two weeks. We've been thinking about adding another vet sometime soon, since the business is growing. Dan Benner is the owner, so he'll have to make the final decision on any hiring. We've not brought it up to him yet, but I wanted to run it by you and see if you would be interested in working for us after you graduate."

I could have hugged the man right then, but that would almost certainly have reduced my chances of landing the job. Instead I smiled and nodded my head enthusiastically, saying, "Yes, I'd definitely be interested! This practice would be a good fit for me, I think. I love the quality of medicine here, and I have an interest in exotic species too. When do you think you'll make a decision?"

"Well, as I said, we have to present the idea to Dr. Benner. He knows that we'll need someone soon. I think he was planning on waiting a little longer, but the time to hire is when new grads come available, not at year's end. I think we'll be able to persuade him."

My heart was doing flips as I tried to contain my excitement. I was barely able to say, "Do you want to call me when you know something? I'll be done with school shortly. Graduation is at the end of the month."

Dr. Johnson smiled and replied, "Yes, that's probably the best way to handle it. Give me your phone number, and I'll contact you after Darin and I talk to the boss. If you don't hear anything by the time you graduate, then give us a call or stop by."

I promised that I would, then I shook his hand and thanked him for his vote of confidence and his tutelage over the previous weeks. After we finished, I walked back down to the treatment room in a happy daze. The rest of the afternoon flashed by like a dream, and I can't even remember any of the cases I saw. At day's end I bid the doctors and staff goodbye. It had been a fun and educational externship, and more than ever I looked forward to practicing veterinary medicine. Several of the staff members wished me luck, and one of the techs said, "I hope you can come back and work for us someday!" That made two of us.

When I walked out the front door, I turned and looked back at the two-story building. Just to the right of the entrance the veterinarians' names were displayed in carved wooden symbols. Each letter was painted a bright gold and stood out in bold relief from the brown cedar wall.

For a moment I smiled as I envisioned my name added to that list. Then I shrugged and reminded myself that nothing was certain. It didn't pay to get one's hopes up too high. Even so, I couldn't suppress the energy inside me, and Cindy got quite an earful when I reached the apartment. It had definitely been a good day.

CHAPTER SEVENTY-NINE

My veterinary school graduation was a quiet ceremony held separately from the rest of the university's student body. On May 31, 1986, we gathered in a small auditorium on campus. The thirty-six students in my class stood at one side of the raised front stage as family and friends sat in folding chairs on the floor level. After waiting for so long, it was hard to believe that we were actually there, ready to receive our degrees and become doctors. This day was the end result of eight years of hard work dating back to our undergraduate days in college. It was also the very last time the senior class would stand together as one.

Cindy, of course, was there to cheer me on. My mom, dad, and younger brother Ted had driven up from Medford to attend as well. Dad had donned his best suit and tie for the occasion, and mom was resplendent in a sky blue dress with pearl jewelry. Ted wore clothes, for which everyone was thankful.

Many faculty were also in attendance that day. Like the graduating students, the professors wore black dress robes with a broad white stripe down the front, and smaller stripes around the upper sleeves. In addition, each faculty member displayed a hood bearing the veterinary colors of orange and grey, which signified the completion of a doctorate. Seeing our teachers in their graduation gowns reminded us that they had once stood in our shoes, and that we were now joining them as peers in the veterinary profession.

When I had first rented my robe and hood, I had donned them in the apartment, turning this way and that in front of the mirror to see how they looked. The velvety cloth with its deep rich colors was far more beautiful than the thin material of my undergraduate gown.

The hood was tied at the neck and worn hanging down the back of the robe, not covering one's head. Its splash of orange added a nice touch of color to the ensemble. Topping it all off was the usual square graduation cap decorated with a grey tassel. At the ceremony, the students gathered on stage wearing gowns and caps but not the hoods; those would be placed on each of us when we received our diplomas.

Dr. Hudson, the dean of the vet school, took the podium and made a short speech. His silvery hair and blue eyes offset the color scheme of his robes as if it were planned that way. "Good afternoon to you all, and welcome," he began, looking out at the assembled crowd and then over to his left at my classmates and I. "This day has been a long time coming, as I'm sure these students can attest to." Laughter drifted up from the crowd as he smiled at us. "But suddenly the time is upon us, the time to recognize and congratulate this fine group of young men and women on the completion of their journey. I remember four years ago when a class of eager freshmen sat in McNairy's lecture hall looking star-struck at just being there. Now they are ready to step beyond those doors and go out into the world as doctors of medicine. Let us applaud their accomplishments on this day. They have certainly earned it."

With that he began clapping, and the rest of the faculty and audience joined in. My classmates and I stood grinning as we accepted the ovation. When at last it died down, Dr. Hudson again spoke to the audience. He told of the challenges of the previous four years, the ups and downs of mastering a difficult curriculum, the strain of living away from family and loved ones, of having to move out of state for a year and a half. As he spoke, my eyes wandered over the crowd in the auditorium, searching for the faces of Cindy and my family. At last I found them about ten rows back on the left side of the room. My mom smiled and waved when she caught my gaze on her; I grinned back before returning my attention to Dr. Hudson.

"...so now it is time to finish my speech and let the proceedings begin," he was saying, and he turned and motioned for another faculty member to come up on stage. It was Dr. Brenda Babick, one of the surgeons at the veterinary hospital. She would do the honors of placing the hood on each student, right before he or she walked across stage to receive a diploma from the dean.

Dr. Babick took her position near the students while two photographers moved in front of the stage to cover her and Dr. Hudson. This way each graduate would receive a picture of the hood-donning ceremony, and also of the conferring of the diploma.

When everyone was in place, the dean cleared his throat and said, "Let us begin. I'll read the names of the graduating class of 1986 in alphabetical order, and each student will step up for Dr. Babick to place the doctoral hood on his or her shoulders. Then I will hand that student the diploma."

He paused as he looked over to us, and then said, "Amy Baker."

Looking excited and smiling nervously, Amy stepped forward, her blonde curls sticking out from under her black cap. Dr. Babick came up behind her and fastened the hood around her neck, arranging it so that it fell in neat folds down Amy's back. The strobe light of a camera flash went off as they stood there.

Amy then walked over to Dr. Hudson, who shook her hand and gave her the diploma bound in a protective black cover. More bright flashes as she took the document, and when she held it up in her left hand the audience erupted into applause. She grinned widely and walked off the other side of the stage.

The dean looked at his list and said, "Molly Boyer." She went through the same routine as Amy, walking off to applause at the end with a smile that was full of relief.

Then it was my turn. "Mark Bridges," Dr. Hudson called out.

I forced my legs into motion and walked out into the open stage in front of the audience. Dr. Babick stepped up close behind me, and her hands reached around front to fasten the hood at my neck. While she arranged the cloth, she spoke in low tones only I could hear. "Congratulations, Mark," she said. "You've done well! Enjoy this day, and good luck out there!"

I smiled and murmured a thank you. When she said I was ready, I walked slowly across the stage toward Dr. Hudson, remembering to look out toward my family and smile as I did so. When I reached the dean, I extended my right hand to clasp his as my left took the diploma. I clutched the smooth binder, feeling its solid reality between my fingers. The truth of it then hit me: I was at that moment a Doctor of Veterinary Medicine. I was barely aware of the camera flashes going off as the crowd applauded and a thrill rushed through me. It was done! I waved and smiled once again at my family, and then walked carefully off the stage to the right.

One by one each of my fellow students walked forward to receive their diploma. Not surprisingly, Trina Caldwell managed to stand out, injecting some laughs into the otherwise solemn ceremony by pumping her fist and yelling, *"Yeah, baby!"* when she received her diploma. I shook my head and chuckled as she sashayed off stage; that was vintage Trina, nonconformist to the end.

The rest of the ceremony was a blur; I remember few details as I watched the other students filing across the stage. After the last student's name had been called and the final applause had faded away, it was time to relax and socialize. Graduates and their loved ones mingled with faculty, talking and sharing stories, and every face I encountered wore a smile. I found Cindy and my family, and approached them with my diploma in hand. Mom looked so happy and excited that you would have thought she was the one graduating. She called out, "There's my son the doctor! You're the first doctor in the family!" I laughed and then she wrapped me in a big hug. When she finally released me, I turned to dad and was surprised to get a hug from him as well. When he stepped back, he said, "Your mom and I are very proud of you, son. This is quite an accomplishment."

"Thank you," I told him. "And thanks for all the help you've given me; I couldn't have done it without you." He smiled and nodded, his face beaming with satisfaction at seeing this day become a reality.

Brother Ted was his typical undemonstrative self, giving me a thumbs-up and a quick, "Nice job, Mark." Lastly I turned to Cindy. She looked at me demurely for a moment, and then squealed and threw her arms wide as she engulfed me in a tight embrace. "You did it, hon!" she murmured in my ear as she pressed tight against me. "I'm very proud of you too!" We stepped back and I told her how much I appreciated her support, putting up with all the time we had spent apart while I pursued my education. She held my hand and we chatted with my family for awhile, watching as other students and their loved ones enacted similar scenes around us.

After awhile Mom said, "You should go say hello to some of your friends, dear. This may be the last time you see some of them." Cindy seconded the motion, so I told them I wouldn't be long and headed out into the press of bodies.

In a moment I spotted Stan Hulbert's head above the crowd and worked my way over to him. He saw me approaching and said, "Dr. Bridges! It's good to see you!"

"Likewise, Dr. Hulbert!" I replied—and then we both started laughing. "I told you that you'd make it here if you just kept the faith," I said to him.

"You certainly helped, many times," Stan answered. "Thank you for all the advice and moral support."

"You are very welcome," I said. "It's been really fun having you as a classmate; I'm going to miss you."

"Me, too," he said somberly. Then his expression lightened and he said, "Hey, I'd like you to meet my dad," as he gestured to the gentleman standing at his right. I reached out to shake the senior Hulbert's hand, and then I had to stop and look again, because he was an almost identical copy of his son. Take away the silver creeping into his black curls and smooth out the age lines around his mouth and eyes, and you had Stan all over again.

"You're a veterinarian, too, aren't you?" I asked him.

"Yes, that's right," he replied in a deep, Stan-like voice. "Stan's going to join me in my practice; I'm very proud of him."

"I know he'll make a great veterinarian," I said. "He's very modest, but he's got a good grasp of medicine, and he's also one of the nicest people I've met in vet school. That's a wonderful combination for any doctor to have."

"Okay, that's enough you guys," Stan said to us, shaking his head. "We'll see what you think when I'm struggling through a two-hour dog spay."

We all laughed at that; I suspected many of us would encounter such difficulties in our first months out of school. I wished Stan and his father all the best, and moved on to find Amy Baker. I found her talking with Ed Martinelli, and stepped forward to congratulate them both. While we chatted, I also got to meet Amy's mom. She was a sweet little gray-haired lady whose head barely came up to my shoulder. I had never seen her before, but she smiled kindly at me and said, "It's so good to meet you, Mark. I've heard so much about you from Amy! Thank you for being her friend while she's been away from home."

"It's been a real pleasure knowing Amy, Mrs. Baker. She's got a good heart and a great sense of humor. I should be thanking you for raising such a nice daughter."

She blushed and smiled even broader, then said in an aside to her daughter, "Oh, this one's a charmer. I can see why you like him." That in turn brought out a similar red hue in Amy's face, and I laughed at both of them.

"You two are quite a pair," I said jokingly.

"Yes, we've been told that a few times," Amy replied, and her mom nodded in agreement as they both smiled coyly.

"Good luck in the working world," I said to Amy. "I hope you find a job that you really enjoy. Stay in touch, if you can. I'd love to hear from you now and then."

"I will," she replied as she looked me in the eye. "Be happy, Mark. Don't forget to take good care of that sweetheart of yours. Life's not all about work, you know."

"You're right about that," I said. We looked at each other for a moment, and then she came up and gave me a warm hug. I returned it and when we separated I told her, "Have fun."

"You, too," she said.

With that we said goodbye, and I wandered through the crowd, meeting and greeting the people who had been a big part of the last four years of my life. When it was over, my family followed me back to the townhouse. Paul was there, and he kindly consented to taking photos for us. I still have one framed to this day, with mom, dad, Ted, and I clustered around the easy chair in the living room on that perfect day. But the pictures we carry in our hearts are the ones that matter most, and those are too numerous for any photo album to hold.

EPILOGUE

CHAPTER EIGHTY

There was one more small hurdle to overcome, one tiny detail to be addressed. After all the excitement and celebration was over, I still had to find a practical use for my newly acquired degree. In other words, I needed a job.

Be it wise or not, I had to admit that I had my hopes pinned on landing employment at Hampton Hills Hospital. No other practice around Portland seemed to offer the combination of high-quality medicine and exotic animal patients that I wanted. My externship had given me a chance to become comfortable there. It seemed perfect for me, which also meant I was bound for considerable disappointment if they turned me away.

In early June I stopped by the hospital to talk with the doctors. I hadn't heard anything from them since my last chat with Dr. Johnson. Perhaps they had simply misplaced my number or had been too busy to call, but I worried that other new grads could be vying for a spot on their staff. There was no way to know without asking, so I decided to be proactive and show them I was still interested.

When I arrived, the receptionist greeted me warmly, saying, "Hi Mark, it's nice to see you again! Are you a doctor now?"

I nodded self-consciously and said, "Yes, I'm officially a DVM now."

She smiled and said, "Were you here to talk with Dr. Benner? I heard a rumor that you might be coming to work for us."

"Well, that has yet to be determined," I replied. "I'm hoping so, but nothing's certain at this point."

"Let me page him then," she said, adding, "I'll think good thoughts for you."

"Thank you," I said, and I sat down in the waiting room, fidgeting aimlessly as I waited. I had donned slacks with a dress shirt and tie for this impromptu meeting, since it never hurt to look professional. After a few tense minutes the door to the waiting area opened and Dr. Benner stepped through. I stood up to meet him, hopeful that I looked calm and confident as I stepped forward.

"Hello there, Mark!" the doctor declared as he shook my hand. "I'm glad you came by. Tyler was his usual scatter-brained self and misplaced your phone number. We were hoping you'd call or stop in sometime soon. Come in, come in!"

With that he led the way through the door and upstairs to his office. Once there, I sat in the familiar chair in front of his desk and he took his seat behind it. Dr. Benner leaned back in his chair and folded his hands as he regarded me. He began the conversation on a casual note, asking, "How have things been going? Did you have a fun graduation? I'll bet you're glad to be done with school after all these years."

"Yes, I'm ready to do something other than study for awhile, I think," I replied with a smile. "I can't complain, though. Oregon has a great vet school, and it was a fun time despite all the work."

The doctor nodded thoughtfully. "Yes, I remember my school days, hectic and thrilling all at the same time. It's easier to handle the demands placed on you when you're young. I don't think I'd like to tackle it at my age."

I laughed and said, "I wouldn't want to start it all over again at my age either!"

"Once is definitely enough," Dr. Benner agreed. "Well, Mark, I imagine you're not here to talk about vet school. Tyler and Darin tell me that you're interested in working for us."

"Yes, I'd love to join the staff here. You've got a very nice practice and I think I could contribute to that," I answered.

"The other vets had good things to say about you, and I tend to agree. One thing concerns me, however, and that is the need to focus and be serious in your work. The hours can be long in this business and the situations with clients can be stressful. You have to be able to put on a professional face with the public, and sometimes be sympathetic as well. A sense of humor is fine, but it isn't always the right approach in life-and-death situations."

I nodded with what I hoped was an appropriately serious expression. Tyler Johnson had told me that Dr. Benner favored a solemn approach to medical practice. At times he had openly criticized his younger doctors' light-hearted banter in the treatment room. "Clients can hear you from up front," the older doctor would grumble. "It sounds like we're having too much fun back here." That had become a catch phrase with the junior vets, and whenever they caught themselves laughing at something, they would stop and say, "Oh, no! We're having 'too much fun' again!"

All of this flashed through my mind during Dr. Benner's admonishment, but given the importance of the moment I managed to not crack a smile the entire time. When he had said his piece, I nodded and replied, "That all makes perfect sense to me. I understand the importance of being professional on the job."

He regarded me for a moment and then said, "So if we hire you, when can you start work?"

I gulped as I tried to find my voice, and then stammered, "Um, right away I guess!"

"How about June 16th?" the doctor replied.

"Oh, that's fine!" I said, nodding eagerly.

"The starting salary is $22,000.00 a year plus benefits. Your hours would be 8:30 A.M. to 6:00 P.M. five days a week, plus two Saturdays a month. The weekend days are half-days, 9:00 A.M. to 1:00 P.M. After you become proficient, we can switch you from a flat salary to a percentage of your gross production, which can net you more income. That way, the harder you work, the more you take home. Does that sound okay with you?"

Veterinary salaries have never been as high as most other medical professions, and back in the 1980s the figures he quoted were very typical compensation for a new graduate. I smiled and told him, "That all sounds fair to me."

A grin finally broke through Dr. Benner's gruff countenance and he said, "All right then, consider yourself hired, young man. Your first day will be June 16th. We'll get you a contract to sign before then. Welcome aboard!"

Cindy and I celebrated my hiring that night with an upscale dinner out on the town. After that I scrambled to find a couple more medical smocks at local uniform outlets. Hampton Hills favored short-sleeved, waist-length garments with dress pants and a tie. The colors didn't seem to matter, as I saw everything from burgundy to gray to baby blue worn by the doctors working there. I picked out two smocks, a blue and a burgundy, as I figured that these would allow me to color coordinate with various slacks and ties.

The other item I needed was a name tag to pin on the front pocket; all the doctors wore them to make it easier for clients to learn their names. Again, I found a local business that could supply my needs; within a week I received a red plastic name plate with black lettering that read, "Mark Bridges DVM."

I pinned the tag on the left breast pocket of my smock. Into the pocket I put a pair of bandage scissors, a pen, and a small notebook that Cindy had bought me. There I could jot down tidbits of useful information such as drug doses which I would need to remember in daily practice. My stethoscope I coiled and stashed in the lower left pocket where I could easily grab it when needed. When I was finished, I gazed at the image that confronted me in the mirror. With the slacks and dress shirt, professional smock, neatly-groomed hair and beard, it certainly looked like a doctor standing there. The reality would be put to the test soon enough. For now all I could do was wait, and I restlessly counted the days until I could begin my new job.

When the 16th of June finally came, I was so tense I could barely eat breakfast. Cindy and I exchanged kisses as we both left for work and she said, "Good luck on your first day, hon. Go knock 'em dead!"

I raised an eyebrow and she pursed her lips thoughtfully, saying, "Maybe that's not a good choice of words for your profession." I shook my head as I grinned widely, and she said, "Oh, all right! You got the idea though!" We laughed and shared one last kiss before heading to our cars.

When I arrived at the clinic, the receptionists greeted me enthusiastically. "Hi there, doctor!" one of them said. "It's nice to have you working here! Good luck today!"

I thanked them and asked what was scheduled for me that day. "You have some appointments this morning," Nancy the head receptionist said. "Nothing difficult, mostly routine exams and such. Your first appointment is a family with a new kitten that needs his shots." She rolled her eyes and chortled, "Babies vaccinating babies! What will happen next?"

The receptionists all giggled and I answered, "Oh, so that's how it's going to be, eh? Laugh it up; what goes around comes around!"

One of the younger women leaned over and said to the head receptionist, "It looks like he'll fit right in here."

Nancy sighed and replied, "That's what I'm afraid of." Then she winked at me and said, "You'll do fine. Head on back to the treatment room and see if anyone needs help with morning treatments. There are quite a few animals hospitalized right now."

I nodded and headed for the back, hearing more giggling from behind me as I left.

When my first appointment arrived, they put the clients into exam room number one. The chart was waiting in a wall holder by the room's entrance. I opened it up and looked inside. The client information form was completed, but the medical file was mostly blank, since it was the kitten's first trip to the vet.

My patient was listed as a male domestic short hair cat, only eight weeks of age. He was an orange tabby and his name was Whiskers. The reason for the visit was scrawled next to the date on the first line of his chart: "Exam and vaccinations." It sounded simple enough, if it weren't for the fact that this was the very first appointment of my veterinary career.

I closed the chart and took a few deep breaths. This was what I had been striving for since my undergraduate days. Today I would begin a life in medicine that hopefully would span decades. It all started right here, with this patient. I glanced down, straightening my smock and checking my appearance one last time. When I was satisfied, I squared my shoulders and grabbed the doorknob.

As I entered the exam room, a young mother and her toddler son glanced up smiling from the chairs where they sat. Perched on the mom's lap was a cute orange fur ball with big eyes and a swishing tail.

I closed the door gently behind me, and stepped forward into the room. "Good morning," I greeted the kitten's owners with a smile. "I'm Dr. Bridges."

ABOUT THE AUTHOR

DR. MARK E. BURGESS received his DVM from Oregon State University's College of Veterinary Medicine in 1986. Since then he has practiced medicine in the Portland, Oregon area. He developed a fascination for small exotic pet species early in his career. Dr. Burgess opened his own practice, Southwest Animal Hospital, in late 1995. Currently ninety-five percent of his practice is exotic pets, including ferrets, rabbits, rodents, reptiles, and a plethora of other small critters, not to mention the occasional dog and cat. In over twenty-three years treating exotic species he has discovered new diseases, published medical articles, written chapters in textbooks, and presented numerous lectures to other veterinarians and veterinary students. He belongs to several veterinary societies, and teaches exotic pet medicine as part of the student curriculum at his alma mater. Dr. Burgess currently resides in Beaverton, Oregon. His interests include exotic plant gardening, science fiction, hiking, camping, and the universe at large. He is graced with two wonderful daughters, a lovely wife, and two pets, Molly the cat, and Claire the rat.

Printed in Great Britain
by Amazon.co.uk, Ltd.,
Marston Gate.